Surgical Treatment of Ankylosing Spondylitis Deformity

Yan Wang
Editor

Surgical Treatment of Ankylosing Spondylitis Deformity

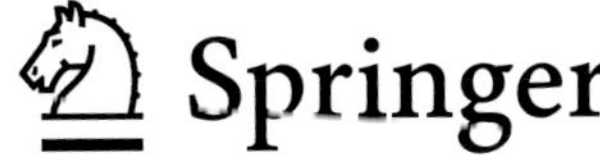

Editor
Yan Wang
Orthopedics department
Chinese PLA General Hospital
Beijing, China

ISBN 978-981-13-6429-7 ISBN 978-981-13-6427-3 (eBook)
https://doi.org/10.1007/978-981-13-6427-3

This Springer imprint is published by the registered company Springer Nature Singapore Pte Ltd.
The registered company address is: 152 Beach Road, #21-01/04 Gateway East, Singapore 189721, Singapore

Preface

Ankylosing spondylitis (AS) characteristically affects the axial skeleton in the spine and bilateral sacroiliac joints, leading to the functional and structural impairments of spine and joint. Spinal deformities such as flattening of the normal lumbar lordosis or a lumbar kyphosis, as well as joint space stenosis, rigidity, and deformity, cause the refractory pain, disability, and complications for AS patients. Appropriate surgery for AS spine and joint deformity lies on providing functional restoration, optimal sagittal balance, retrieve spinal alignment, and horizontal vision for obtaining effective improvement. Consequently, changing times have increased the demands for systematic surgical treatments of AS deformity.

To achieve satisfactory clinical results, following aspects need to be taken into consideration. Initially, for AS patients with spinal flexion or scoliosis deformity causing significant disability, spinal osteotomy is useful for the deformity correction. Various types of corrective osteotomy were performed, while a widely accepted classification system has not been developed, leading to the variation in surgical decision-making. What aspects should be focused on an ideal system in clinical practice? Furthermore, the combination of fixed thoracolumbar kyphosis and severe hip flexion contracture can significantly compromise ambulatory capacity in AS patients with advanced cases. Therefore, the interrelationship between the hip and spine is essential in the evaluation and management of patients with sagittal spinal deformity coexisting with hip joints involvement. For AS patients who have both hips affected as well as a spinal flexion deformity, two operations are required. Determining the surgical sequence that whether to perform spinal realignment correction or total hip arthroplasty first should be based on patient circumstances. Third, in the involved hip of AS patients, different levels of pathological changes result in varying joint deformities and different function damages, subsequently influencing the surgical decision of hip replacement. A new classification of AS involving hip with/without spinal deformity would benefit for making the preoperative plan and select surgical techniques. Additionally, the treatment of hip intraoperative and postoperative complications and surgical techniques of total knee arthroplasty for AS are also important for gaining good outcomes for AS deformity patients.

Understanding the concepts in surgical treatments of AS deformity will allow surgeons to adopt and embed principles into the clinical practice. However, certain inalienable approaches hold true across successful exponents of AS deformity treatments. Based on the experience in thousands of

AS spine and joint deformity surgical cases, I am delighted to recommend our present book of the *Surgical Treatment of Ankylosing Spondylitis Deformity* to all scientists, experts, and students, which would enhance your clinical knowledge and provide new insights into the increasingly rational approaches for AS deformity treatments. From anatomy, pathophysiology, basic research, and surgical techniques of AS deformity treatments, we give overview and build systematic surgery strategy, contributing to the practical guide and extending the future advancements and improvements for AS deformity.

I would like to thank the Springer staff and each of the contributors for their great efforts to create this work. I also dedicate this meticulous and important undertaking to the respective families for their encouragement, endurance, and continued supports.

Beijing, China Yan Wang

Contents

About the Editor

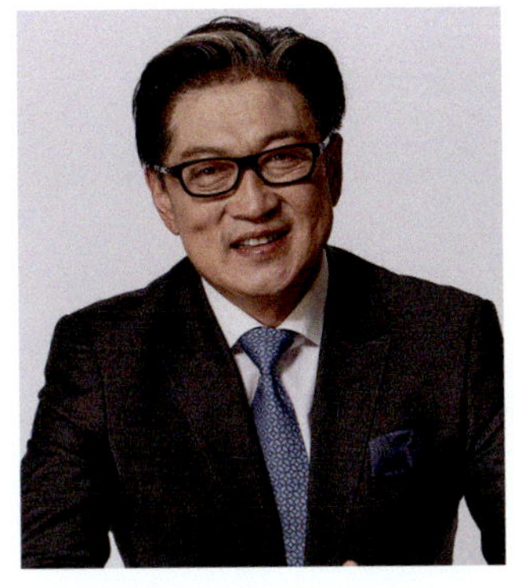

Yan Wang, MD is a professor and chief surgeon in the Department of Orthopedics at 301 Hospital in Beijing, China. He is an orthopedic surgeon dedicated to numerous clinical experiences on correction of spinal deformity, arthroplasty, and surgical treatment of patients with advanced ankylosing spondylitis in particular. Innovatively, He proposed a new spinal osteotomy technique – vertebral column decancellation – and has treated the world's largest number of ankylosing spondylitis patients with kyphotic deformity. He is the deputy editor of *Spine* journal and *Journal of Arthroplasty*. Professor Wang is the president of Chinese Academy of Orthopedic Surgeons and the past president of Chinese Orthopedic Association.

Part I

Overview

1 Ankylosing Spondylitis

Yan Wang and Quanbo Ji

Ankylosing spondylitis (AS) represents a common, highly heritable prototype of an interrelated group of chronic inflammatory rheumatic diseases now referred to as spondyloarthritis (SpA), which characteristically affects the axial skeleton in the spine and bilateral sacroiliac joints, resulting in structural and functional impairments, such as inflammatory back pain, asymmetrical peripheral oligoarthritis (predominantly of lower limbs), enthesitis, and specific organ involvement including psoriasis, acute anterior uveitis (AAU), inflammatory bowel disease (IBD), and the so-called extra-articular manifestations (EAM) [1–4]. The past decade yields major advances in the recognition of AS as an entity, the understanding of genetic and pathophysiological mechanisms, and the management due to the new clinical and imaging techniques or therapies [3]. Proteomic and genomic findings while in an early stage have potential both as diagnostic/prognostic tools to investigate the pathogenesis of AS [5]. The strongest known contributing factor is the main histocompatibility complex (MHC) class I molecule human leukocyte antigen-B27 (HLA-B27); several other genes and genetic regions still remain to be identified [4, 6]. The blockers of tumor necrosis factor (TNF), a major therapeutic advance, have allowed patients refractory to conventional treatment [3]. However, the available nonsteroidal anti-inflammatory drugs and physiotherapy or the other biological treatments are yet unclear [7]. In addition, the development of defining better strategies and techniques for early diagnosis, therapeutic modulation, and induction of drug-free remission remains one of the major challenges in AS for clinical practice for the next decade.

Y. Wang (✉) · Q. Ji
Department of orthopaedics, Chinese PLA General Hospital, Beijing, China

1 Epidemiology

AS, a chronic inflammatory disease, possesses a clear phenomenon of familial aggregation and is roughly related to the prevalence of HLA-B27 in a specific population [3, 6, 8]. AS affects people within the scope of the world and is now regarded as a major subtype of SpA. AS can occur at any age, which usually presents at around 10–40 years old. About 10–20% of patients develop the first symptoms at an age younger than 16 years, and the fastigium of incidence presents at around 18–25 years of age. Men are much more likely than women to be affected, with a ratio of roughly 2–3 to 1. Adults over 40 years old at onset of symptoms is often mild and not be taken seriously [4].

Overall, the prevalence of AS differs in groups with ethnic background. The Indians had the highest incidence, followed by white. The incidence in yellow race is lower than that of white, while black people have the lowest rate. In Europe, the prevalence of AS is between 0.1 and 1.4% per year [4]. In China, the incidence is about 0.3%.

Y. Wang (ed.), *Surgical Treatment of Ankylosing Spondylitis Deformity*,
https://doi.org/10.1007/978-981-13-6427-3_1

HLA-B27 is closely associated with the genetic effect in AS and is most prevalent in some tribes (with up to 50% of cases) and northern countries. The prevalence of HLA-B27 and the distribution of its subtypes contribute to the differences in patients with AS. Over 90% of AS patients are positive for HLA-B27. The risk of AS developing is correlated with the positive rate of HLA-B27 in the population. The rate of individuals who harbor HLA-B27 is about 5–8% in white, 8% in Chinese Han population, 50% in Haida Indians, and 0.5% in Japanese. Studies (in twins) revealed the monozygotic twin concordance rate is 63% compared with dizygotic twin rate of 13% [9]. In addition, HLA-B27-positive groups with a first-degree relative having AS have a rate of 8.2%.

2 Etiology and Pathogenesis

2.1 Genetics

HLA-B27 itself is the major genetic risk factor predisposing to AS. According to the DNA sequence of HLA-B27, over 100 subtypes are currently recognized and are designated HLA-B*2701 to HLA-B*27,106 [6]. All subtypes prefer arginine at the second position of bound peptide and share common amino acid residues. The most common subtype is B*2705, which is recognized as the ancestral subtype. In white Europeans, the common subtypes are B*2705 and B*2702. B*2705 and B*2704 are the main subtypes found closely in people of Chinese descent. In Indonesian and Thai individuals, B*2704 and B*2706 predominate [10–12]. However, <5% of HLA-B27-positive individuals develop AS [13]. Besides, the percentage of HLA-B27-positive relatives of patients with AS who will develop AS is 20%. Family studies show that HLA-B27 explains only 20–40% of the genetic susceptibility to AS, whereas the entire effect of the MHC contributes about 50%, suggesting the clear evidence that other genetic influences are operative in AS [13].

Apart from HLA-B27, other MHC genes, such as HLA-B60 and HLA-DR1, seem to be correlated with AS [4, 13]. Studies also reveal the presence of a non-MHC susceptibility locus, for AS is located on 9q31–34 [14]. The candidate genes are familial Mediterranean fever (MEFV) [15] and signal transducer and activator of transcription 3 (STAT3) [16]. Studies have suggested the identification of potential associations with genes for endoplasmic reticulum aminopeptidase 1 (ERAP1), interleukin-1A (IL-1A), interleukin 1 receptor 2 (IL1R2), interleukin-4 (IL-4), interleukin-12B (IL-12B), interleukin-13 (IL-13), interleukin-23A (IL-23A), interleukin-23 receptor (IL23R), tumor necrosis factor (TNF) receptor superfamily member 1A (TNFRSF1A), T-box 21 (TBX21), TNF receptor 1-associated death domain protein (TRADD), transforming growth factor-β (TGF-β), vascular morphogenesis protein gene anthrax toxin receptor 2 (ANTXR2), caspase recruitment domain family member 9 (CARD9), nucleotide-binding oligomerization domain-containing protein 2 (NOD2), and autophagy-related protein 6 (Atg6) [13, 17].

2.2 Environmental Effects

About 10–20% of HLA-B27-positive individuals develop the full clinical picture of AS, suggesting the environmental effect is also on strong susceptibility [18]. Bacteria play a possibly central role in the pathogenesis of AS [4, 19]. Studies of the synovium of AS patients revealed that microbial antigen persistence could be involved in continuing joint inflammation. Arthritis infected with *Chlamydia trachomatis* and gram-negative enterobacteria, such as *Yersinia*, *Salmonella*, *Shigella*, or *Campylobacter* spp., presents a firm background [20]. Inflammation caused by colitis results in the leakage of the gut mucosa, leading to an interaction between gut flora and immune system and changes in joint inflammation [4, 21]. Additionally, animals also indicate B27-bacteria interaction is important. Studies show HLA-B27 transgenic rats develop AS-like features; however, when HLA-B27 transgenic rats bred in a germ-free environment, they do not develop AS, indicating gut flora is closely related with the colitis and environmental trigger(s) are likely to be essential [22]. Many studies have suggested that AS is associated with infection. However, persistence of pathogenic bacteria seems unlikely to be related to initiation of AS, and the role of microbial antigens in AS is as yet unclear.

2.3 Cytokines and Biomarkers

Studies have investigated inflammation protein profiles in synovial samples from AS patients to reflect the disease state. As with cytokine profiling studies, inflammatory cytokines, such as TNF-α, IL-1b, IL-4, IL-6, IL-8, IL-15, IL-17, and IFN-c, were higher in AS [23–25]. There is also a definite contribution of cell subsets to the state of AS. M2 macrophage activation markers, previously associated with AS and correlated with tissue remodeling and immune regulation, are likely to be promoted by synovial fluid from AS patients [26, 27]. In addition, serum samples have been more widely used to develop biomarkers. Erythrocyte sedimentation rate (ESR) and C-reactive protein (CRP), two standard serum biomarkers, are widely identified as well-established inflammation markers and are thus not particularly useful for AS [28]. Study also indicated that the key markers distinguishing AS were CD69 in CD4 T cells, CD1c in B cells, and CXCR4 in CD8+ T cells (CCR7, CD45RA positive) and a subset of NK cells (CD62, CD45RA positive) by using a multiplexing fluorescence-associated cell sorting (FACS)-based approach [29], which looks promising potentially as a tool for AS investigation.

3 Pathophysiology

Inflammation triggers the formation of ectopic of new bone, especially in the spine. The development of square vertebral bodies of AS is based on a combination of destruction and repair of the spongiosa and cortex of the vertebral bodies [4, 30]. Bone morphogenetic protein (BMP) signaling is shown to be the potential molecular pathways associated with these pathological changes [31, 32]. Furthermore, both innate and adaptive immune responses could have effects in AS. Collagen type II and proteoglycan, two components of cartilaginous structures, have been investigated as possible targets of an autoimmune response in AS. Several findings revealed that cartilaginous structures of intervertebral discs and sacroiliac joints could be invaded by mononuclear cells, causing articular cartilage and even ankylosis or joint fusion [33]. Besides, $CD4^+$ and $CD8^+$ T-cell responses to collagen and aggrecan-derived peptides have also been reported in peripheral blood and synovial fluid samples of AS patients, indicating they're relevant for outcome measurement and targeted treatment [34, 35].

4 Clinical Features

The main clinical manifestations of AS are predominal axial symptoms, such as inflammatory back pain, spinal stiffness, sacroiliitis, anterior chest wall inflammation, morning stiffness, and loss of spinal mobility, which are mainly caused by structural damage, spinal inflammation, or both, leading to spondylodiscitis, spondylitis, and structural osteoproliferation [36–38]. The most characteristic features of AS are syndesmophytes and ankylosis [39]. Also low bone density, increases in fracture, and osteoporosis have also been predominantly seen in hyperkyphosis in AS populations and increased the burden.

Inflammations at other locations are peripheral arthritis, enthesitis, uveitis, and colitis, whereas manifestations in other organs, such as the kidney and heart, are rare [39]. The incidence of peripheral arthritis is usually related to the age of the patients. Peripheral arthritis in individuals of younger age is obviously severe. The main manifestations of peripheral arthritis are monoarticular or oligoarticular, asymmetric than symmetrical, and affect mainly but not exclusively the lower limbs [40]. Enthesitis, inflammation of entheseal sites, takes place not only at classic sites of attachment of tendon or ligaments to the bone but at many locations, including the spine [41]. Uveitis regarded as a kind of eye inflammation usually occurs unilaterally but can also be bilateral alternation. Other manifestations, such as psoriasis and colitis, are also closely correlated with IBD in AS.

5 Laboratory Tests

Currently, the serological examinations of significance for AS-specific diagnosis are very limited. HLA-B27, CRP, and ESR are three main potential examination indices for AS diagnosis [42, 43]. Although HLA-B27 has a high sensitivity and specificity for diagnosis of early AS, the laboratory tests rely on the prevalence of HLA-B27 in the population of different races, thus affecting the possibility of accurate diagnosis. ESR, an old and practical acute phase index, is increased in about 50–80% of AS patients while reduced to normal in the quiescent or late phase [44]. ESR increased in patients with mild anemia is not correlated with disease activity. Detection of ESR can be regarded as a reference index to judge the activity of AS and evaluation of the clinical curative effect. CRP is an acute phase protein and can be significantly raised during the acute phase of AS. When the clinical symptoms of AS are controlled, the concentrations of CRP were also decreased. CRP is more sensitive than ESR in the development and outcome of reactive inflammation for AS, and the values are not likely to be affected by anemia or hypergammaglobulinemia. Therefore, the detection of CRP is helpful to evaluate the activity and clinical efficacy of AS. Other indices, such as platelet and immunoglobulin, can also provide potential assessment for AS in some cases [45–48].

6 Radiography

Sacroiliitis, a hallmark of AS, takes place in the early phase of AS, causing chronic structural changes in the sacroiliac joints and spine, such as costovertebral joints, ischial tuberosity, vertebral endplate, and intervertebral disc annulus fibrosus attachment [49]. Therefore, the detection of sacroiliitis could be useful for diagnosis and classification in individual patients. Conventional radiography is still sufficiently sensitive and the gold standard for the quantitative assessment of structural damages in the spine and sacroiliac joints because of its very high prevalence in patients with AS. According to the last modification of the New York criteria, the radiograph of a healthy sacroiliac joint was categorized as grade 0, suspicious changes as 1, minor changes as 2, moderate changes as 3, and ankylosis as 4. This modified grading system is the most useful scoring method and has changed the criteria limit of chest expansion and the normal values of age and sex adjustment [50]. Furthermore, radiographic damages at baseline can predict the future structural changes in AS [51].

The possible osteoproliferative changes of the sacroiliac joints, however, could appear normal in the early course of AS. Therefore, radiographs might become apparent only after months even some years. At present, CT technique allows for detection of early damages in the sacroiliac joint due to the high spatial resolution and density resolution. Because of the higher radiation dose required and cartilage lesions unable to be displayed, the widespread use of CT was limited [52].

MRI, with its capacity to detect structural changes and active inflammation, has been proved especially useful for assessment and diagnostic benefit of early sacroiliitis and spondylitis when short T1 inversion recovery (STIR) and a field strength of T2 for fat saturated or a field strength of T1 after application of contrast agents are used [53, 54]. MRI is sensitive to active and acute change in AS patients with inflammatory back pain and can predict the development of radiographic changes before they occur. Besides, MRI is also useful for detection and localization of inflammation in peripheral joints and enthuses [55].

Ultrasonography has been so far used to assess the synovitis, tendonitis, bursitis, and damages of the cartilage and bone. For diagnostic examinations, such as histological biopsy, ultrasonography is currently considered a powerful tool to visualize the disease activity and prognosis and treatment effects by screening persistence, improvement, or new onset in AS [56, 57].

7 Diagnosis and Classification

Currently, it's not suitable for conventional radiography to be regarded as a prerequisite for the early diagnosis and treatment of AS. Besides, compared with patients diagnosed by AS, individuals without radiographs of sacroiliitis have no obvious differences in disease activities, pain evaluation, treatment needs, and the influence to life quality, indicating radiology changes of sacroiliac joints are just the manifestations of different periods for the SpA patients with axial symptoms [58, 59]. Furthermore, radiographs of changes in sacroiliac joints can reveal the chronicity and severity of diseases, but they are not necessary [60]. Therefore, the concept of axial spondyloarthritis (axSpA) was developed on the basis of the fact showing SpA and AS are characterized with the same axial symptoms. The axSpA includes AS and the previous concept of SpA with axial symptoms. As a result, it's necessary to establish a new diagnostic and classification criteria with both high sensitivity and high specificity, thus guiding care of the individual patient. According to the ASAS criteria, radiographs of sacroiliitis are parts required but not requisite. For those patients without radiographic changes in sacroiliac joint inflammation, MRI is an important reference index [61–63]. Besides, a combination with various clinical grounds, such as inflammatory back pain, arthritis, and tendonitis, and the laboratory tests, for instance, HLA-B27 and CRP, suggested that MRI is more beneficial for the early diagnosis of AS [41, 59, 60].

A novel set of ASAS classification criteria for axSpA has been proposed, which allows a diagnosis of patient with chronic (>3 months) low back pain and age at onset younger than 45 years who either has sacroiliitis shown by imaging, carries HLA-B27, or has the clinical symptom of inflammatory back pain [58, 63].

The diagnosis criteria for peripheral spondyloarthritis were also established, suggesting that patients should be younger than 45 years with chronic low back pain. Moreover, criteria also includes arthritis or enthesitis, added by at least one clinical feature of SpA, such as uveitis, psoriasis, Crohn's disease, colitis, history of past infection, HLA-B27, and sacroiliitis shown by imaging, or added by at least two clinical characteristics, for instance, arthritis, enthesitis, inflammatory back pain, or family history of SpA [58, 63].

8 Treatment

The appropriate treatment of patients with AS has consisted of a combination of non-pharmacological and pharmacological treatment approaches, including education, physical therapy, drugs, regular exercise, joint replacement, and spine surgery [64–67]. Disease activity, symptoms, and other features like function and expectations should be considered.

8.1 Non-pharmacological Therapy

Structured exercise programs were recommended. Non-pharmacological treatment methods include education, spa treatment, self-help groups, and physical therapy [68–70]. A Cochrane systematic review identified that an individual supervised or home-based exercise program is better than no intervention, while the supervised physical therapy is better than home programs, and that combined inpatient spondyloarthritis-exercise therapy with subsequent group physiotherapy is better than group physiotherapy alone [71]. Whether and to what extent exercise and physical therapy are useful in every stage of AS and beneficial during the painful inflammatory flares, however, has not been fully elucidated.

8.2 Pharmacological Therapy

Briefly, NSAIDs, as a top priority, can rapidly improve the patients' symptoms, such as low back pain, stiffness, and joint swelling, and increase the range of activities in early and late stage of AS. Besides, NSAID has also been regarded as a useful diagnostic method for AS because of its rapid effects and symptom relief. Clinical experience suggests that patients with AS should be given NSAIDs before bed in order to control the nocturnal pain. However, these drugs also have the most common side effects, such as gastrointestinal discomfort. COX-2 inhibitors may have the minimal reaction to the gastrointestinal tract [64, 65]. Therefore, the patients should refer to the physicians for appropriate dose of NSAIDs [72].

Long-term oral treatment of glucocorticoid cannot prevent the development of the disease, which also brings many adverse effects. For low back pain uncontrolled by other treatments, CT-guided glucocorticoid injection in sacroiliac joints can improve symptoms of some patients. For AS individuals with long-term single joint effusion, glucocorticoid is recommended for intra-articular injection [73, 74].

Sulfasalazine (SSZ), the most widely used anti-rheumatic drugs for AS treatment, improves joint pain, swelling, and stiffness and suppresses the serum IgA level as well as other laboratory activity indices, especially for those patients with peripheral arthritis. Besides, SSZ can also prevent recurrence and reduce the lesions of uveitis. So far, the effect of this drug on axial joint lesions and the exact prognosis of AS are still difficult to evaluate [75].

Methotrexate (MTX), a folic acid inhibitor, is generally used in patients with rheumatoid arthritis, as well as Crohn's disease, malignant tumor, and psoriasis. MTX is also applied to the treatment of AS but lacks sufficient proof of evidence-based medicine. Studies have revealed that patients with AS show some improvement of peripheral arthritis and inflammatory back pain [76, 77]. However, any effect in axial joint lesions shown by imaging is not seen. MTX dose is recommended 7.5–15 mg per week and more for severe cases [78].

Thalidomide was also widely used for the treatment of AS with specific immune regulation but is considered as too toxic for widespread use [79]. Leflunomide, a low molecular weight synthesis of oral immunosuppressive drugs, is beneficial in treatment of symptoms and suppressing radiographic changes of peripheral arthritis [80, 81]. Bisphosphonates are also reported that are useful for spinal symptoms for AS patients [82].

8.3 Biological Agents

Recent decades have witnessed the novel development and progress in research fields of cytology and molecular biology, allowing the application of biological agents for the treatment of autoimmune diseases, such as AS. Biological agent, a monoclonal antibody or recombinant product of natural inhibitory molecules, takes the molecule or receptor which participates in the immune response or inflammatory process as a target [58, 83]. For the pathogenesis of rheumatic diseases, theoretically, biological agents have a higher specificity to control the disease fundamentally when compared with the conventional immunosuppressive therapy, making the treatment of AS and other diseases enter a completely new phase. Clinical practices have demonstrated that TNF blockers now approved for AS, such as infliximab, etanercept, and adalimumab, were significantly effective in improving the functions of patients [41, 84, 85]. On the other side, possible side effects and the high costs of these drugs also merit attention.

Infliximab, an IgG1 monoclonal chimeric antibody (a chimera of human constant and mouse variable regions), is given intravenously in a dose of 3–5 mg/kg every 6–8 weeks (approved dosage is 5 mg/kg every 6–8 weeks). As approved for Crohn's disease and ulcerative colitis, infliximab has also shown effectiveness. Besides, studies also indicated that infliximab suppressed the active spinal inflammation, and no substantial radiological progression was seen which was assessed by the modified Stoke Ankylosing Spondylitis Spine Score (SASSS) using MRI [86, 87].

Etanercept is a recombinant soluble 75 kD TNF-α receptor fusion protein that binds to TNF-alpha and has also been proved effective for rheumatic manifestations and peripheral joint and skin symptom but not gut symptoms in patients with AS, indicating it is not recommended for the small spondyloarthritis subgroup with concomitant inflammatory bowel disease [87, 88]. Moreover, individuals without etanercept treatment several months later all have developed a relapse of disease activity; however, reintroduction of the therapy was effective [89]. In addition, etanercept is given subcutaneously in a dose of 50 mg once per week or 25 mg twice per week.

As a fully humanized monoclonal antibody, adalimumab has been proven efficacious in the treatment of active AS and is approved in Europe and the USA [90, 91]. Adalimumab is given subcutaneously in a dose of 40 mg every other week, which can significantly reduce clinical disease activity and spinal inflammation as evaluated by MRI. Besides, this result is confirmed in a randomized controlled trial [92].

Anakinra, a recombinant human interleukin-1 receptor antagonist, responses to a different cytokine in the inflammation than TNF blockers. However, evidence that this treatment works well in AS are deficient, and whether anakinra is able to stop radiographic progression of sacroiliac joints has not yet been fully elucidated [65, 93].

Other biological agents, such as human anti-IL-12/IL-23 monoclonal antibody ustekinumab, anti-LFA3 antibody alefacept, and the CTLA4-Ig construct abatacept, showed only slight but significantly efficient clinical improvement of psoriatic arthritis [64, 65, 94, 95]. However, rituximab, the anti-CD20 antibody, did not show significant efficacy in AS, although some response appeared among TNF blocker-naive patients [95].

8.4 Surgery

Joint space stenosis, rigidity, and deformity caused by hip involvement are the main causes of refractory pain and disability in this disease. In order to improve the joint function and quality of life of the patients, the total hip arthroplasty has to be considered in patients with obvious stenosis or necrosis of the femoral head [96, 97]. After replacement, the majority of patients can return to normal.

For patients with spinal flexion or scoliosis deformity causing significant disability, spinal osteotomy is useful in the correction of deformity [68, 98, 99]. Surgical techniques, such as Smith-Petersen osteotomy (SPO), pedicle subtraction osteotomy (PSO), and vertebral column resection (VCR), are beneficial and useful strategies utilized in complex spine deformity [100–103]. Besides, vertebral column decancellation (VCD) firstly named modified VCR and described by Yan Wang in his series study for 13 adult patients with severe rigid congenital kyphoscoliosis also combines the advantages of SPO, PSO, VCR, and eggshell techniques, showing less spine cord shortening and a better bony fusion in the treatments [104–106]. Moreover, the cervical extension osteotomy is mainly useful in correction of sagittal balance of cervical-thoracic junction in patients with severe AS flexion deformity [107–109]. However, complications, such as neurological risks, still exist, but these are likely be minimized in the future.

9 Prognosis and Future Prospects

Based on the present state, the severity of the clinical manifestations of AS is relatively various. Some patients are with recrudescence, while some are in a relatively quiescent state. Patients of younger age of onset, or early hip involvement, or diagnosis delayed and treatment unreasonable, cannot achieve an effective prognosis. Despite the prognosis greatly improved by the presence of biological agents, patients should be under the guidance of a specialist in long-term follow-up because of AS still being a chronic progressive disease. Besides, the development of validation of better clinical or biological markers for early diagnosis and anti-inflammatory assessment and therapies now appears overwhelming. Furthermore, our efforts of AS research, as well as clinical strategies targeting tissue remodeling, will also open the new gateways for AS treatment over the coming years.

References

1. Stolwijk C, van Tubergen A, Castillo-Ortiz JD, et al. Prevalence of extra-articular manifestations in patients with ankylosing spondylitis: a systematic review and meta-analysis. Ann Rheum Dis. 2015;74(1):65–73.
2. Elewaut D, Matucci-Cerinic M. Treatment of ankylosing spondylitis and extra-articular manifestations in everyday rheumatology practice. Rheumatology (Oxford). 2009;48(9):1029–35.
3. Dougados M, Baeten D. Spondyloarthritis. Lancet. 2011;377(9783):2127–37.
4. Braun J, Sieper J. Ankylosing spondylitis. Lancet. 2007;369(9570):1379–90.

5. Thomas GP, Brown MA. Genetics and genomics of ankylosing spondylitis. Immunol Rev. 2010;233(1):162–80.
6. Bowness P. Hla-B27. Annu Rev Immunol. 2015;33:29–48.
7. Braun J, Baraliakos X. Imaging of axial spondyloarthritis including ankylosing spondylitis. Ann Rheum Dis. 2011;70(Suppl 1):i97–103.
8. Costantino F, Talpin A, Said-Nahal R, et al. Prevalence of spondyloarthritis in reference to HLA-B27 in the French population: results of the GAZEL cohort. Ann Rheum Dis. 2015;74(4):689–93.
9. Brown MA, Laval SH, Brophy S, et al. Recurrence risk modelling of the genetic susceptibility to ankylosing spondylitis. Ann Rheum Dis. 2000;59(11):883–6.
10. Liu Y, Jiang L, Cai Q, et al. Predominant association of HLA-B*2704 with ankylosing spondylitis in Chinese Han patients. Tissue Antigens. 2010;75(1):61–4.
11. Lopez-Larrea C, Sujirachato K, Mehra NK, et al. HLA-B27 subtypes in Asian patients with ankylosing spondylitis. Evidence for new associations. Tissue Antigens. 1995;45(3):169–76.
12. Rana MK, Luthra-Guptasarma M. Multi-modal binding of a 'Self' peptide by HLA-B*27:04 and B*27:05 allelic variants, but not B*27:09 or B*27:06 variants: fresh support for some theories explaining differential disease association. Protein J. 2016;35(5):346–53.
13. Reveille JD. The genetic basis of spondyloarthritis. Ann Rheum Dis. 2011;70(Suppl 1):i44–50.
14. Miceli-Richard C, Zouali H, Said-Nahal R, et al. Significant linkage to spondyloarthropathy on 9q31-34. Hum Mol Genet. 2004;13(15):1641–8.
15. Guncan S, Bilge NS, Cansu DU, et al. The role of MEFV mutations in the concurrent disorders observed in patients with familial Mediterranean fever. Eur J Rheumatol. 2016;3(3):118–21.
16. Davidson SI, Liu Y, Danoy PA, et al. Association of STAT3 and TNFRSF1A with ankylosing spondylitis in Han Chinese. Ann Rheum Dis. 2011;70(2):289–92.
17. Lau MC, Keith P, Costello ME, et al. Genetic association of ankylosing spondylitis with TBX21 influences T-bet and pro-inflammatory cytokine expression in humans and SKG mice as a model of spondyloarthritis. Ann Rheum Dis. 2017;76(1):261–9.
18. Sieper J, Braun J, Rudwaleit M, et al. Ankylosing spondylitis: an overview. Ann Rheum Dis. 2002;61(Suppl 3):iii8–18.
19. Chen DY, Chen YM, Hung WT, et al. Immunogenicity, drug trough levels and therapeutic response in patients with rheumatoid arthritis or ankylosing spondylitis after 24-week golimumab treatment. Ann Rheum Dis. 2015;74(12):2261–4.
20. Sieper J, Braun J, Kingsley GH. Report on the fourth international workshop on reactive arthritis. Arthritis Rheum. 2000;43(4):720–34.
21. Ciccia F, Accardo-Palumbo A, Rizzo A, et al. Evidence that autophagy, but not the unfolded protein response, regulates the expression of IL-23 in the gut of patients with ankylosing spondylitis and subclinical gut inflammation. Ann Rheum Dis. 2014;73(8):1566–74.
22. Onderdonk AB, Richardson JA, Hammer RE, et al. Correlation of cecal microflora of HLA-B27 transgenic rats with inflammatory bowel disease. Infect Immun. 1998;66(12):6022–3.
23. Hunter CA, Jones SA. IL-6 as a keystone cytokine in health and disease. Nat Immunol. 2015;16(5):448–57.
24. Evans DM, Spencer CC, Pointon JJ, et al. Interaction between ERAP1 and HLA-B27 in ankylosing spondylitis implicates peptide handling in the mechanism for HLA-B27 in disease susceptibility. Nat Genet. 2011;43(8):761–7.
25. Ciccia F, Guggino G, Rizzo A, et al. Type 3 innate lymphoid cells producing IL-17 and IL-22 are expanded in the gut, in the peripheral blood, synovial fluid and bone marrow of patients with ankylosing spondylitis. Ann Rheum Dis. 2015;74(9):1739–47.
26. Lin S, Qiu M, Chen J. IL-4 modulates macrophage polarization in ankylosing spondylitis. Cell Physiol Biochem. 2015;35(6):2213–22.
27. Ciccia F, Alessandro R, Rizzo A, et al. Macrophage phenotype in the subclinical gut inflammation of patients with ankylosing spondylitis. Rheumatology (Oxford). 2014;53(1):104–13.
28. Sezgin M, Tecer D, Kanik A, et al. Serum RDW and MPV in ankylosing spondylitis: can they show the disease activity? Clin Hemorheol Microcirc. 2017;65(1):1–10.
29. Steinbrich-Zollner M, Grun JR, Kaiser T, et al. From transcriptome to cytome: integrating cytometric profiling, multivariate cluster, and prediction analyses for a phenotypical classification of inflammatory diseases. Cytometry A. 2008;73(4):333–40.
30. Aufdermaur M. Pathogenesis of square bodies in ankylosing spondylitis. Ann Rheum Dis. 1989;48(8):628–31.
31. Wendling D, Claudepierre P. New bone formation in axial spondyloarthritis. Joint Bone Spine. 2013;80(5):454–8.
32. Chen HA, Chen CH, Lin YJ, et al. Association of bone morphogenetic proteins with spinal fusion in ankylosing spondylitis. J Rheumatol. 2010;37(10):2126–32.
33. Lv Q, Li Q, Zhang P, et al. Disorders of MicroRNAs in peripheral blood mononuclear cells: as novel biomarkers of ankylosing spondylitis and provocative therapeutic targets. Biomed Res Int. 2015;2015:504208.
34. Appel H, Wu P, Scheer R, et al. Synovial and peripheral blood CD4+FoxP3+ T cells in spondyloarthritis. J Rheumatol. 2011;38(11):2445–51.
35. Atagunduz P, Appel H, Kuon W, et al. HLA-B27-restricted CD8+ T cell response to cartilage-derived self peptides in ankylosing spondylitis. Arthritis Rheum. 2005;52(3):892–901.
36. del Rio-Martinez P, Navarro-Compan V, Diaz-Miguel C, et al. Similarities and differences between

patients fulfilling axial and peripheral ASAS criteria for spondyloarthritis: results from the Esperanza cohort. Semin Arthritis Rheum. 2016;45(4):400–3.
37. Baraliakos X, Braun J. Spondyloarthritides. Best Pract Res Clin Rheumatol. 2011;25(6):825–42.
38. Braun J, Sieper J. Classification criteria for rheumatoid arthritis and ankylosing spondylitis. Clin Exp Rheumatol. 2009;27(4 Suppl 55):S68–73.
39. Tan S, Wang R, Ward MM. Syndesmophyte growth in ankylosing spondylitis. Curr Opin Rheumatol. 2015;27(4):326–32.
40. Dougados M, van der Linden S, Juhlin R, et al. The european spondylarthropathy study group preliminary criteria for the classification of spondylarthropathy. Arthritis Rheum. 1991;34(10):1218–27.
41. Sieper J, Poddubnyy D. New evidence on the management of spondyloarthritis. Nat Rev Rheumatol. 2016;12(5):282–95.
42. Prajzlerova K, Grobelna K, Pavelka K, et al. An update on biomarkers in axial spondyloarthritis. Autoimmun Rev. 2016;15(6):501–9.
43. Maksymowych WP. Biomarkers in axial spondyloarthritis. Curr Opin Rheumatol. 2015;27(4):343–8.
44. de Vlam K. Soluble and tissue biomarkers in ankylosing spondylitis. Best Pract Res Clin Rheumatol. 2010;24(5):671–82.
45. Chen CH, Yu DT, Chou CT. Biomarkers in spondyloarthropathies. Adv Exp Med Biol. 2009;649:122–32.
46. Di Minno MN, Iervolino S, Zincarelli C, et al. Cardiovascular effects of Etanercept in patients with psoriatic arthritis: evidence from the cardiovascular risk in rheumatic diseases database. Expert Opin Drug Saf. 2015;14(12):1905–13.
47. Durham LE, Taams LS, Kirkham BW. Psoriatic arthritis. Br J Hosp Med. 2016;77(7):C102–8.
48. Dal Pont E, D'Inca R, Caruso A, et al. Non-invasive investigation in patients with inflammatory joint disease. World J Gastroenterol. 2009;15(20):2463–8.
49. Deodhar A, Strand V, Kay J, et al. The term 'non-radiographic axial spondyloarthritis' is much more important to classify than to diagnose patients with axial spondyloarthritis. Ann Rheum Dis. 2016;75(5):791–4.
50. van der Linden S, Valkenburg HA, Cats A. Evaluation of diagnostic criteria for ankylosing spondylitis. A proposal for modification of the New York criteria. Arthritis Rheum. 1984;27(4):361–8.
51. Baraliakos X, Listing J, Rudwaleit M, et al. Progression of radiographic damage in patients with ankylosing spondylitis: defining the central role of syndesmophytes. Ann Rheum Dis. 2007;66(7):910–5.
52. Yang CH, Wu TH, Chiou YY, et al. Imaging quality and diagnostic reliability of low-dose computed tomography lumbar spine for evaluating patients with spinal disorders. Spine J. 2014;14(11):2682–90.
53. Baraliakos X, Hermann KG, Landewe R, et al. Assessment of acute spinal inflammation in patients with ankylosing spondylitis by magnetic resonance imaging: a comparison between contrast enhanced T1 and short tau inversion recovery (STIR) sequences. Ann Rheum Dis. 2005;64(8):1141–4.
54. Braun J, Golder W, Bollow M, et al. Imaging and scoring in ankylosing spondylitis. Clin Exp Rheumatol. 2002;20(6 Suppl 28):S178–84.
55. Weber U, Jurik AG, Lambert RG, et al. Imaging in spondyloarthritis: controversies in recognition of early disease. Curr Rheumatol Rep. 2016;18(9):58.
56. Toprak H, Kilic E, Serter A, et al. Doppler US in rheumatic diseases with special emphasis on rheumatoid arthritis and spondyloarthritis. Diagn Interv Radiol. 2014;20(1):72–7.
57. Arend CF. Role of sonography and magnetic resonance imaging in detecting deltoideal acromial enthesopathy: an early finding in the diagnosis of spondyloarthritis and an under-recognized cause of posterior shoulder pain. J Ultrasound Med. 2014;33(4):557–61.
58. Taurog JD, Chhabra A, Colbert RA. Ankylosing spondylitis and axial spondyloarthritis. N Engl J Med. 2016;374(26):2563–74.
59. Slobodin G, Eshed I. Non-radiographic axial spondyloarthritis. IMAJ. 2015;17(12):770–6.
60. Kok HK, Mumtaz A, O'Brien C, et al. Imaging the patient with sacroiliac pain. Can Assoc Radiol J. 2016;67(1):41–51.
61. van der Linden S, Akkoc N, Brown MA, et al. The ASAS criteria for axial Spondyloarthritis: strengths, weaknesses, and proposals for a way forward. Curr Rheumatol Rep. 2015;17(9):62.
62. Lubrano E, Parsons WJ, Marchesoni A, et al. The definition and measurement of axial psoriatic arthritis. J Rheumatol Suppl. 2015;93:40–2.
63. Akkoc N, Khan MA. ASAS classification criteria for axial spondyloarthritis: time to modify. Clin Rheumatol. 2016;35(6):1415–23.
64. Wendling D. An overview of investigational new drugs for treating ankylosing spondylitis. Expert Opin Investig Drugs. 2016;25(1):95–104.
65. Palazzi C, D'Angelo S, Gilio M, et al. Pharmacological therapy of spondyloarthritis. Expert Opin Pharmacother. 2015;16(10):1495–504.
66. Del Rosso A, Maddali-Bongi S. Mind body therapies in rehabilitation of patients with rheumatic diseases. Complement Ther Clin Pract. 2016;22:80–6.
67. Moon KH, Kim YT. Medical treatment of ankylosing spondylitis. Hip Pelvis. 2014;26(3):129–35.
68. Lubrano E, Astorri D, Taddeo M, et al. Rehabilitation and surgical management of ankylosing spondylitis. Musculoskelet Surg. 2013;97(Suppl 2):S191–5.
69. Hoving JL, Lacaille D, Urquhart DM, et al. Non-pharmacological interventions for preventing job loss in workers with inflammatory arthritis. Cochrane Database Syst Rev. 2014;11:CD010208.
70. Van Tubergen A, Boonen A, Landewe R, et al. Cost effectiveness of combined spa-exercise therapy in ankylosing spondylitis: a randomized controlled trial. Arthritis Rheum. 2002;47(5):459–67.
71. Dagfinrud H, Kvien TK, Hagen KB. The Cochrane review of physiotherapy interventions for ankylosing spondylitis. J Rheumatol. 2005;32(10):1899–906.

72. Kroon FP, van der Burg LR, Ramiro S, et al. Nonsteroidal anti-inflammatory drugs (NSAIDs) for axial spondyloarthritis (ankylosing spondylitis and non-radiographic axial spondyloarthritis). Cochrane Database Syst Rev. 2015;7:CD010952.
73. Fendler C, Baraliakos X, Braun J. Glucocorticoid treatment in spondyloarthritis. Clin Exp Rheumatol. 2011;29(5 Suppl 68):S139–42.
74. Siu S, Haraoui B, Bissonnette R, et al. Meta-analysis of tumor necrosis factor inhibitors and glucocorticoids on bone density in rheumatoid arthritis and ankylosing spondylitis trials. Arthritis Care Res. 2015;67(6):754–64.
75. Chen J, Lin S, Liu C. Sulfasalazine for ankylosing spondylitis. Cochrane Database Syst Rev. 2014;11:CD004800.
76. Cipriani P, Ruscitti P, Carubbi F, et al. Methotrexate: an old new drug in autoimmune disease. Expert Rev Clin Immunol. 2014;10(11):1519–30.
77. Yang Z, Zhao W, Liu W, et al. Efficacy evaluation of methotrexate in the treatment of ankylosing spondylitis using meta-analysis. Int J Clin Pharmacol Ther. 2014;52(5):346–51.
78. Chen J, Veras MM, Liu C, et al. Methotrexate for ankylosing spondylitis. Cochrane Database Syst Rev. 2013;2:CD004524.
79. Davis JC Jr, Huang F, Maksymowych W. New therapies for ankylosing spondylitis: etanercept, thalidomide, and pamidronate. Rheum Dis Clin N Am. 2003;29(3):481–94.
80. Haibel H, Rudwaleit M, Braun J, et al. Six months open label trial of leflunomide in active ankylosing spondylitis. Ann Rheum Dis. 2005;64(1):124–6.
81. Kaltwasser JP, Nash P, Gladman D, et al. Efficacy and safety of leflunomide in the treatment of psoriatic arthritis and psoriasis: a multinational, double-blind, randomized, placebo-controlled clinical trial. Arthritis Rheum. 2004;50(6):1939–50.
82. Viapiana O, Gatti D, Idolazzi L, et al. Bisphosphonates vs infliximab in ankylosing spondylitis treatment. Rheumatology (Oxford). 2014;53(1):90–4.
83. Katsicas MM, Russo R. Biologic agents in juvenile spondyloarthropathies. Pediatr Rheumatol Online J. 2016;14(1):17.
84. Callhoff J, Sieper J, Weiss A, et al. Efficacy of TNF alpha blockers in patients with ankylosing spondylitis and non-radiographic axial spondyloarthritis: a meta-analysis. Ann Rheum Dis. 2015;74(6):1241–8.
85. Machado MA, Barbosa MM, Almeida AM, et al. Treatment of ankylosing spondylitis with TNF blockers: a meta-analysis. Rheumatol Int. 2013;33(9):2199–213.
86. Elalouf O, Elkayam O. Long-term safety and efficacy of infliximab for the treatment of ankylosing spondylitis. Ther Clin Risk Manag. 2015;11:1719–26.
87. Maxwell LJ, Zochling J, Boonen A, et al. TNF-alpha inhibitors for ankylosing spondylitis. Cochrane Database Syst Rev. 2015;4:CD005468.
88. Murdaca G, Spano F, Contatore M, et al. Pharmacogenetics of etanercept: role of TNF-alpha gene polymorphisms in improving its efficacy. Expert Opin Drug Metab Toxicol. 2014;10(12):1703–10.
89. Scott LJ. Etanercept: a review of its use in autoimmune inflammatory diseases. Drugs. 2014;74(12):1379–410.
90. Murdaca G, Spano F, Contatore M, et al. Immunogenicity of infliximab and adalimumab: what is its role in hypersensitivity and modulation of therapeutic efficacy and safety? Expert Opin Drug Saf. 2016;15(1):43–52.
91. Lapadula G, Marchesoni A, Armuzzi A, et al. Adalimumab in the treatment of immune-mediated diseases. Int J Immunopathol Pharmacol. 2014;27(1 Suppl):33–48.
92. Wang H, Zuo D, Sun M, et al. Randomized, placebo controlled and double-blind trials of efficacy and safety of adalimumab for treating ankylosing spondylitis: a meta-analysis. Int J Rheum Dis. 2014;17(2):142–8.
93. Goh L, Samanta A. A systematic MEDLINE analysis of therapeutic approaches in ankylosing spondylitis. Rheumatol Int. 2009;29(10):1123–35.
94. Bonafede M, Fox KM, Watson C, et al. Treatment patterns in the first year after initiating tumor necrosis factor blockers in real-world settings. Adv Ther. 2012;29(8):664–74.
95. Heredia S, Aparicio M, Armengol E, et al. Rituximab therapy for ankylosing spondylitis associated to demyelinating disease of the central nervous system. Joint Bone Spine. 2016;83(1):105–6.
96. Fu D, Sun W, Shen J, et al. Inflammatory pseudotumor around metal-on-polyethylene total hip arthroplasty in patients with ankylosing spondylitis: description of two cases and review of literature. World J Surg Oncol. 2015;13:57.
97. Guan M, Wang J, Zhao L, et al. Management of hip involvement in ankylosing spondylitis. Clin Rheumatol. 2013;32(8):1115–20.
98. Van Royen BJ, De Gast A. Lumbar osteotomy for correction of thoracolumbar kyphotic deformity in ankylosing spondylitis. A structured review of three methods of treatment. Ann Rheum Dis. 1999;58(7):399–406.
99. Mundwiler ML, Siddique K, Dym JM, et al. Complications of the spine in ankylosing spondylitis with a focus on deformity correction. Neurosurg Focus. 2008;24(1):E6.
100. Burton DC. Smith-Petersen osteotomy of the spine. Instr Course Lect. 2006;55:577–82.
101. Gill JB, Levin A, Burd T, et al. Corrective osteotomies in spine surgery. J Bone Joint Surg Am. 2008;90(11):2509–20.
102. Liu H, Yang C, Zheng Z, et al. Comparison of smith-petersen osteotomy and pedicle subtraction osteotomy for the correction of thoracolumbar kyphotic deformity in ankylosing spondylitis: a systematic review and meta-analysis. Spine. 2015;40(8):570–9.
103. Boachie-Adjei O. Role and technique of eggshell osteotomies and vertebral column resections in the

treatment of fixed sagittal imbalance. Instr Course Lect. 2006;55:583–9.
104. Zhang X, Zhang Z, Wang J, et al. Vertebral column decancellation: a new spinal osteotomy technique for correcting rigid thoracolumbar kyphosis in patients with ankylosing spondylitis. Bone Joint J. 2016;98-B(5):672–8.
105. Wang Y, Lenke LG. Vertebral column decancellation for the management of sharp angular spinal deformity. Eur Spine J. 2011;20(10):1703–10.
106. Wang Y, Zhang Y, Zhang X, et al. A single posterior approach for multilevel modified vertebral column resection in adults with severe rigid congenital kyphoscoliosis: a retrospective study of 13 cases. Eur Spine J. 2008;17(3):361–72.
107. Wang Y, Zhang Y, Mao K, et al. Transpedicular bivertebrae wedge osteotomy and discectomy in lumbar spine for severe ankylosing spondylitis. J Spinal Disord Tech. 2010;23(3):186–91.
108. Hoh DJ, Khoueir P, Wang MY. Management of cervical deformity in ankylosing spondylitis. Neurosurg Focus. 2008;24(1):E9.
109. Chin KR, Ahn J. Controlled cervical extension osteotomy for ankylosing spondylitis utilizing the Jackson operating table: technical note. Spine. 2007;32(17):1926–9.

Part II

History and Basic Research

2 History of Spinal Osteotomy of Ankylosing Spondylitis Kyphosis

Xuesong Zhang and Yao Wang

Ankylosing spondylitis (AS) is a chronic inflammatory disease that predominantly affects the axial skeleton. Without treatment, ankylosing spondylitis may lead to thoracolumbar kyphotic deformity, which affects over 30% of patients in the late phase [1]. Severe spinal kyphosis may result in sagittal imbalance and limitation of psychosocial activities and physical exercises [2, 3]. Corrective spinal osteotomy is necessary for these patients to improve their appearance and daily life function. Since 1945, a variety of surgical techniques have been proposed for the treatment of ankylosing spondylitis kyphosis. The safety and effectiveness of surgery had been significantly improved by the development of instrumentation, surgical details, and anesthesiologic techniques [4].

The aim of this chapter is to historically review the common spinal osteotomy techniques utilized in ankylosing spondylitis kyphotic deformity.

1 In the 1940s

The Smith-Petersen osteotomy (SPO) was firstly described by Smith-Petersen in 1945 [5] to treat global AS kyphosis. In SPO osteotomy, facet joints of lumbar spine were narrowly resected, while ligamentum flavum from the inferior margin of the lamina and inferior articular process were detached. Deformity correction during this procedure is achieved by shortening the posterior column and lengthening the anterior column by opening a disk through manual extension.

The Dutch orthopedic surgeon La Chapelle, in 1946, introduced a two-stage opening-wedge osteotomy through anterior approach for correction of thoracic-lumbar kyphosis in one case of AS [6]. The L2 lamina was firstly removed under local anesthesia, and the L2/L3 disk was anteriorly released and resected 2 weeks later. Then, the anterior and medium columns were wedged open and filled with bone graft. After that, several modifications of this opening-wedge osteotomy have been raised [7–11].

However, this maneuver was assumed to be associated with some severe complications such as aortic rupture because of the huge elongation of the anterior column [12, 13].

Several years later, Briggs et al. [14] and Wilson and Turkell [15] reported a posterior wedge osteotomy with bilateral intervertebral foraminotomy. This method modified SPO to a gradual correction without rupturing of the anterior longitudinal ligament.

2 In the 1950s

In 1958, Urist [16] first described extension osteotomy of the cervical spine for correction of cervical deformity. The indications for cervical extension osteotomy include horizontal gaze lost

X. Zhang (✉) · Y. Wang
PLA General Hospital (301 Hospital), Beijing, China

Y. Wang (ed.), *Surgical Treatment of Ankylosing Spondylitis Deformity*,
https://doi.org/10.1007/978-981-13-6427-3_2

and difficulties with attending to personal hygiene with function and with swallowing due to cervical flexion deformity.

Urist's procedure was performed in the sitting position, under local anesthesia with the patient awake to facilitate neurologic monitoring during the reduction, and consisted of a laminar resection followed by correction obtained gradually over several days using a plaster jacket that incorporated the head and neck [13]. Because the canal is relatively wide and the vertebral artery does not pass through the lateral mass at C7–T1 segments, the correction center is usually located at this level [1].

3 In the 1960s to 1990s

Scudese and Calabro in 1963 [17] and later Ziwjan in 1982 [18] and Thomasen in 1985 [3] described the pedicle subtraction osteotomy (PSO), a three-column posterior osteotomy as a closing-wedge osteotomy (CWO) for the management of fixed sagittal plane deformities in patients with ankylosing spondylitis. Typically, pedicle subtraction osteotomy is performed at either L2 or L3, as these vertebrae are the normal apex of lumbar lordosis and safer because they are caudal to the conus medullaris. During this procedure, posterior elements and a V-shaped bony wedge of the vertebral body are resected, and the middle column is shortened without lengthening the anterior column [19]. Pedicle subtraction osteotomies are typically indicated for fixed sagittal deformities with sharp or angular kyphosis and are often applied for the treatment of ankylosing spondylitis kyphosis deformities that lack anterior flexibility [20].

In the 1970s, Simmons [21, 22] modified the Urist's extension osteotomy of the cervical spine involving the performance of the osteotomy at C7–Tl. McMaster reviewed 15 patients who underwent the original Simmons' osteotomy under general anesthesia while in the prone position [23]. Belanger et al. and Langeloo began to utilize internal fixation with Simmons' techniques [24, 25].

The Ponte osteotomy (PO) was described in 1984 by Alberto Ponte, which consists of a wide resection of thoracic facet joints as well as of lamina and in a complete removal of the ligamentum flavum [26]. Gradual segmental compression is obtained by closure of the posterior column in thoracic kyphosis patients with mobile disks with the Ponte osteotomy. The main differences between Ponte osteotomy and SPO are not related to the osseous resection but to the corrective mechanism [27]. The Ponte osteotomy as a modified technique advanced the SPO one step further as indicated for Scheuermann's kyphosis and adolescent idiopathic scoliosis [19, 28].

Hehne et al. improved the SPO technique to polysegmental opening-wedge osteotomies (POWs) in 1990 [29]. It changed from one level to multiple levels, and the hinge changed to posterior fiber ring. Not too much elongation in each level would happen because one level only obtained about 10° correction. When multilevel osteotomy was done, the correction curve is smooth rather than sharp. At the same time, complications reduce significantly [30]. Though recent study noted that SPOs might lead to correction lost [31], it is still a safe and effective method.

4 In the Twenty-First Century

Compared with SPO, PSO is classified as a higher-grade osteotomy and is technically more demanding [32]. On average, classical PSO can achieve approximately 30–40° of lordosis at each level when it is performed [33]. Many modifications of this closing-wedge osteotomy have been described.

Chen et al. [34] removed the bone and the upper disk through the pedicle, and this technique was performed as a safe and reliable surgical option in 13 patients with failed short-segment pedicle instrumentation after thoracolumbar fracture. Zhang et al. [35] obtained favorable results by modified PSO in treating Kümmell disease. If most of the lamina and upper and/or lower end plates were removed, modified PSO through a single level may achieve 60° correction as maximum [36]. Recently, pedicle subtraction osteotomy has become a more favorable method to correct spinal kyphosis. Several spinal deformities are usually candidates for pedicle subtraction osteotomy, including sharp angular kyphosis, severe global kyphosis, concomitant coronal imbalance, etc. More structures would be resected during PSO, which may theoretically cause increase of operation time, blood loss, and risk of neural complications. Sometimes, sagittal translation (ST) may occur during procedures of folding the osteotomy area.

The bone–disk–bone osteotomy, which was further developed from pedicle subtraction osteotomy by extending the resection to the cranial disk with its adjacent end plates, improved the corrective angle by single CWO [37]. This technique guaranteed anterior column fusion by bone-on-bone contact [37].

The posterior-only VCR technique, which was firstly described by MacLennan in 1922 [38] and considered as the most powerful method for the correction of spinal deformity, is retained for rare cases since the risk of neurological complication is high [39]. In 2012, Kim et al. performed pVCR to correct the major deformity in the thoracolumbar junction of a patient with ankylosing spondylitis.

Vertebral column decancellation was firstly named modified VCR and described by Yan Wang in 2008 in his series study for 13 adult patients with severe rigid congenital kyphoscoliosis [40]. This technique was designed to combine advantages of eggshell technique, SPO, PSO, and VCR. Basic procedures of VCD osteotomy include resection of the elements anterior to the spinal cord as less as possible to decrease the complications of shortening the spinal cord, and enough posterior elements must be removed to accommodate the spinal cord to avoid new compression. The partial and selective decancellation of deformed vertebrae may facilitate realignment of the angular spine, and the residual bone of deformed vertebrae may take the place of metal mesh described in the VCR technique, serving as a "bony cage" [41, 42].

VCD techniques were later developed by Wang and his colleagues to a Y-shaped osteotomy, which preserved the middle vertebral column [43, 44]. It is characterized by controllably opening the anterior column and closing the posterior column and preserving the middle column as a hinge. The essential procedures of the "Y"-shaped VCD technique include the resection of a relatively limited posterior part of the column and enough preservation of the middle column as a hinge, which would provide more stability and better fusion. A greater correction could be achieved by opening the anterior column, while the requirement to shorten the posterior column was decreased, which would diminish the danger of sagittal translation and neurological deficits. Moreover, the osteoclasis of the anterior column cortex would be appropriate for correction of ankylosing spondylitis kyphosis.

References

1. Kubiak EN, Moskovich R, Errico TJ, Di Cesare PE. Orthopaedic management of ankylosing spondylitis. J Am Acad Orthop Surg. 2005;13:267–78.
2. Thiranont N, Netrawichien P. Transpedicular decancellation closed wedge vertebral osteotomy for treatment of fixed flexion deformity of spine in ankylosing spondylitis. Spine (Phila Pa 1976). 1993;18:2517–22.
3. Thomasen E. Vertebral osteotomy for correction of kyphosis in ankylosing spondylitis. Clin Orthop Relat Res. 1985;194:142–52.
4. Koller H, Koller J, Mayer M, Hempfing A, Hitzl W. Osteotomies in ankylosing spondylitis: where, how many, and how much? Eur Spine J. 2018;27(Suppl 1):70–100.
5. Smith-Petersen MF, Larson CB, Aufranc OE. Osteotomy of the spine for correction of flexion deformity in rheumatoid arthritis. JBJS. 1945; 27(1):1–11.
6. La Chapelle EH. Osteotomy of the lumbar spine for correction of kyphosis in a case of ankylosing spondylarthritis. JBJS. 1946;28(4):851–8.
7. Bossers GT. Columnotomy in severe Bechterew kyphosis. Acta Orthop Belg. 1972;58:47–54.
8. McMaster MJ, Coventry MB. Spinal osteotomy in ankylosing spondylitis. Technique, complications, and long-term results. Mayo Clin Proc. 1973;48:476–86.
9. McMaster MJ. A technique for lumbar spinal osteotomy in ankylosing spondylitis. J Bone Joint Surg Br. 1985;67:204–10.
10. Adams JC. Technique, dangers and safeguards in osteotomy of the spine. J Bone Joint Surg Br. 1952;34: 226–32.

11. Goel MK. Vertebral osteotomy for correction of fixed flexion deformity of the spine. J Bone Joint Surg Am. 1968;50:287–94.
12. Camargo FP, Cordeiro EN, Napoli MM. Corrective osteotomy of the spine in ankylosing spondylitis. Experience with 66 cases. Clin Orthop Relat Res. 1986;208:157–67.
13. Klems H, Friedebold G. Rupture of the abdominal aorta following a corrective spinal operation for ankylopoeitic spondylitis. Z Orthop Ihre Grenzgeb. 1971;108:554–63.
14. Briggs H, Keats S, Schlesinger PT. Wedge osteotomy of the spine with bilateral intervertebral foraminotomy; correction of flexion deformity in five cases of ankylosing arthritis of the spine. J Bone Joint Surg Am. 1947;29:1075–82.
15. Wilson MJ, Turkell JH. Multiple spinal wedge osteotomy; its use in a case of Marie-Strumpell spondylitis. Am J Surg. 1949;77:777–82.
16. Urist MR. Osteotomy of the cervical spine; report of a case of ankylosing rheumatoid spondylitis. J Bone Joint Surg Am. 1958;40:833–43.
17. Scudese VA, Calabro JJ. Vertebral wedge osteotomy. Correction of rheumatoid (ankylosing) spondylitis. JAMA. 1963;186:627–31.
18. Ziwjan JL. The treatment of flexion deformities of the spine in Bechterew disease. Beitr Orthop Traumatol. 1982;29:195–9.
19. Hu WH, Wang Y. Osteotomy techniques for spinal deformity. Chin Med J. 2016;129:2639–41.
20. Cho KJ, Bridwell KH, Lenke LG, Berra A, Baldus C. Comparison of Smith-Petersen versus pedicle subtraction osteotomy for the correction of fixed sagittal imbalance. Spine (Phila Pa 1976). 2005;30:2030–7; discussion 2038.
21. Simmons EH. The surgical correction of flexion deformity of the cervical spine in ankylosing spondylitis. Clin Orthop Relat Res. 1972;86:132–43.
22. Simmons EH. Kyphotic deformity of the spine in ankylosing spondylitis. Clin Orthop Relat Res. 1977; 128:65–77.
23. McMaster MJ. Osteotomy of the cervical spine in ankylosing spondylitis. J Bone Joint Surg Br. 1997; 79:197–203.
24. Langeloo DD, Journee HL, Pavlov PW, de Kleuver M. Cervical osteotomy in ankylosing spondylitis: evaluation of new developments. Eur Spine J. 2006;15:493–500.
25. Lazennec JY, d'Astorg H, Rousseau MA. Cervical spine surgery in ankylosing spondylitis: review and current concept. Orthop Traumatol Surg Res. 2015;101:507–13.
26. Ponte A, Orlando G, Siccardi GL. The true Ponte osteotomy: by the one who developed it. Spine Deform. 2018;6:2–11.
27. Dorward IG, Lenke LG, Stoker GE, Cho W, Koester LA, Sides BA. Radiographical and clinical outcomes of posterior column osteotomies in spinal deformity correction. Spine (Phila Pa 1976). 2014;39:870–80.
28. Pizones J, Sanchez-Mariscal F, Zuniga L, Izquierdo E. Ponte osteotomies to treat major thoracic adolescent idiopathic scoliosis curves allow more effective corrective maneuvers. Eur Spine J. 2015;24:1540–6.
29. Hehne HJ, Zielke K, Bohm H. Polysegmental lumbar osteotomies and transpedicled fixation for correction of long-curved kyphotic deformities in ankylosing spondylitis. Report on 177 cases. Clin Orthop Relat Res. 1990;258:49–55.
30. van Royen BJ, de Kleuver M, Slot GH. Polysegmental lumbar posterior wedge osteotomies for correction of kyphosis in ankylosing spondylitis. Eur Spine J. 1998;7:104–10.
31. Zhu Z, Wang X, Qian B, Wang B, Yu Y, Zhao Q, Qiu Y. Loss of correction in the treatment of thoracolumbar kyphosis secondary to ankylosing spondylitis: a comparison between Smith-Petersen osteotomies and pedicle subtraction osteotomy. J Spinal Disord Tech. 2012;25:383–90.
32. Diebo B, Liu S, Fau-Lafage V, Lafage V, Fau-Schwab F, Schwab F. Osteotomies in the treatment of spinal deformities: indications, classification, and surgical planning. Eur J Orthop Surg Traumatol. 2014;24(1):11–20.
33. Jaffray D, Becker V, Eisenstein S. Closing wedge osteotomy with transpedicular fixation in ankylosing spondylitis. Clin Orthop Relat Res. 1992;279:122–6.
34. Chen F, Kang Y, Li H, Lv G, Lu C, Li J, Wang B, Chen W, Liao Y, Dai Z. Modified pedicle subtraction osteotomy as a salvage method for failed short-segment pedicle instrumentation in the treatment of thoracolumbar fracture. Clin Spine Surg. 2016;29:E120–6.
35. Zhang X, Hu W, Yu J, Wang Z, Wang Y. An effective treatment option for Kummell disease with neurological deficits: modified Transpedicular subtraction and disc osteotomy combined with long-segment fixation. Spine (Phila Pa 1976). 2016;41(15):E923–30.
36. Xi YM, Pan M, Wang Z-J, Zhang G-Q, Shan R, Shan R, Liu Y-J, Chen B-H, Hu Y-G. Correction of post-traumatic thoracolumbar kyphosis using pedicle subtraction osteotomy. Eur J Orthop Surg Traumatol. 2013;23(Suppl 1):S59–66.
37. Enercan M, Ozturk C, Kahraman S, Sarıer M, Hamzaoglu A, Alanay A. Osteotomies/spinal column resections in adult deformity. Eur Spine J. 2013;22(Suppl 2):S254–64.
38. Meredith DS, Vaccaro AR. History of spinal osteotomy. Eur J Orthop Surg Traumatol. 2014;24(Suppl 1):S69–72.
39. Kim KT, Lee SH, Son ES, Kwack YH, Chun YS, Lee JH. Surgical treatment of "chin-on-pubis" deformity in a patient with ankylosing spondylitis: a case report of consecutive cervical, thoracic, and lumbar corrective osteotomies. Spine (Phila Pa 1976). 2012;37(16):E1017–21.
40. Wang Y, Zhang Y, Zhang X, Huang P, Xiao S, Wang Z, Liu Z, Liu B, Lu N, Mao K. A single posterior approach for multilevel modified vertebral column resection in adults with severe rigid congenital

kyphoscoliosis: a retrospective study of 13 cases. Eur Spine J. 2008;17:361–72.
41. Wang Y, Lenke LG. Vertebral column decancellation for the management of sharp angular spinal deformity. Eur Spine J. 2011;20:1703–10.
42. Wang Y, Zhang YG, Zheng GQ, Xiao SH, Zhang XS, Wang Z. Vertebral column decancellation for the management of rigid scoliosis: the effectiveness and safety analysis. Zhonghua Wai Ke Za Zhi. 2010;48(22):1701–4.
43. Hu W, Yu J, Liu H, Zhang X, Wang Y. Y shape osteotomy in ankylosing spondylitis, a prospective case series with minimum 2 year follow-up. PLoS One. 2016;11(12):e0167792.
44. Zhang X, Zhang Z, Wang J, Lu M, Hu W, Wang Y, Wang Y. Vertebral column decancellation: a new spinal osteotomy technique for correcting rigid thoracolumbar kyphosis in patients with ankylosing spondylitis. Bone Joint J. 2016;98-B:672–8.

3

Cardiopulmonary and Gastrointestinal Manifestations of Patients with Ankylosing Spondylitis

Jun Fu and Zheng Wang

1 Cardiac Manifestations of Ankylosing Spondylitis

Many previous publications have reported that cardiac manifestations were involved in 2–10% of AS patients, such as aortitis, cardiomyopathy, conduction disorders, and valvular regurgitation, and were associated with AS. What is more, human leukocyte antigen (HLA)-B27 is found in most AS patients and is demonstrated to contribute to the pathophysiologic changes of the aforementioned conditions [1].

The onset of aortic root and valve disease in AS patients is associated with the duration of the underlying disease. Aortic disease and aortic regurgitation may predict the presence of any articular symptoms, and the onset of AS as a potential cause may be initially overlooked. Bulkley and Roberts [2] noted aortic root fibrous proliferation along the intima. Further examination revealed cellular inflammatory processes and platelet aggregation resulted in endarteritis around the aortic root and valve. This in turn stimulates hyperactivity of fibroblast, which leads to tissue thickening, including aortic valve annulus and cusps, aortomitral junction along with the conduction system.

Roldan et al. [3] researched the aortic roots and valves in AS patients using transthoracic echocardiography (TEE), and their research results showed morbidity rate of aortic root and valve diseases (Fig. 3.1) was 82% in AS patients compared with control (27%). And valvular regurgitation was common in these cases (Fig. 3.2). According to the follow-up data, 20% patients developed heart failure and received valve replacement.

Conduction dysfunction is one of the most common cardiac manifestations of AS patients that usually precede other cardiac manifestations such as valvular defects [4]. It has been reported two popular theories about the etiology of conduction abnormalities in AS patients: abnormalities in the aortic valve nodal artery leading to aortic valve node dysfunction versus inflammation in the intraventricular septum resulting in lesion. Recently, Toussirot et al. [5] found that autonomic disturbances may bring on arrhythmias and conduction dysfunction, therefore negatively affecting prognosis of these AS patients.

It is widely reported in many studies that the diastolic disorder not the systolic is the most common myocardial dysfunction in AS patients, which was demonstrated by means of echocardiography with the results that the statistically significant lower E-wave peak (early diastolic filling), higher A-wave peak (late diastolic filling), and overall low E/A ratio represent as diastolic dysfunction in AS patients. And these research results also sustain an overall decrease in compliance and hence a reduction in diastolic function.

J. Fu · Z. Wang (✉)
Chinese PLA General Hospital, Beijing, China

Y. Wang (ed.), *Surgical Treatment of Ankylosing Spondylitis Deformity*,
https://doi.org/10.1007/978-981-13-6427-3_3

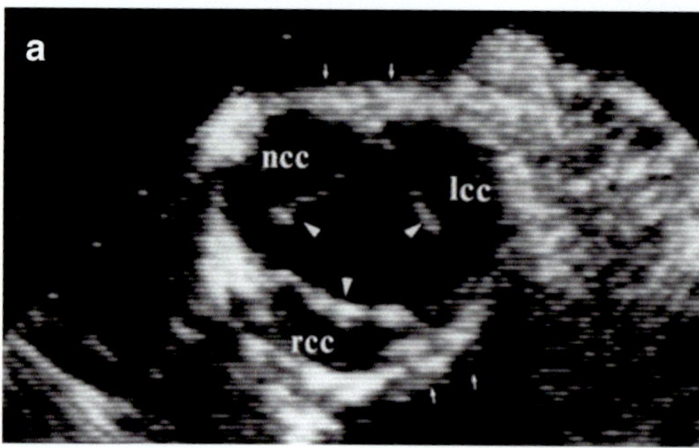

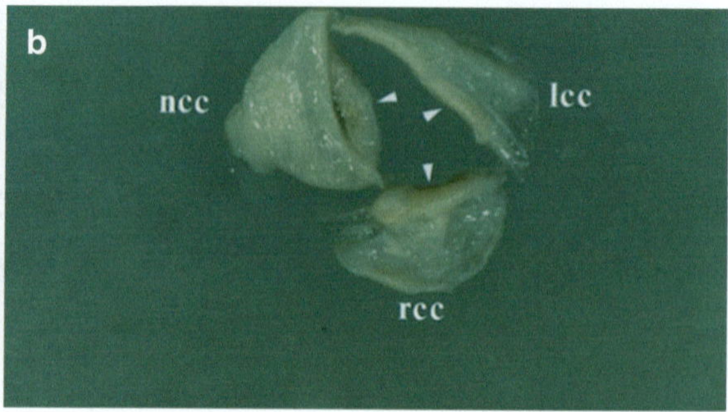

Fig. 3.1 (**a**) A 34-year-old patient with severe aortic regurgitation, transesophageal echocardiography image of the aortic valve which showed thickening of the aortic root walls (small arrows) and irregular thickening of the three aortic cusp tips (arrowheads). (**b**) The specimen showed a central regurgitant orifice, resulting in retracted and rolled noncoronary cusp (ncc) and right coronary cusp (rcc), along with the irregularly thickened fringes of three aortic cusps (arrowheads). *lcc* left coronary cusp. (*Reprint with permission from reference: Carlos A. Roldan, Aortic root disease and valve disease associated with ankylosing spondylitis 32:5, 1998*)

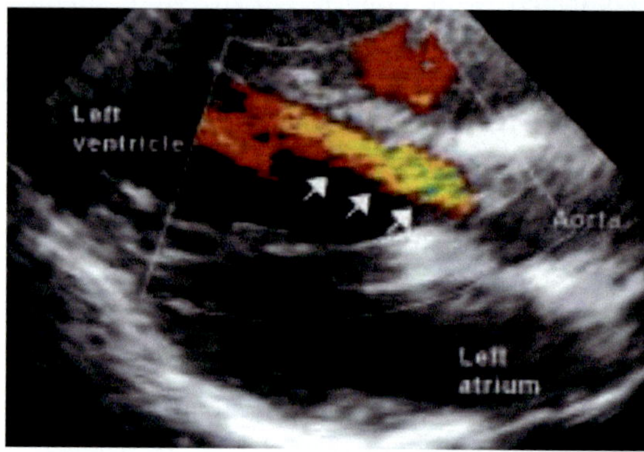

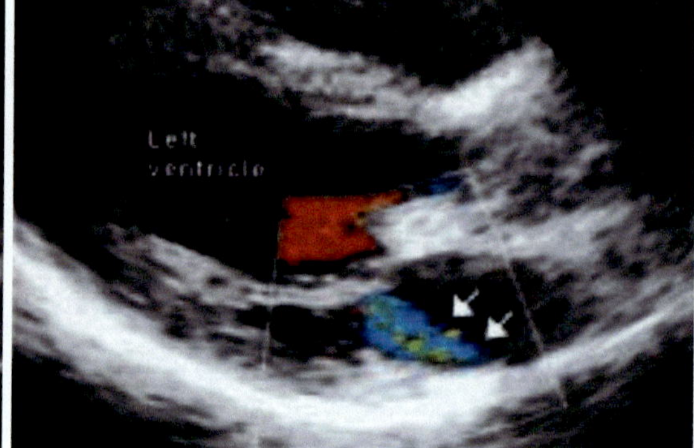

Fig. 3.2 The color Doppler echocardiography image showed valve disorders: grade II aortic valve regurgitation (left) and grade I/II mitral valve regurgitation (right). (*Reprint with permission from reference: S J Lee, HLA-B27 positive juvenile arthritis with cardiac involvement preceding sacroiliac joint changes 86:6, 2001*)

What is more, Fu et al. [6] compared the differences in cardiovascular performance between AS patients with and without kyphosis, and they found a statistically increased incidence of cardiovascular complications in patients with kyphosis including left ventricular diastolic dysfunction, left ventricular high voltage, and increased heart rate. Another prospective study by the same author measured the cardiac function changes in AS patients with kyphosis after pedicle subtraction osteotomy (PSO). The clinical improvement was 15/20 (75.0%): cardiac function in AS patients with kyphosis undergoing PSO surgery was significantly improved [7]. After PSO, sagittal balance of AS patients was improved so the abdominal organs are not any longer compressed, and the moving range of diaphragm is consequently larger, increasing the thoracic volume and resulting in more normal ventricular function during cardiac diastole (Fig. 3.3).

2 Pulmonary Manifestations of Ankylosing Spondylitis

Pulmonary abnormality in AS patients is a common extra-articular manifestation of the disease that was first demonstrated in 1941 [8]. The pulmonary abnormalities of AS patients include

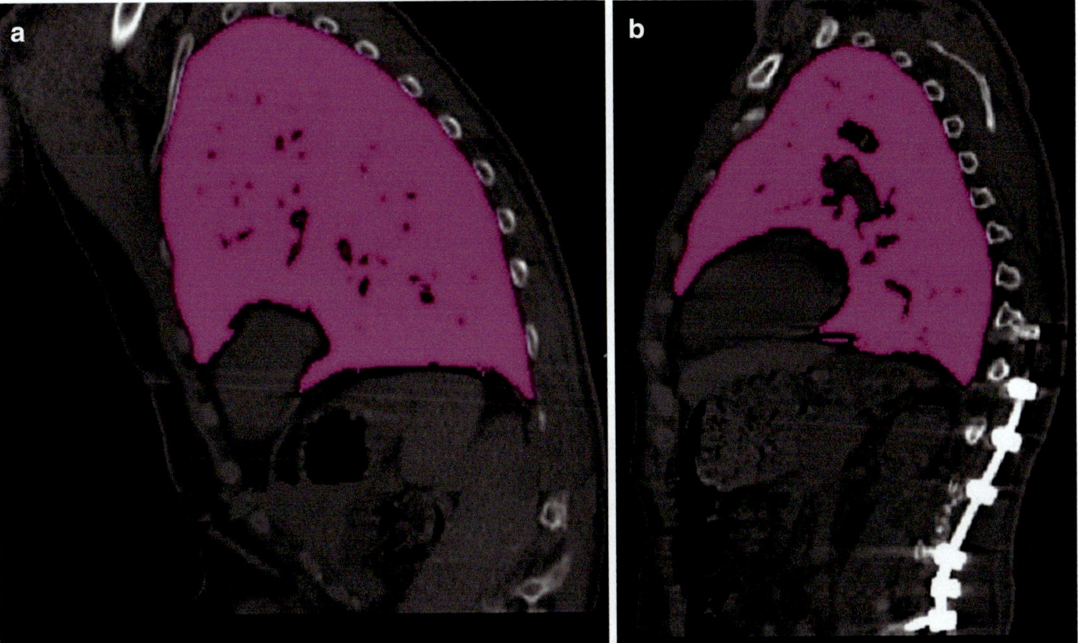

Fig. 3.3 The sagittal position changes in heart, lung, and abdominal viscera. (**a**) preoperation, (**b**) postoperation

upper lobe fibrosis, interstitial lung disease, and obstructive ventilation due to chest wall restriction, sleep apnea, and spontaneous pneumothorax. The incidence of pulmonary abnormalities in AS patients has increased with the development of high-resolution computed tomography (HRCT).

Upper lobe fibrosis has been determined as lung abnormality associated with AS for a long time. The incidence of apical fibrosis in AS is low with an estimated range from 1.3% to 30% and is associated with a longer disease duration [9]. Apical fibrosis (Fig. 3.4) usually occurs greater than 5 years after the onset of the arthritic symptoms associated with the disease. The cause of fibrosis is not clear, but repeated aspiration leading to ventilation dysfunction in aspiration pneumonitis, changes in apical mechanical stress from a stiff thoracic spine, and recurrent cough impairment due to alterations in respiratory mechanics have been proposed [10, 11]. The pulmonary parenchymal abnormality is a fertile bed for multiple biological reinfections including atypical *Mycobacterium*, *Mycobacterium tuberculosis*, *Aspergillus*, and *Metschnikowia pulcherrima*. In the past, the abnormal distribution and appearance of the upper lobe in AS patients led many physicians to misdiagnose these patients with *Mycobacterium tuberculosis*.

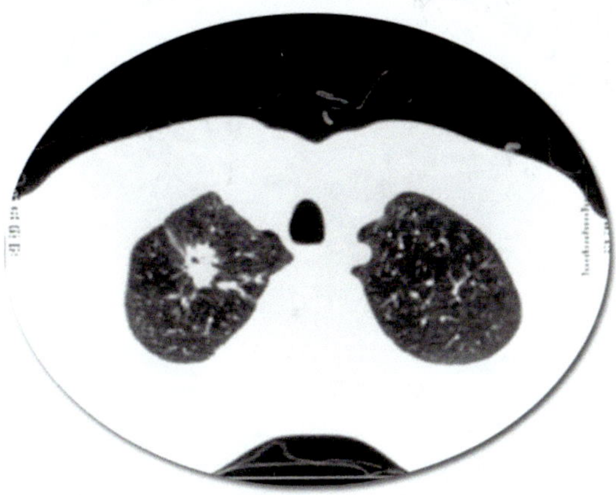

Fig. 3.4 HRCT scan of a patient with right-sided apical fibrosis. Cavity formation is accompanied by substantial distortion. (*Reprint with permission from reference: Ozlem Senocak, Lung parenchyma changes in ankylosing spondylitis: demonstration with high resolution CT and correlation with disease duration 45:2, 2003*)

Interstitial lung disease (ILD), beyond apical fibrosis, is now an established feature of pulmonary abnormality in AS patients owing to reinforced visualization of the lung parenchyma with HRCT. Due to the relative lack of autopsy studies, there is few pathologic diagnosis of ILD in AS patients, and the cause of the ILD with AS is still unknown. Lung needle biopsy and lobectomy examinations revealed infiltration of chronic inflammatory cell and protruding interstitial fibrosis with collagen elastic degeneration. Several studies have shown the correlation between ILD and AS [12–14]. The parenchymal abnormalities were extensive including bronchiectasis, emphysema, ground glass opacities, parenchymal micronodules, pleural thickening, parenchymal bands, and septal thickening (Fig. 3.5).

Multiple studies widely reported that the incidence of pulmonary dysfunction in AS patients was 20% to 57%, and the classifications of pulmonary dysfunction were restrictive pulmonary dysfunction, obstructive pulmonary dysfunction, or mixed pulmonary dysfunction, of which the most common type in AS patients was the restrictive pulmonary dysfunction [12, 15]. Spine kyphosis secondary to involvement of the thoracic spine and sternomanubrial, sternoclavicular, and costovertebral joints brings on impairment of chest wall expansion and respiratory disorder. And kyphosis angle is negatively correlated with the impaired pulmonary function.

Zhang et al. [16] investigated the change of pulmonary volume in patients with AS kyphosis after the pedicle subtraction osteotomy (PSO) surgery and found pulmonary volume was increased significantly after the osteotomy. A computed tomography (CT)-based method (Fig. 3.6) was used to measure accurate pulmonary volume change during the PSO surgery. What is more, Fu et al. [17] observe postoperative

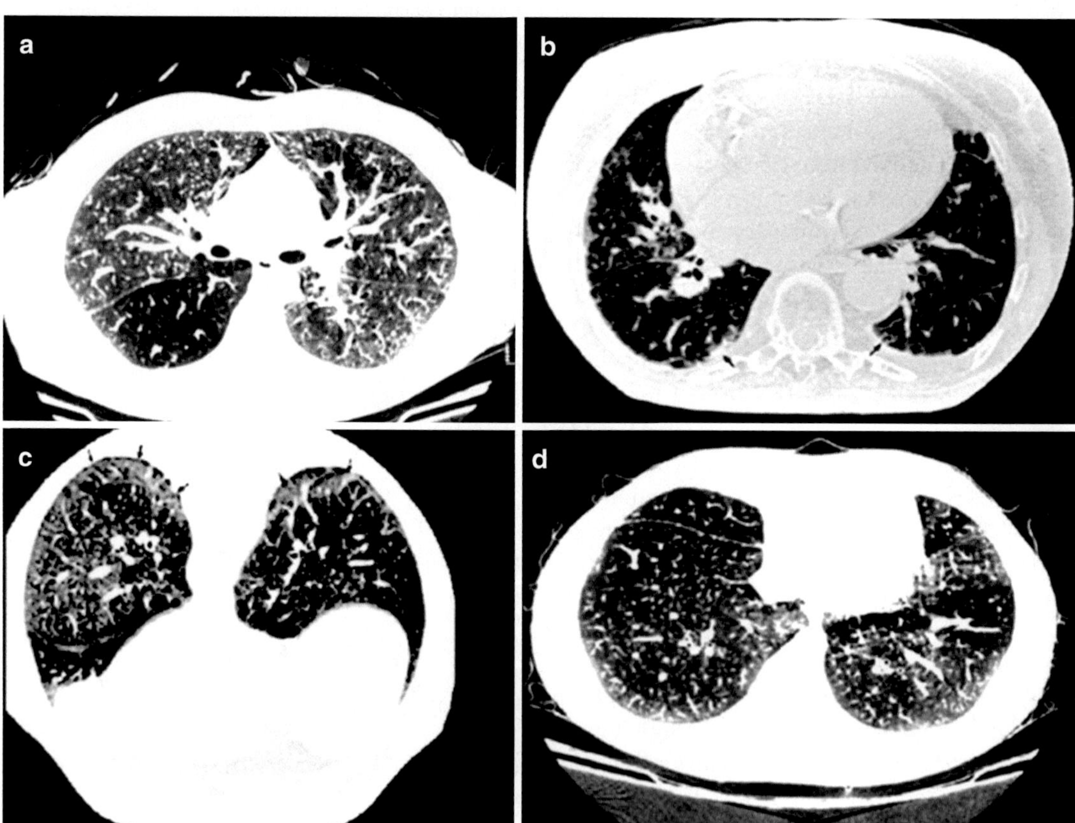

Fig. 3.5 HRCT image diagnosis of parenchymal abnormalities. (**a**) emphysema, (**b**) parenchymal bands, (**c**) septal and pleural thickening, (**d**) bronchiectasis. (*Reprint with permission from reference: Ozlem Senocak, Lung parenchyma changes in ankylosing spondylitis: demonstration with high resolution CT and correlation with disease duration 45:2, 2003*)

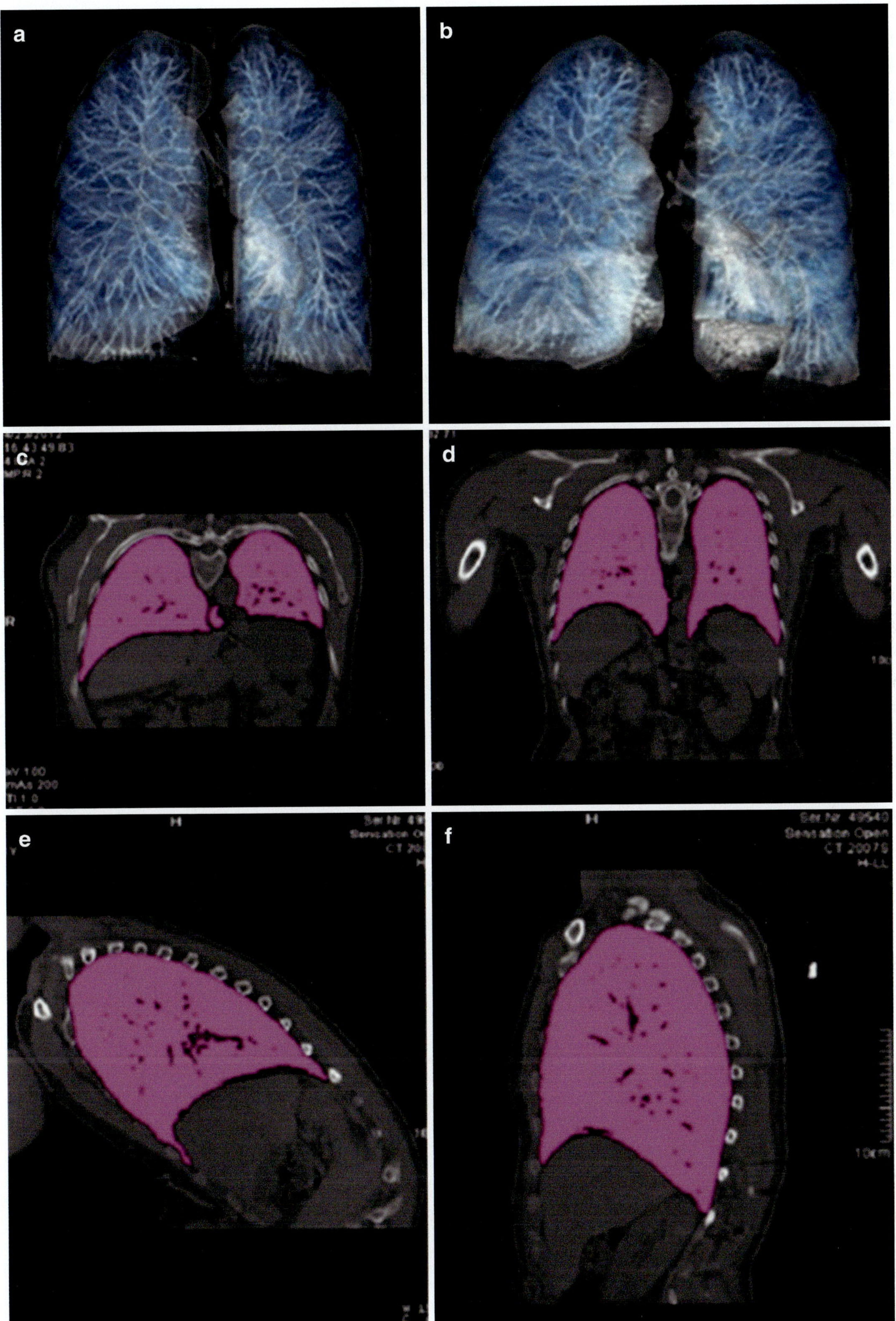

Fig. 3.6 Three-dimensional reconstruction, coronal and sagittal LV images. (**a**, **c**, **e**) preoperation, (**b**, **d**, **f**) postoperation

changes of pulmonary function tests and breath-holding time in patients with AS kyphosis after PSO. They concluded the pulmonary function in patients with AS kyphosis including pulmonary volume and ventilatory function had significantly improved after 2-year PSO surgery. And, the improved pulmonary function was positively correlated with the kyphosis correction.

3 Gastrointestinal Manifestations of Ankylosing Spondylitis

A close connection between AS and the gastrointestinal disorders has been demonstrated for a long time. Clinically diagnosed inflammatory bowel disease (IBD), whether Crohn's disease or ulcerative colitis, was reported to be present in 5–10% of AS patients [18, 19]. And subclinical gut inflammation was found by ileocolonoscopy in 25–49% of AS patients (Fig. 3.7). These findings have hypothesized that the initiating and/or ongoing events in the pathogenesis may be a disorder of the gut/blood barrier that promotes the interaction of bacteria and immune systems. Although there are confounding factors in both cases, such as the use of NSAIDs in AS patients and the inflammation in IBD, both of which may lead to increased intestinal permeability. For the 10–60% of healthy relatives of patients with either disease who did not use NSAIDs, the observation of increased intestinal permeability provides convincing evidence, suggesting that the underlying causes associated with AS and IBD are possible [20, 21].

In the later stage of AS, severe thoracic or thoracolumbar kyphotic deformity can cause extrusion of viscera owing to trunk flexion and decreased abdominal cavity volume, lowering the gastrointestinal function and gastrointestinal motility. The gastrointestinal symptom developed with deterioration of digestive function and weight loss, such as the decrease in food intake and the change in frequency of defecation. Spinal osteotomy is the only way to restore the spinal sagittal balance for AS patients. This study has proved that, theoretically, spinal osteotomy in patients with AS can improve the digestive function of patients with AS, thereby reducing the abdominal volume and viscera compression and changing the shape of the organs caused by kyphosis deformity. The study of Liu et al. [22] showed that MD (minimum distance) and AMSPA (acreage of the abdominal median sagittal plane) were significantly improved after PSO surgery. What is more, the spinal osteotomy improved trunk flexion and extrusion of viscera and decreased abdominal cavity volume and abnormal abdominal viscera position during the follow-up, leading to improved digestive function [23] (Fig. 3.8).

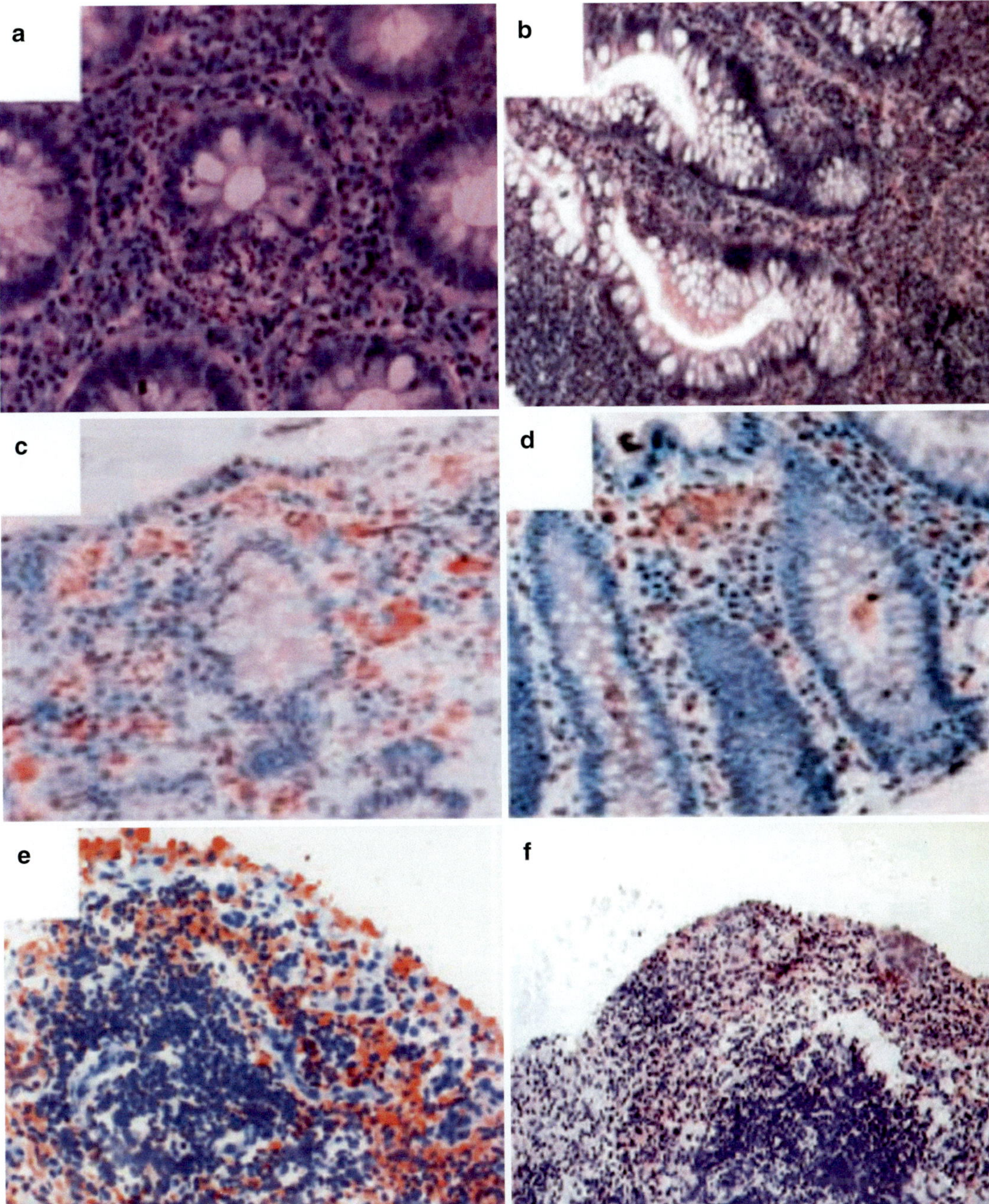

Fig. 3.7 Representative histologic images of gut and joint inflammation in ankylosing spondylitis (AS). (**a**) Acute gut inflammation in an AS patient, just as in that case of bacterial infection. (**b**) Chronic gut inflammation in an AS patient, just as in that case of inflammatory bowel disease (IBD). (**c**) CD163-positive macrophage stain in the gut of an AS patient. (**d**) CD163-positive macrophage stain in the gut of a patient with Crohn's disease. (**e**) CD163-positive macrophage stain in the inflamed synovium of an AS patient. (**f**) CD163-positive macrophage stain in the inflamed synovium of a patient with rheumatoid arthritis. (*Reprint with permission from reference: M. Rudwaleit, Ankylosing spondylitis and bowel disease 20:3, 2006*)

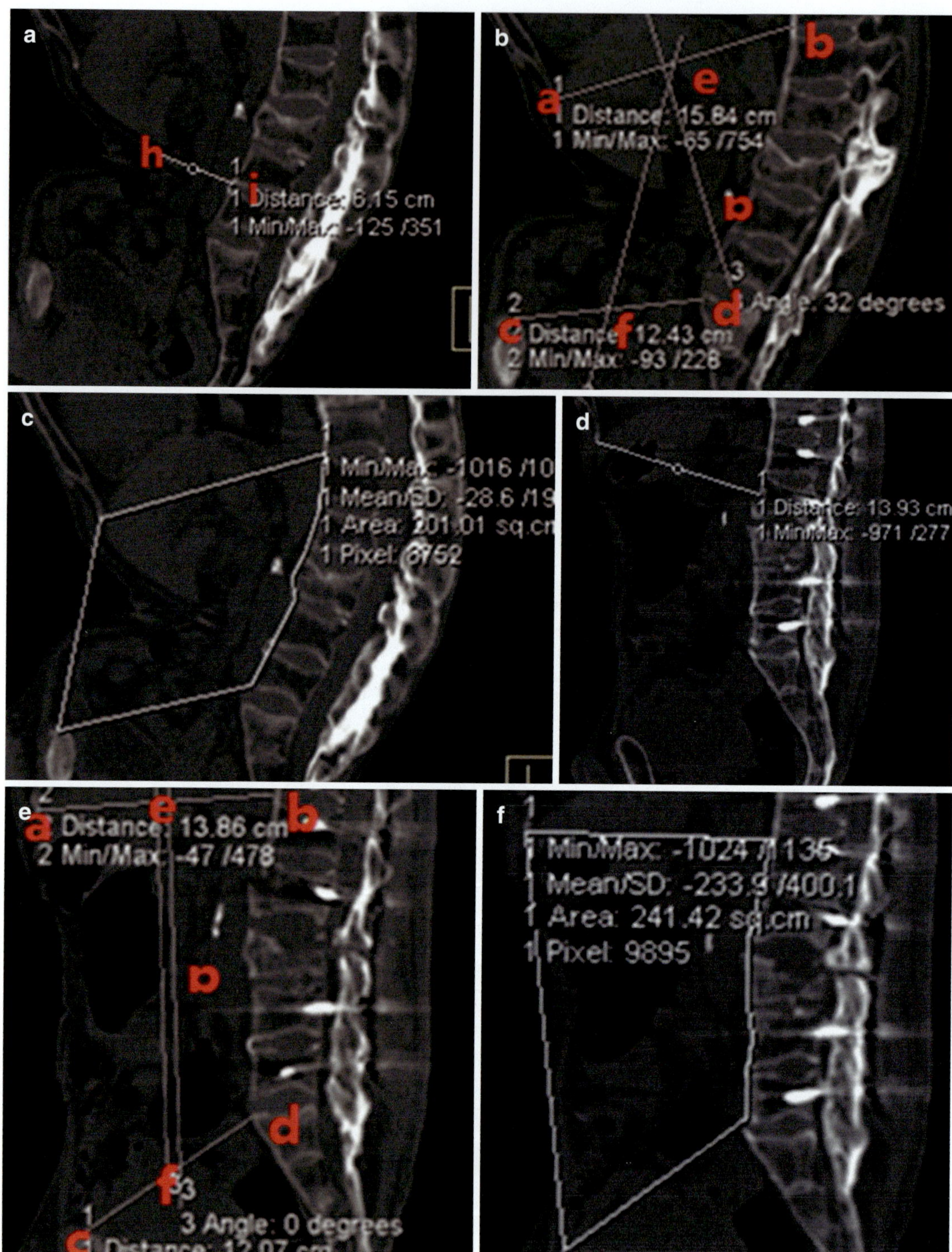

Fig. 3.8 MD indicates the minimum distance from the midsagittal plane of the abdomen, the minimum distance between the xiphoid process and the spine (**d**) or that between the abdominal wall and the spine when the abdominal wall was folded into abdomen (**a**, line h–i). AMSPA indicates acreage of the abdominal midsagittal plane; the acreage is enclosed by the following four peripheral lines (**b**, **c**, **e**, **f**): (1) a straight line from the xiphoid process to the inferior edge of T12, (2) a straight line between the xiphoid process and the superior edge of the pubis, (3) a straight line from the superior edge of the pubis to the anterosuperior corner of the sacrum, and (4) the anterior edge line of T12-S1

References

1. Moyssakis I, Gialafos E, Vassiliou VA, et al. Myocardial performance and aortic elasticity are impaired in patients with ankylosing spondylitis. Scand J Rheumatol. 2009;38(3):216–21.
2. Bulkley BH, Roberts WC. Ankylosing spondylitis and aortic regurgitation: description of the characteristic cardiovascular lesion from study of eight necropsy patients. Circulation. 1973;48(5):1014–27.
3. Roldan CA, Chavez J, Wiest PW, et al. Aortic root disease and valve disease associated with ankylosing spondylitis. J Am Coll Cardiol. 1998;32(5):1397–404.
4. Kaźmierczak J, Peregud-Pogorzelska M, Biernawska J, et al. Cardiac arrhythmias and conduction disturbances in patients with ankylosing spondylitis. Angiology. 2008;58(6):751–6.
5. Toussirot E, Bahjaoui-Bouhaddi M, Poncet JC, et al. Abnormal autonomic cardiovascular control in ankylosing spondylitis. Ann Rheum Dis. 1999;58(8):481–7.
6. Fu J, Wu MY, Liang Y, et al. Differences in cardiovascular manifestations between ankylosing spondylitis patients with and without kyphosis. Clin Rheumatol. 2016;35(8):2003–8.
7. Fu J, Song K, Zhang YG, et al. Changes in cardiac function after pedicle subtraction osteotomy in patients with a kyphosis due to ankylosing spondylitis. Bone Joint J. 2015;97-B(10):1405–10.
8. Dunham C, Kautz F. Sondylarthritis ankylopoietica, a review and report of twenty cases. Am J Med Sci. 1941;201:232–50.
9. Kanathur N, Lee-Chiong T. Pulmonary manifestations of ankylosing spondylitis. Clin Chest Med. 2010;31(3):547–54.
10. Davies D. Lung fibrosis in ankylosing spondylitis. Thorax. 1972;27(2):262.
11. Thai D, Ratani RS, Salama S, Steiner RM. Upper lobe fibrocavitary disease in a patient with back pain and stiffness. Chest. 2000;118(6):1814–6.
12. Baser S, Cubukcu S, Ozkurt S, et al. Pulmonary involvement starts in early stage ankylosing spondylitis. Scand J Rheumatol. 2006;35(4):325–7.
13. Casserly IP, Fenlon HM, Breatnach E, Sant SM. Lung findings on high-resolution computed tomography in idiopathic ankylosing spondylitis-correlation with clinical findings, pulmonary function testing and plain radiography. Br J Rheumatol. 1997;36(6):677–82.
14. Souza AS, Müller NL, Marchiori E, et al. Pulmonary abnormalities in ankylosing spondylitis: inspiratory and expiratory high-resolution CT findings in 17 patients. J Thorac Imaging. 2004;19(4):259–63.
15. Senocak O, Manisali M, Ozaksoy D, et al. Lung parenchyma changes in ankylosing spondylitis: demonstration with high resolution CT and correlation with disease duration. Eur J Radiol. 2003;45:117–22.
16. Zhang GY, Fu J, Zhang YG, et al. Lung volume change after pedicle subtraction osteotomy in patients with ankylosing spondylitis with thoracolumbar kyphosis. Spine (Phila Pa 1976). 2015;40(4):233–7.
17. Fu J, Zhang GY, Zhang YG, et al. Pulmonary function improvement in patients with ankylosing spondylitis kyphosis following pedicle subtraction osteotomy. Spine (Phila Pa 1976). 2014;39(18):E1116–22.
18. de Vlam K, Mielants H, Cuvelier C, et al. Spondyloarthropathy is underestimated in inflammatory bowel disease: prevalence and HLA association. J Rheumatol. 2000;27:2860–5.
19. Brophy S, Pavy S, Lewis P, et al. Inflammatory eye, skin, and bowel disease in spondyloarthritis: genetic, phenotypic, and environmental factors. J Rheumatol. 2001;28:2667–73.
20. Smale S, Natt RS, Orchard TR, et al. Inflammatory bowel disease and spondylarthropathy. Arthritis Rheum. 2001;44:2728–36.
21. Vaile JH, Meddings JB, Yacyshyn BR, et al. Bowel permeability and CD45RO expression on circulating CD20CB cells in patients with ankylosing spondylitis and their relatives. J Rheumatol. 1999;26:128–35.
22. Liu C, Song K, Zhang YG, et al. Changes of the abdomen in patients with ankylosing spondylitis kyphosis. Spine. 2014;40:E43–8.
23. Liu C, Zheng GQ, Zhang YG, et al. The radiologic, clinical results and digestive function improvement in patients with ankylosing spondylitis kyphosis after pedicle subtraction osteotomy. Spine J. 2015;15:1988–93.

4 Clinical and Radiographic Evaluation

Ziming Yao and Yan Wang

This chapter covers virtually all aspects of the general musculoskeletal and neuromuscular examination and radiographic evaluation of ankylosing spondylitis (AS) patients. The orthopedist is frequently the first to be consulted for lumbosacral pain or stiffness of hip joint, conditions that may be due to sacroiliitis.

The spinal involvement is more extensive in AS and may result in a lot of complications, including deformity, fracture, and neurologic compromise in some patients [1, 2]. Thus, the orthopedist must not only be familiar with examination of the musculoskeletal system but also knowledgeable about the neurologic examination.

1 Physical Examination

Besides the general physical examination, the physical examinations for AS focus on the spine, hips, peripheral joints, and entheses.

1.1 Cervical Spine

AS may cause forward curve of the thoracic spine and cervical spine. This deformity could be measured by asking the patient to stand erectly with buttocks and heels against a wall and to extend his or her neck as possible as he/she can, trying to touch the wall by the occiput. Most of the normal people can touch the wall with the occiput. The distances between the occiput and the wall reflect the degree of cervical and thoracic spinal deformity. What's more, the range of extension, flexion, rotation, and lateral flexion should also be recorded.

1.2 Thoracic Spine

Chest expansion could be reflected by the range of motion of the costovertebral joints. Chest expansion is measured at the level of the xiphoid. The patients are asked to exert a maximal forced expiration followed by a maximal inspiration while raising their arms above their heads. Normal motion of costovertebral joints is usually >2 cm.

1.3 Lower Spine

Schober test is used to measure the sagittal range of motion of the lower spine, and lateral spinal flexion is used to measure the coronal range of motion.

1.3.1 Schober Test

Schober test measures the forward flexion of the lumbar spine. The midpoint of a line joining the posterior superior iliac spines (dimples of Venus)

Z. Yao
Beijing Children's Hospital, Capital Medical University, National Center for Children's Health, Beijing, China

Y. Wang (✉)
Chinese PLA General Hospital, Beijing, China

Y. Wang (ed.), *Surgical Treatment of Ankylosing Spondylitis Deformity*,
https://doi.org/10.1007/978-981-13-6427-3_4

is marked when the patient stands erectly; another point is marked 10 cm above it in the midline. The patient bends forward maximally without bending the knees, and the distance is measured again. In normal person, the difference between the two measurements should be more than 2 cm.

1.3.2 Lateral Spinal Flexion

When the patient stands erectly with the heel and back against a wall and knees and hands extended, the distance between the tip of the middle finger and the floor is measured. Then, the patient is instructed to bend sideways without bending the knees or lifting the heels. The second measurement is made, and the difference between the two is recorded. The averaged measurements of right and left flexion are taken as the final result. In normal individuals, the measurements should be more than 10 cm.

1.4 Sacroiliac Joint (SI) Tenderness

Patients who have pain in the region of the sacroiliac joints or the buttock may have tenderness elicited by direct pressure over the sacroiliac joint. In addition, three physical maneuvers can be used to exert stress on the sacroiliac joint and to bring out sacroiliac pain. However, none of these physical examinations for sacroiliac involvement have been demonstrated to be specific for sacroiliitis. These include the following:

- With the patient lying supine, direct pressure is exerted by the examiner on the anterior superior iliac spine, and, at the same time, the iliac spine is forced laterally.
- With the patient lying on the side, pressure is exerted by the examiner to compress the pelvis.
- With the patient lying supine, he or she is instructed to flex one of the knees and then to abduct as well as externally rotate the corresponding hip. Pressure on the flexed knee causes pain at the corresponding sacroiliac joint.

1.5 Hip Joint

Hip involvement should be suspected when a patient shows an abnormal gait. It is necessary to test comprehensively whether there is limitation of flexion, external and internal rotation, or pain at the extremes of these joint motions. Destruction caused by AS at the hip joints can lead to flexion deformities. However, a unilateral flexion deformity is frequently hard to be verified because of the compensatory motion of the spine. To eliminate this problem during physical examination, the patient is introduced to lie supine and maximally flex one hip (Fig. 4.1). If there is a flexion deformity of the contralateral hip, the knee of the contralateral limb will be raised, and the degree of flexion deformity can be measured by the angle of the contralateral thigh. Some patients with severe stiffed hip joint are difficult to be evaluated; we called these people "folding-knife man" (Fig. 4.2).

1.6 Peripheral Joint Count

Peripheral joint count involves a 44-joint count of the number of tender or swollen joints, including counts of the ankles, feet, and sternoclavicular joints.

1.7 Sausage Digit (Dactylitis)

The number of digits that have sausage appearance should be recognized and recorded.

1.8 Enthesitis Count

At least 18 entheseal sites are evaluated during clinical trials. The minimum should be at the heel, at the sites where the Achilles tendon and the plantar fascia are each attached to the calcaneus.

2 Scoring Instruments

AS is thought to be the most common and typical form of spondyloarthropathy. Pain and spinal stiffness gradually leading to severe impairment

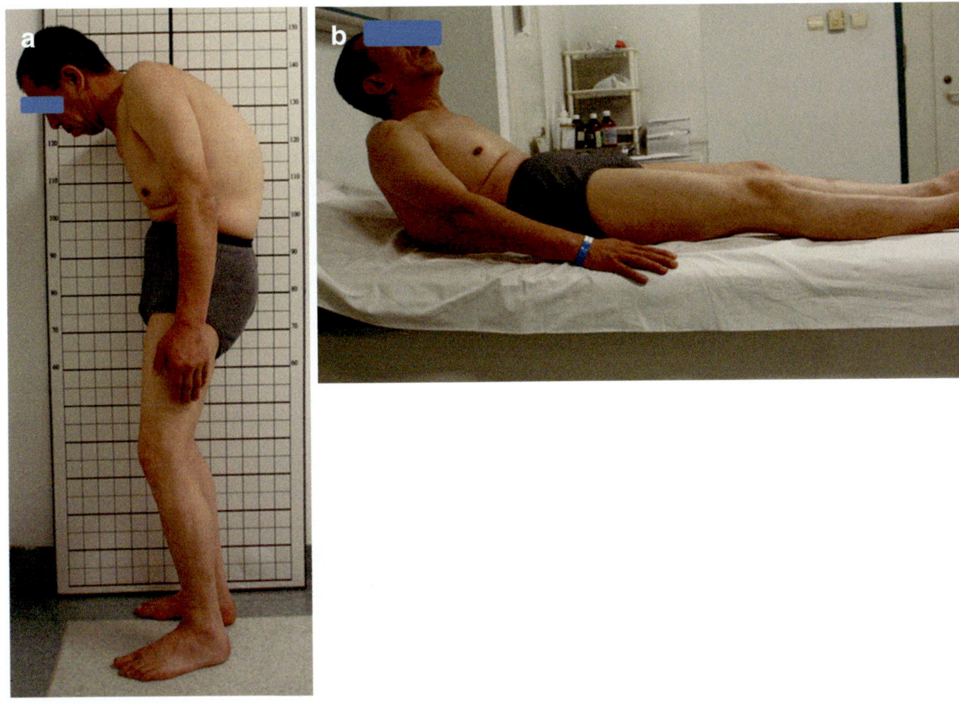

Fig. 4.1 The lateral image of standing (**a**) and lying down (**b**) of a typical AS patient

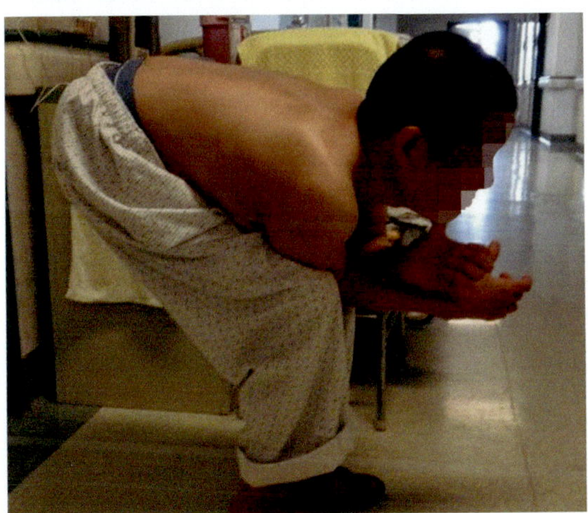

Fig. 4.2 The lateral image of a "folding-knife man"

in physical function and quality of life are regarded as the most important complaints and therapeutic targets in this disease.

Instruments currently available for AS focus on symptoms (impairment) and function (disability) and are used to assess outcome in these terms. Recommended core measures for disability include the Bath Ankylosing Spondylitis Functional Index (BASFI), the Dougados Functional Index (DFI), the Health Assessment Questionnaire modified for the spondyloarthropathies (HAQ-S), the Revised Leeds Disability Questionnaire (RLDQ), the MOS 36-Item Short-Form Health Survey (SF-36), and the modified Arthritis Impact Measurement Scale (mAIMS) [3–6].

2.1 BASFI

The BASFI is a self-administered, disease-specific instrument for AS, designed by a multi-professional expert team of rheumatologists, physiotherapists, and research associates with a major input from patients. The final version, first published in 1994, consists of ten questions altogether. Eight items concern activities referring to the functional anatomy of the patients and two additional questions assessing the patients' ability to cope with daily life.

2.2 DFI

The DFI is a self-administered, disease-specific instrument for AS designed by rheumatologists with special interest on AS and originally applied as an interview. The revised self-administered questionnaire contains 20 items corresponding to activities of daily living.

2.3 HAQ-S

The HAQ-S is a self-administered, disease-specific instrument for ankylosing spondylitis. It was built on the standard HAQ designed for rheumatoid arthritis by adding five questions relating to neck and back functioning. Those were identified in a 1985-mailed survey of 300 British patients with ankylosing spondylitis. The HAQ-S consists of 25 items.

2.4 RLDQ

The RLDQ is a self-administered, disease-specific instrument for ankylosing spondylitis. During the revision process of the questionnaire, a group of 12 patients with ankylosing spondylitis was interviewed; all of them were attending a 3-week inpatient rehabilitation course. The RLDQ includes 16 items grouped into four areas: "mobility," "bending down," "reaching up and neck mobility," and "posture."

2.5 SF-36

SF-36 contains 36 items and could be grouped into eight domains: physical function (PF), role physical (RP), bodily pain (BP), general health (GH), vitality (VT), social function (SF), role emotional (RE), and mental health (MH), respectively, of which the first four domains reflect the physical health and the remaining psychological health. Scores of each domain were added up and transformed into the eight 0–100 scales, with higher value representing better health status. What's more, since the SF-36, as a commonly applied instrument, could be used both in the general population and various diseased populations, especially in different rheumatic disease patients, this enables us to make a comparison of health-related quality of life among individuals of different diseases and health conditions.

2.6 mAIMS

It is a questionnaire measuring changes in physical function, indoor activity, outdoor activity, psychosocial activity, pain, and patient's satisfaction with the surgery. The modified Arthritis Impact Measurement Scale in this study consisted of three simple questions and six subscales: function (five items), indoor activity (nine items), outdoor activity (six items), psychosocial activity (ten items), pain (five items), and overall subjective results (five items). Each item had a score of 5 grades (0 = markedly worse than preoperative state, 1 = slightly worse than preoperative state, 2 = no change, 3 = slightly improved, 4 = markedly improved). Compared with other instruments, mAIMS is well established and comprehensive for measuring physical and psychosocial function in ankylosing spondylitis patients who accepted the corrective surgery.

3 Radiographic Evaluation

3.1 X-ray

The earliest changes in the sacroiliac joints (SI) demonstrable by plain X-ray shows erosions and sclerosis. Progression of the erosions leads to pseudo-widening of the joint space and bony ankylosis. X-ray spine can reveal squaring of vertebrae with spine ossification with fibrous band run longitudinally called syndesmophyte while producing bamboo spine appearance [7].

The SI joint abnormalities are typically graded from 0 (normal) to 4 (total ankylosis) to identify the nature and severity of involvement, and such grading is used to determine the degree

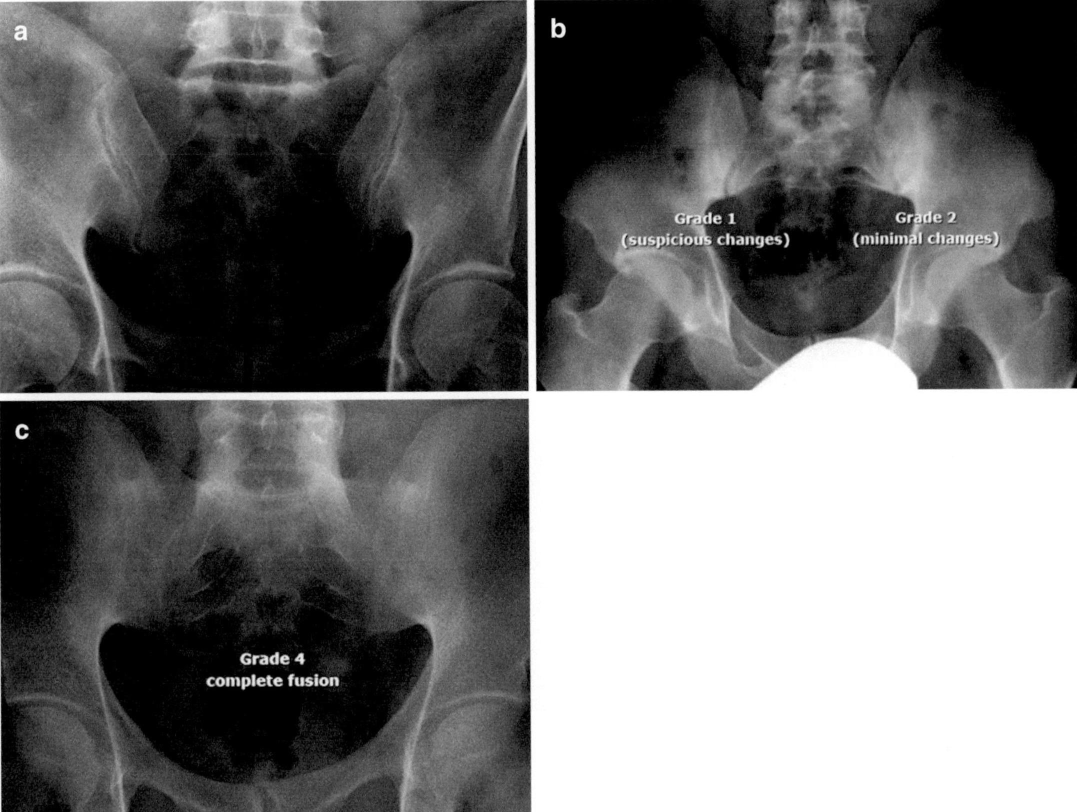

Fig. 4.3 Examples for sacroiliitis grade 0 (**a**), 1 and 2 (**b**), and 4 (**c**)

of confidence that the changes seen reflect sacroiliitis (Fig. 4.3). The findings that characterize each grade are:

- Grade 0: Normal
- Grade 1: Suspicious (but not definite) changes
- Grade 2: Minimal abnormality—Small localized areas with erosions or sclerosis, without alteration in the joint width
- Grade 3: Unequivocal abnormality—Moderate or advanced sacroiliitis with one or more of the following: Erosions, sclerosis, joint-space widening, narrowing, or partial ankylosis
- Grade 4: Total ankylosis of joints

A fixed thoracolumbar kyphosis is the most common deformity that causes difficulty standing, walking, looking horizontally, and lying flat on ones back in advanced patients (Fig. 4.1b). The common radiographic parameters were available in picture archiving and communication system and measured on the lateral X-ray plain of the full spine (Fig. 4.4), including:

- GK (global kyphosis)—The angle between the superior endplate of the maximally tiled upper end vertebra and the inferior endplate of the maximally tilted lower end vertebra.
- TLK (thoracolumbar kyphosis)—The angle between the upper endplate of the T11 vertebra and the lower endplate of the L2 vertebra.
- LL (lumbar lordosis)—The angle between the superior endplate of L1 and S1; positive value indicates lumbar kyphosis and negative value indicates lumbar lordosis.
- SVA (sagittal vertical axis)—The distance measured between the C7 plumb line and the posterosuperior corner of S1 vertebra.

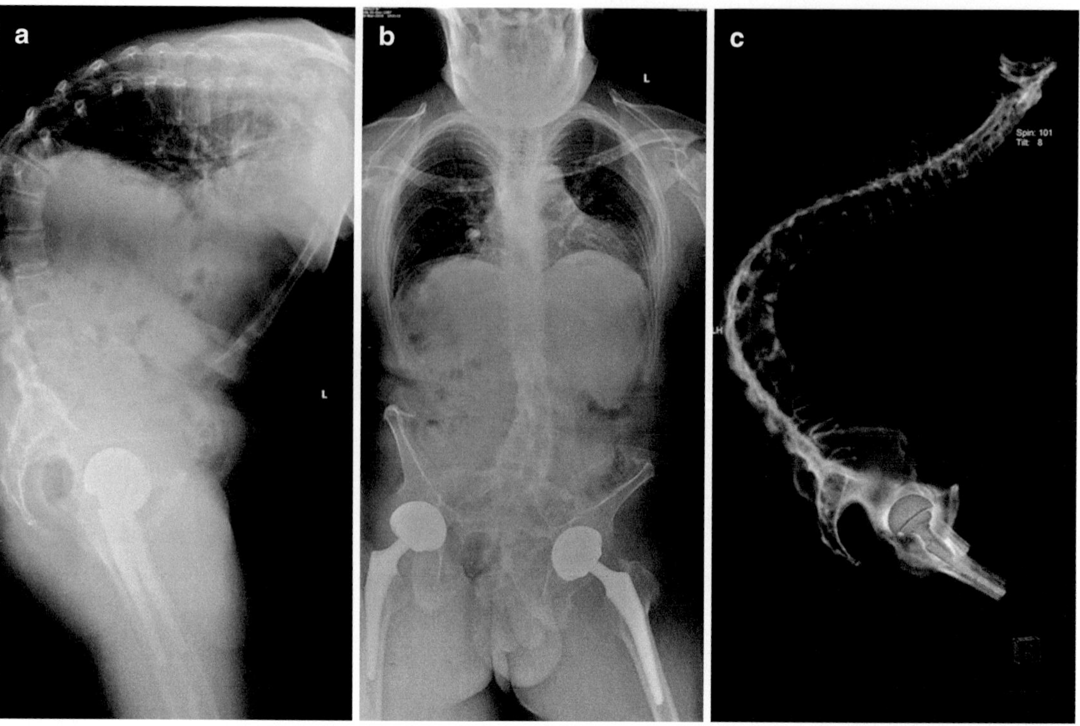

Fig. 4.4 The lateral and anteroposterior X-ray of the full spine (**a**, **b**) and sagittal reconstruction of CT scan (**c**) which shows the Andersson lesions from T11 to L2

- PI (pelvic incidence)—The angle between the line perpendicular to the sacral plate at its midpoint and the line connecting this point to the axis of the hip (Fig. 4.5).
- PT (pelvic tilt)—The vertical angle of the line connecting the hip axis and the midpoint of the sacral plate (Fig. 4.5).
- SS (sacral slope)—The angle between the sacral endplate and the horizontal plane (Fig. 4.5).
- CBVA (chin-brow vertical angle)—Defined as an angle measured between the line from the brow to the chin and a vertical plumb line while the patient stood with knee joint extension on an appearance image.
- C7PL (C7 plumb line)—Distance measured between the C7 plumb line and the center sacral vertical line on the coronal plane.

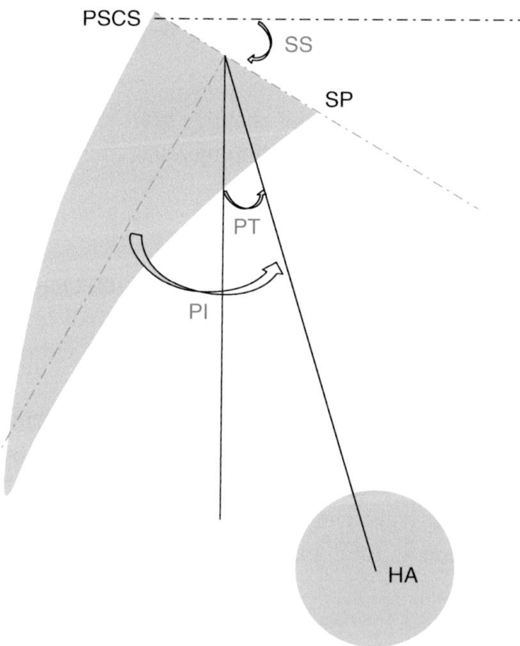

Fig. 4.5 Diagrammatic sketch for spinopelvic parameters. *PI* pelvic incidence, *PT* pelvic tilt, *SS* sacral slope, *PSCS* posterosuperior corner of sacrum, *SP* sacral plate

3.2 CT (Computed Tomography)

It should be used when it is the most appropriate imaging modality to answer a clinical question.

Potential indications include preoperative assessment of complex bony spine anomalies, bony involvement in chronic osteomyelitis, and evaluation of malpositioned hardware. For AS patients, it's very important to detect the occult fracture and Andersson lesion which are difficult to be detected on the X-ray (Fig. 4.4c). The earliest changes in the sacroiliac joints and pseudoarthrosis demonstrated by CT are more clear than plain X-ray. In advanced disease, sagittal CT of the spine will reveal "bamboo spine" with virtually complete fusion of the vertebral column.

3.3 MRI (Magnetic Resonance Imaging)

MRI, unlike plain radiography, can reveal inflammatory changes, fatty changes, and subtle structural abnormalities. MRI has had a significant impact on the imaging and diagnosis of musculoskeletal disorders since its development. It has not replaced CT in musculoskeletal imaging but has influenced the practitioner's ability to identify normal anatomy and a multitude of pathologic processes confidently. Its capability to demonstrate anatomy and disease states in varied planes without the use of ionizing radiation is extremely advantageous when evaluating the AS patient. Structural AS abnormalities (e.g., erosions, bony ankylosis, fat metaplasia, or sclerosis) alone may be seen but can be nonspecific as well, as are inflammatory lesions such as synovitis, enthesitis, or capsulitis, which may also be present.

A number of imaging abnormalities, particularly those affecting the sacroiliac (SI) joints and spine, are characteristic of axial spondyloarthritis (axSpA) which may be evident by MRI. For AS patients, MRI is very important to detect the occult fracture and early pseudoarthrosis.

MRI of the lumbar spine may show changes other than those visible in plain radiographs and infrequently even in the absence of SI joint inflammation; spinal changes in the absence of significant SI joint inflammation were more frequent in a study population of patients with clinically active, long-standing nr-axSpA. The spinal lesions of anterior/posterior spondylitis result in either bone marrow edema, which is observed with the STIR or the T2-weighted sequences with fat suppression, or areas of fatty deposition observed as high-intensity lesions in the T1-weighted sequences, especially in younger adults and in the presence of "healthy" discs (bright signal on STIR). Findings of single or only a few vertebral lesions are relatively nonspecific.

References

1. Vosse D, Feldtkeller E, Erlendsson J, et al. Clinical vertebral fractures in patients with ankylosing spondylitis. J Rheumatol. 2004;31:1981.
2. Carette S, Graham D, Little H, et al. The natural disease course of ankylosing spondylitis. Arthritis Rheum. 1983;26:186.
3. Madsen OR. Stability of fatigue, pain, patient global assessment and the bath ankylosing spondylitis functional index (BASFI) in spondyloarthropathy patients with stable disease according to the bath ankylosing spondylitis disease activity index (BASDAI). Rheumatol Int. 2018;38(3):425–32.
4. Zochling J. Measures of symptoms and disease status in ankylosing spondylitis: ankylosing spondylitis disease activity score (ASDAS), ankylosing spondylitis quality of life scale (ASQoL), bath ankylosing spondylitis disease activity index (BASDAI), bath ankylosing spondylitis functional index (BASFI), Bath ankylosing spondylitis global score (BAS-G), bath ankylosing spondylitis metrology index (BASMI), dougados functional index (DFI), and health assessment questionnaire for the Spondylarthropathies (HAQ-S). Arthritis Care Res (Hoboken). 2011;63(Suppl 11):S47–58.
5. Lubrano E, Sarzi Puttini P, Parsons WJ, et al. Validity and reliability of an Italian version of the revised Leeds disability questionnaire for patients with ankylosing spondylitis. Rheumatology (Oxford). 2005;44(5):666–9.
6. Vosse D, van der Heijde D, Landewé R, et al. Determinants of hyperkyphosis in patients with ankylosing spondylitis. Ann Rheum Dis. 2006;65:770.
7. Jang JH, Ward MM, Rucker AN, et al. Ankylosing spondylitis: patterns of radiographic involvement--a re-examination of accepted principles in a cohort of 769 patients. Radiology. 2011;258:192.

Part III

Strategy and Technical

Classification and Surgical Decision-Making for Ankylosing Spondylitis Kyphosis

5

Guoquan Zheng, Yonggang Zhang, Diyu Song, and Yan Wang

1 Introduction

Ankylosing spondylitis (AS) is a kind of chronic inflammatory disease, which usually results in spinal deformity. The feature of this deformity is a combination of severe thoracic kyphosis and flattening of the lumbar lordosis, accompanied with the head and neck thrust forward. As a consequence, patient's truncal center of the body shifts downward and forward. When deformity aggravating, the patient has to extension hips, flex knees and plantar flexes ankles in order to maintain sagittal balance. AS patients cannot move the other spinal segment compensate. Patients in sagittal imbalance condition are hard to walk or stand erect without overwork of musculature. The compromised position leads to muscle fatigue and activity-related pain, restricts activities of daily living, and causes intra-abdominal complications [1–3]. The goal of surgical correction of these patients is to restore an optimal sagittal balance and retrieve spinal alignment and horizontal vision for obtaining satisfactory clinical results besides appearance [4–6].

Various osteotomy techniques were used to correct AS kyphosis [6]. Smith-Petersen first described opening wedge osteotomy (OWO), in 1945, by removing the posterior elements and extending the anterior column at the level of the disc space [7]. Pedicle subtraction osteotomy (PSO), which is a closing wedge osteotomy (CWO), is another osteotomy technique. In PSO, the posterior elements, the pedicles, and the vertebral body are carefully wedged removed with correcting hinge at the anterior cortex [8, 9].

The classification system for AS deformity contributing to the variation in surgical decision-making is lack of widespread recognition. An ideal system should be easy to learn and applied in clinical practice. For AS kyphotic deformity, to decide appropriate surgery procedures should be focused on the following:

- The ideal location of osteotomy(ies)
- The number of osteotomy(ies)
- The anchor points of instrumentation

2 Classification

This classification just focuses on sagittal deformity of the spine; the other conditions, such as coronal deformity and dislocation of sacroiliac joints, hip joints, etc., were not included. The diagnosis of AS was made by radiographic features, laboratory tests, and clinical features according to New York Standard. We have divided the kyphosis into four types according to the location of kyphotic apex:

G. Zheng (✉) · Y. Zhang · D. Song · Y. Wang
Chinese PLA General Hospital, Beijing, China

Y. Wang (ed.), *Surgical Treatment of Ankylosing Spondylitis Deformity*,
https://doi.org/10.1007/978-981-13-6427-3_5

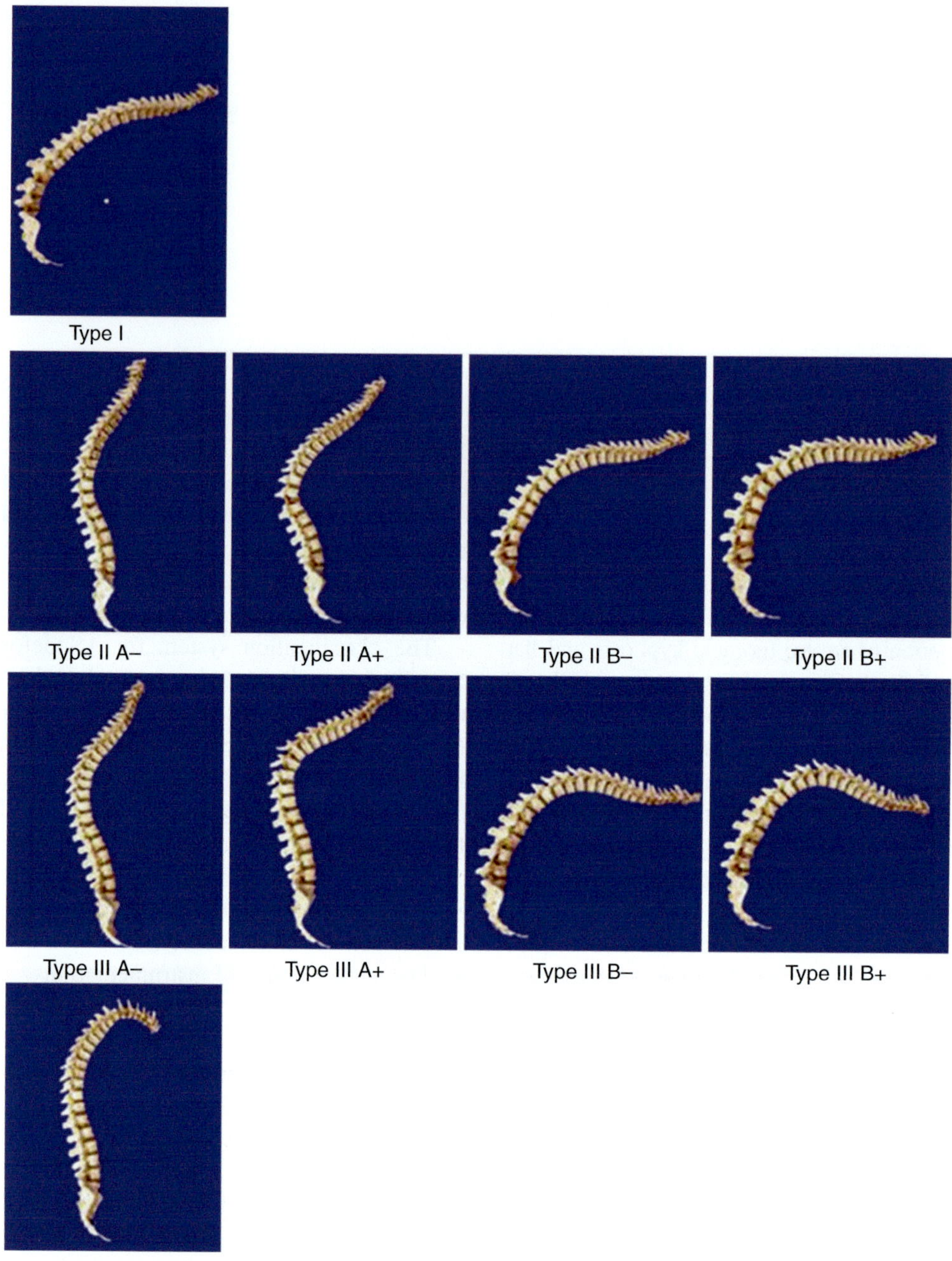

Fig. 5.1 This AS kyphosis classification just focuses on sagittal deformity, which divided the kyphosis into four types according to the location of kyphotic apex. The thoracic/thoracolumbar kyphosis severity modifier divided type II and type III into four subtypes. Reprint with permission from reference Wang Y, Zheng GQ, Zhang YG, et al. Proposal of a New Treatment-Oriented Classification System for Spinal Deformity in Ankylosing Spondylitis. Spine Deformity, 2018, 6(4):366–372

- Lumbar kyphosis (type I)
- Thoracolumbar hyperkyphosis (type II)
- Thoracic hyperkyphosis (type III)
- Cervical or cervicothoracic junction kyphosis (type IV)

Every type except type 1 has two subtypes:

- With relative normal lumbar lordosis (A)
- With lumbar kyphosis (B) (Fig. 5.1, Table 5.1)

Table 5.1 Classification of AS kyphosis

Type	Description
Type I	Lumbar kyphosis
Type II	Thoracolumbar kyphosis A with relative normal lumbar lordosis – thoracolumbar kyphosis (20–40°) + thoracolumbar kyphosis >40° B with lumbar kyphosis – thoracolumbar hypokyphosis (20–40°) + thoracolumbar hypokyphosis >40°
Type III	Thoracic kyphosis A with relative normal lumbar lordosis – thoracic kyphosis (50–70°) + thoracic kyphosis >70° B with lumbar kyphosis – thoracic kyphosis (50–70°) + thoracic kyphosis >70°
Type IV	Cervical kyphosis

Table 5.2 Surgical decision-making according to classification

Type	Surgical plan
Type I	One- or two-level spinal osteotomy at the lumbar spine
Type II A-	Non-operative or thoracolumbar SPOs
Type II A+	L2 or L3 osteotomy
Type II B-	L3 or L2 osteotomy +/or thoracolumbar SPOs
Type II B+	Two-level spinal osteotomy (L1 + L3 or T12 + L2)
Type III A-	Non-operative or thoracic SPOs
Type III A+	L2 spinal osteotomy
Type III B-	L2 +/or T12 osteotomy
Type III A+	L2 + T12 osteotomy
Type IV	C7 spinal osteotomy

3 Surgical Decision-Making

Surgical decision-making for AS kyphosis should focus on the location of osteotomy sites and number of osteotomy. Before this, the following question must be answered:

- What are the patient's need?
- What is the risk of surgery?
- What osteotomy type is suitable to the patient's conditions?

According to the classification mentioned above, patients are divided into four types by identifying the apex of kyphosis. It contributes most to the deformity that performs osteotomy at the apex of the deformity. The suggested operative treatments are listed in the following table (Table 5.2).

For patients with type I kyphosis, which is characterized by kyphotic lumbar spine with normal thoracic kyphosis, it is usually enough to perform one- or two-level osteotomy at the lumbar spine. For this type of kyphosis, performing osteotomy at the lumbar spine is not only able to correct kyphotic deformity but also able to reconstruct the lumbar lordosis. The accurate correction angle of osteotomy was calculated by shifting the gravity center over the hip axis. Usually, if the required angle is <60°, or more than 60° with unfused anterior intervertebral disc, one-level osteotomy is enough (Fig. 5.2). However, if the required angle is more than 60° but the intervertebral discs are fused, we recommend to perform two-level spinal osteotomy (L1 and L3) (Fig. 5.3).

For patients with classification of type II A−, treatment involves non-operative or multilevel thoracolumbar SPOs. But for type II A+, we recommend osteotomy at L2 (Fig. 5.4). For patients with subtype B, reconstructing lumbar lordosis is necessary, which means performing osteotomy at L3 or L2 is recommended (Fig. 5.5). Additional one-level PSO or multilevel SPOs are alternative according to thoracolumbar kyphosis.

For patients with type III, who are characterized by severe thoracic hyperkyphosis, it is recommended to perform spinal osteotomy at the lumbar spine (non-spinal cord regions) to avoid the restriction of thoracic cage and to decrease the risk of spinal cord or nerve injury. The correction of deformity was mainly achieved by retrieving the global alignment rather than correcting the local kyphotic curve (Figs. 5.6 and 5.7).

As for type IV, cervical kyphosis or cervicothoracic junction kyphosis (usually is described as chin-on-chest deformity), C7 spinal osteotomy is the widely acceptable in literatures (Fig. 5.8).

4 Conclusion

Currently, the osteotomy techniques for AS kyphosis mainly include OWO, CWO, and closing-opening wedge osteotomy [6–9]. Most of

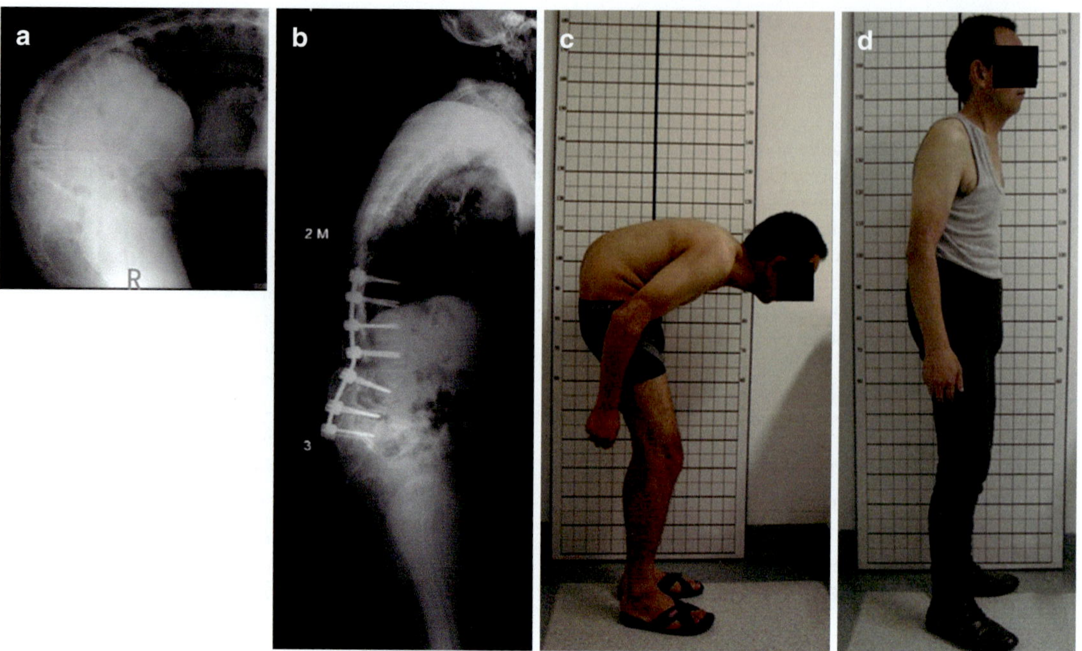

Fig. 5.2 A type I deformity. (**a**) The preoperative X-ray shows the apex of kyphotic curvature is located at the lumbar spine. The lumbar kyphosis is 41° preoperatively. (**b**) One-level osteotomy was performed at L3. The postoperative lumbar lordosis is 30°. A correction angle of 71° was achieved. This correction angle equals to two SPOs and one PSO at the same level, because total laminectomy at L3 and partial laminectomy below and above were performed and the anterior intervertebral discs are not fused. (**c**, **d**) Pre/postoperative clinical appearances show that the sagittal imbalance was improved largely. Reprint with permission from reference Wang Y, Zheng GQ, Zhang YG, et al. Proposal of a New Treatment-Oriented Classification System for Spinal Deformity in Ankylosing Spondylitis. Spine Deformity, 2018, 6(4):366–372

them were performed at one level, and only a little number of authors reported two- or multilevel osteotomy [10–12]. Differences in strategy management for AS kyphotic deformity are owing to the lack of a classification system which is universally accepted. An ideal system to classify AS should take several key variables into consideration which influence decision-making and clinical outcomes such as determining the osteotomy site and the number of osteotomies.

Our classification has divided the curvature of AS kyphosis into four types according to the location of the apex, which is very easy to learn. The sequent consideration is whether the classification can be served as a reference in surgical planning. As we know, performing osteotomy at the apex of the deformity contributes to restoring alignment most. Therefore, identifying the apex of the kyphotic curve is the first step to make surgical decision. For AS patients with type I kyphosis, performing osteotomy at the lumbar spine is no doubt. The second step is to decide the optimal number of osteotomy and the osteotomy sites, which is highly related to the required angle of osteotomy with the aim of shifting the gravity center over the hip axis as well as the movability of intervertebral disc. Though achieving 60° correction at one level is very easy for lumbar osteotomy with unfused anterior intervertebral disc (Fig. 5.2), two-level osteotomy (L1 and L3) is recommended to bring a more smooth lordosis when the required angle is more than 60° or with fused anterior intervertebral disc.

But for patients with type II and III, the curvature of the patient's spine is like a letter "C."

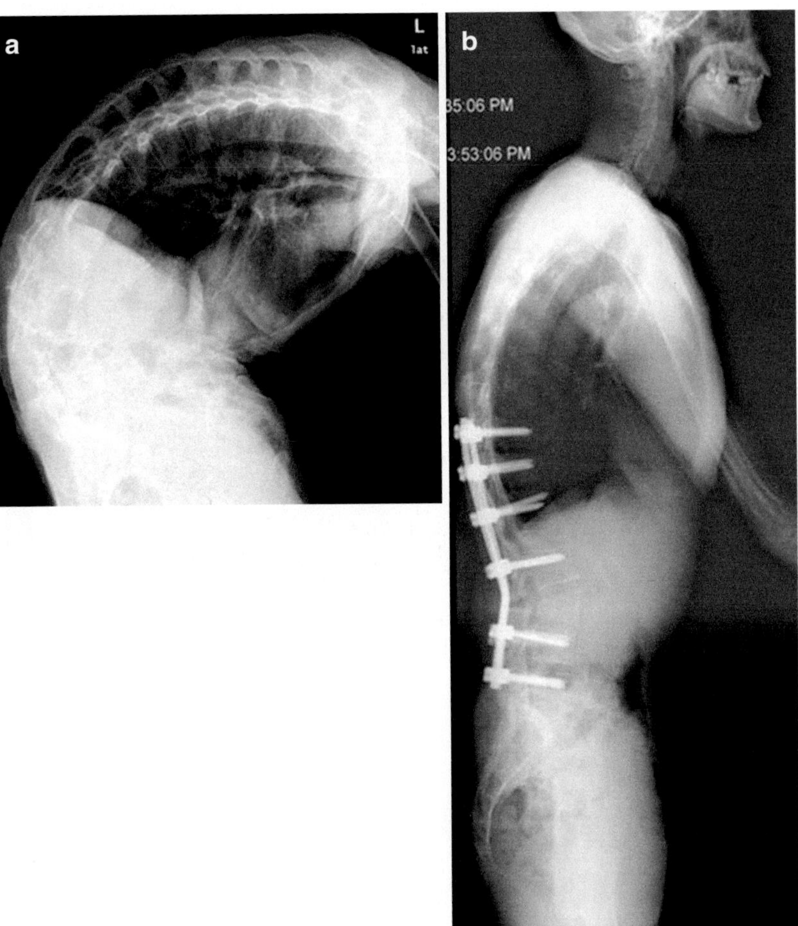

Fig. 5.3 A type I deformity. (**a**) Preoperative X-ray shows L2/L3 disc is the apex of kyphosis. (**b**) Two-level spinal osteotomies were performed at L1 and L3. Postoperative X-ray shows that a lumbar lordosis was re-achieved and the whole alignment is very good. Reprint with permission from reference Wang Y, Zheng GQ, Zhang YG, et al. Proposal of a New Treatment-Oriented Classification System for Spinal Deformity in Ankylosing Spondylitis. Spine Deformity, 2018, 6(4):366–372

In this type of patients, the loss of lumbar lordosis or even lumbar kyphosis is coexistent with hyperkyphosis of thoracolumbar and thoracic spine. The loss of lumbar lordosis has to be taken into consideration, because the physiological curve of the spine is like a letter "S." So, L2 or L3 can be regarded as a potential apex. Therefore, two subtypes of the lumbar spine in this classification were proposed. For subtype B, we recommend to perform osteotomy at L2 or L3 for restoring lumbar lordosis. Then, one-level PSO or multilevel SPOs are recommended for alternative according to thoracolumbar kyphosis, additionally.

It is well known that the hip axis plays a leading role in the hinge center of the upper body for a fixed spine, such as ankylosing spine of AS patients. The lumbar spine theoretically has a shorter arm of force than the thoracic spine, and the degree of loss in lumbar lordosis may lead to greater sagittal imbalance than the equal degree of hyperkyphosis in the thoracic spine [13, 14]. In other words, the lower vertebral body is chosen as the osteotomy site, the greater capability of deformity correction acquired for the whole sagittal imbalance. Besides, it is very easy and safe for reconstruction of the lumbar lordosis, which can compensate the thoracic hyperkyphosis.

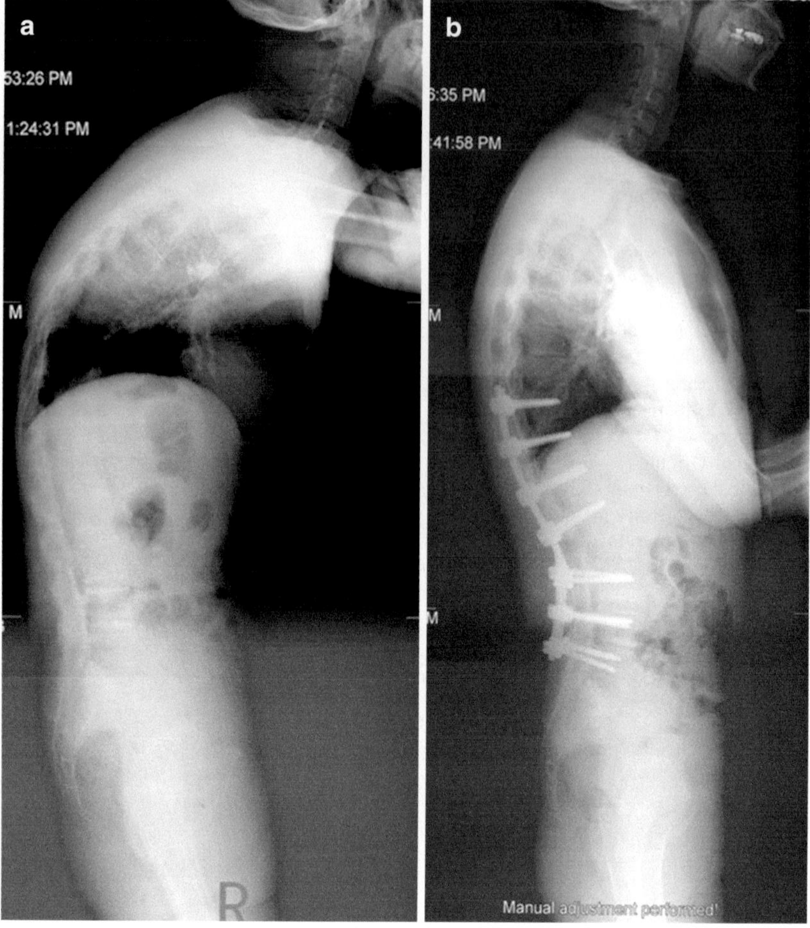

Fig. 5.4 A type II A deformity. (**a**) Preoperative X-ray shows the apex of the kyphosis is located at T11. The lumbar lordosis is 15°. (**b**) Spinal osteotomy was performed at L2. Postoperative X-ray shows the whole alignment is very good. Reprint with permission from reference Wang Y, Zheng GQ, Zhang YG, et al. Proposal of a New Treatment-Oriented Classification System for Spinal Deformity in Ankylosing Spondylitis. Spine Deformity, 2018, 6(4):366–372

Therefore, only a few of patients with type III kyphosis need osteotomy at the deformity position. Van Royen and Slot [15] suggested that the site of corrective osteotomy should be selected in the lower lumbar spine, which may make the process safer and more correction. This procedure also has other advantages, such as no restriction of thorax and no risk of spinal cord injury. On the account of the whole ankylosing spine of AS, the goal of surgery is to achieve a global balance of the spine and pelvic, not the correction of the local spinal deformity. Because the vertebral canal at L2 is relatively spacious, in which there is already no spinal cord, L2 is usually chosen as the site of osteotomy instead of L3 [6]. In type III A kyphosis, if L3 is chosen as the site of osteotomy to correct the hyperkyphosis of thoracic spine, the process may result in larger lumbar lordosis and impair the whole balance.

Cervical or cervicothoracic junctional kyphosis, namely, chin-on-chest deformity, may cause and interfere with forward vision, swallowing, chewing, skin care under the chin, functionality, etc. Traditionally, performing extension osteotomy at C7 is widely accepted for these patients, which is a technically demanding procedure with high risk of neurological deficit [16–20]. Patient satisfaction rate and functional outcomes are increasingly better with development of anesthesia,

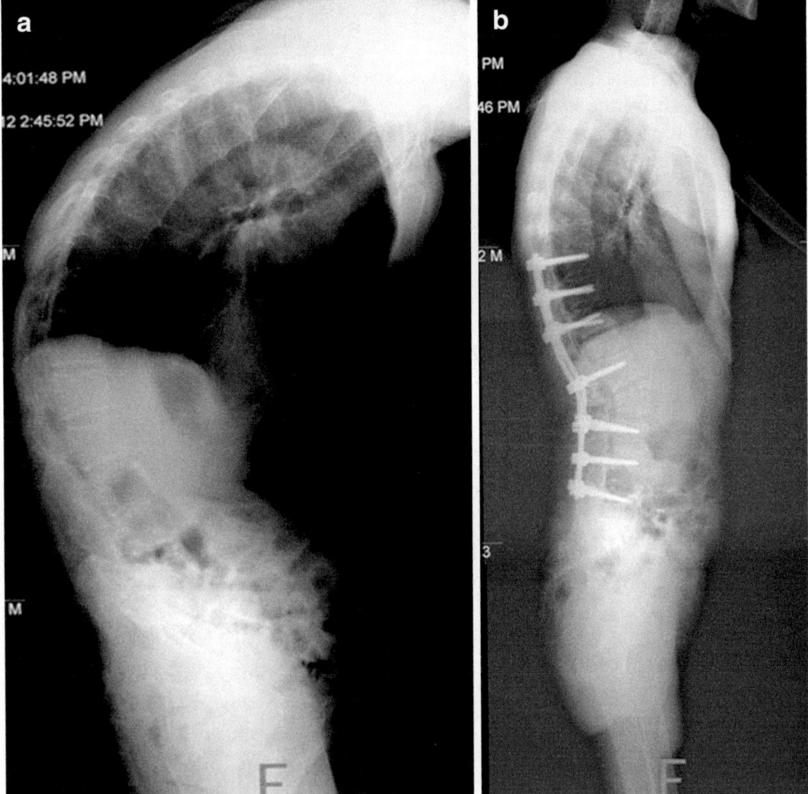

Fig. 5.5 A type II B deformity. (**a**) Preoperative X-ray shows the apex of thoracolumbar kyphosis is located at T12. The lumbar lordosis was lost. (**b**) Two-level spinal osteotomies were performed at T12 and L2. Postoperative X-ray shows the whole alignment is very good. Reprint with permission from reference Wang Y, Zheng GQ, Zhang YG, et al. Proposal of a New Treatment-Oriented Classification System for Spinal Deformity in Ankylosing Spondylitis. Spine Deformity, 2018, 6(4):366–372

internal fixation system, and intraoperative neural monitoring [21]. Though no such patients were treated in our hospital, undoubtedly, it is an independent type of kyphosis. So, we classified these patients into type IV.

Due to the fusion of the whole spine, the segments without instrumentation cannot realign after surgery. Osteotomy is the unique means to achieve the balance of whole sagittal plane. The main role of instrumentation is just to maintain the correction after the surgery. The anchor points should be chosen according to the osteotomy type, the location of spinal osteotomy, and the conditions of kyphosis. Usually, two pair pedicle screws below the osteotomy are enough to maintain the stability, because the interface between vertebrae and pedicle screws is compressive stress after the lordosis was reconstructed. To decrease the occurrence of proximal junction kyphosis (PJK), we recommend that two or three pair pedicle screws or even more pedicles screws should be implanted above the osteotomy site, because the interface between vertebrae and pedicle screws is tensile stress. The basic principle is that the upper instrumentation should not be stopped at the apex of kyphosis.

In conclusion, this classification outlines four types of AS kyphosis according to the location of the apex and two subtypes according to the condition of the lumbar spine. It is very easy to learn and to be applied in clinical practice, helping to descript the curvature type and to make a surgical decision.

Fig. 5.6 A type III A deformity. (**a**) Preoperative X-ray shows there is a thoracic hyperkyphosis causing sever sagittal imbalance. (**b**) Two-level spinal osteotomies were performed at T12 and L2. Postoperative X-ray shows the sagittal balance was restored by retrieving global alignment. Reprint with permission from reference Wang Y, Zheng GQ, Zhang YG, et al. Proposal of a New Treatment-Oriented Classification System for Spinal Deformity in Ankylosing Spondylitis. Spine Deformity, 2018, 6(4):366–372

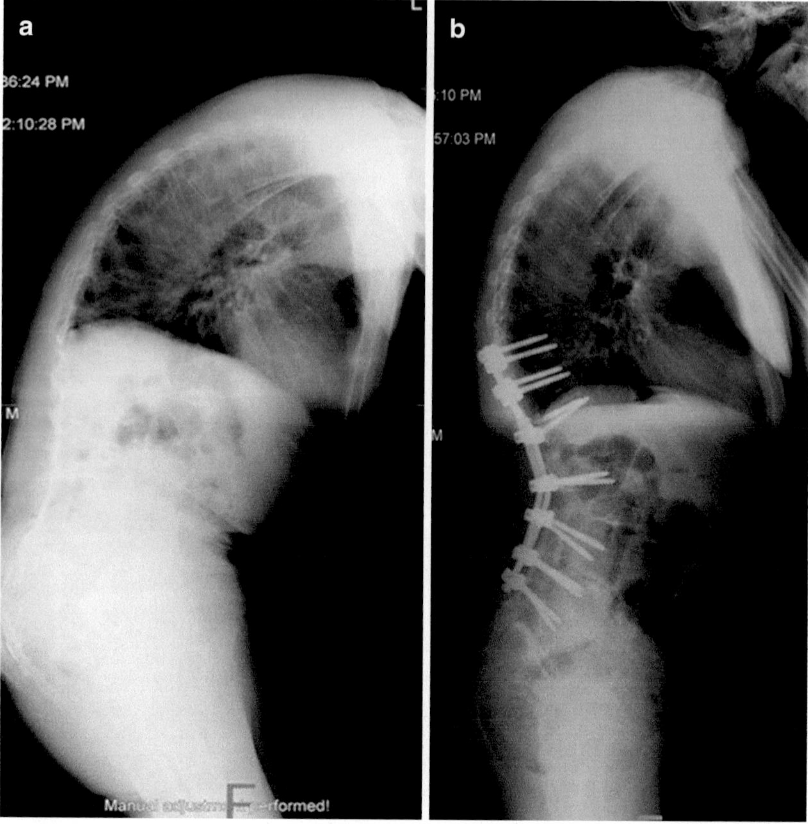

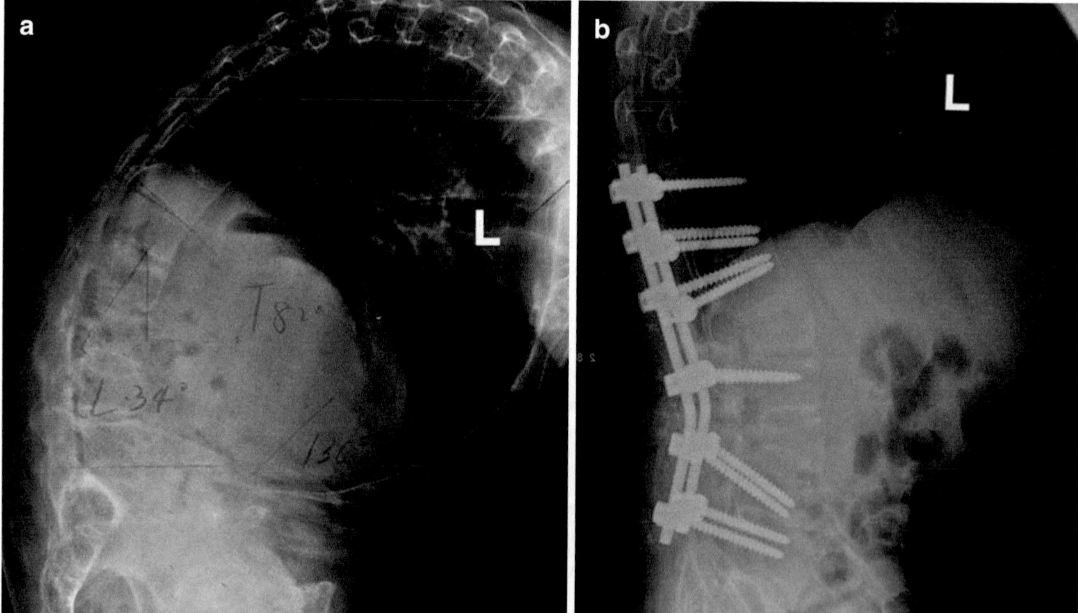

Fig. 5.7 A type III B deformity. (**a**) Preoperative X-ray shows the thoracic hyperkyphosis coexisted with the lumbar kyphosis. (**b**) Two-level spinal osteotomies were performed at L1 and L3. Postoperative X-ray shows sagittal balance was achieved. Reprint with permission from reference Wang Y, Zheng GQ, Zhang YG, et al. Proposal of a New Treatment-Oriented Classification System for Spinal Deformity in Ankylosing Spondylitis. Spine Deformity, 2018, 6(4):366–372

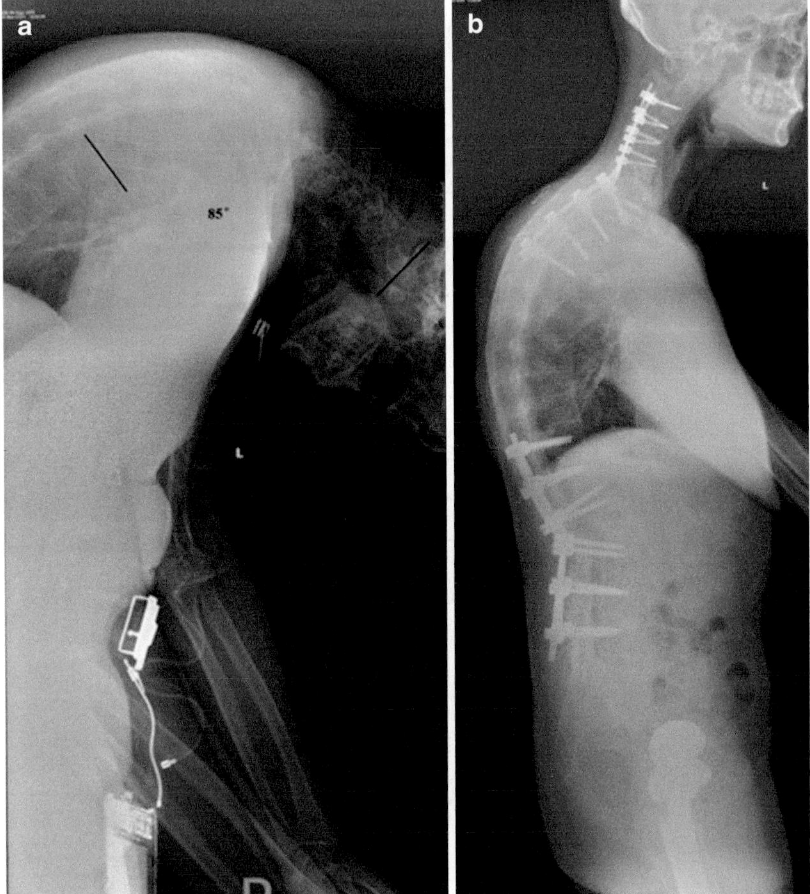

Fig. 5.8 A Type IV deformity. (**a**) Preoperative X-ray shows chin-on-chest deformity and lumbar kyphosis. (**b**) Spinal osteotomies were performed at C7 and L2. Postoperative X-ray shows sagittal balance was achieved. Reprint with permission from reference Wang Y, Zheng GQ, Zhang YG, et al. Proposal of a New Treatment-Oriented Classification System for Spinal Deformity in Ankylosing Spondylitis. Spine Deformity, 2018, 6(4):366–372

References

1. Kubiak EN, Moskovich R, Errico TJ, et al. Orthopaedic management of ankylosing spondylitis. J Am Acad Orthop Surg. 2005;13(4):267–78.
2. McGonagle D, Khan MA, Marzo-Ortega H, et al. Enthesitis in spondyloarthropathy. Curr Opin Rheumatol. 1999;11:244–50.
3. Chang KW. Quality control of reconstructed sagittal balance for sagittal imbalance. Spine. 2011;36:E186–97.
4. Mac-Thiong JM, Transfeldt EE, Mehbod AA, et al. Can C7 plumbline and gravity line predict health related quality of life in adult scoliosis? Spine. 2009;34:E519–27.
5. Glassman SD, Bridwell K, Dimar JR, et al. The impact of positive sagittal balance in adult spinal deformity. Spine. 2005;30:2024–9.
6. Chang KW, Chen YY, Lin CC, et al. Closing wedge osteotomy versus opening wedge osteotomy in ankylosing spondylitis with thoracolumbar kyphotic deformity. Spine (Phila Pa 1976). 2005;30:1584–93.
7. Smith-Peterson M, Larson C, Aufranc O. Osteotomy of the spine for correction of flexion deformity in rheumatoid arthritis. J Bone Joint Surg Am. 1945;27:1–11.
8. Boachie-Adjei O, Ferguson JI, Pigeon RG, et al. Transpedicular lumbar wedge resection osteotomy for fixed sagittal imbalance: surgical technique and farly results. Spine. 2006;31:485–92.
9. Van Royen BJ, De Gast A. Lumbar osteotomy for correction of thoracolumbar kyphotic deformity in ankylosing spondylitis: a structured review of three methods of treatment. Ann Rheum Dis. 1999;58:399–406.
10. Chen IH, Chien JT, Yu TC. Transpedicular wedge osteotomy for correction of thoracolumbar kyphosis in ankylosing spondylitis experience with 78 patients. Spine (Phila Pa 1976). 2001;26(16):E354–60.
11. Hehne H-J, Zielke K, Böhm H. Polysegmental lumbar osteotomies and transpedicled fixation for correction of long-curved kyphotic deformities in ankylosing spondylitis. Report on 177 cases. Clin Orthop. 1990;258:49–55.
12. Wang Y, Zhang Y, Mao K, et al. Transpedicular bivertebrae wedge osteotomy and discectomy in lumbar spine for severe ankylosing spondylitis. J Spinal Disord Tech. 2010;23:186–91.
13. Kiaer T, Gehrchen M. Transpedicular closed wedge osteotomy in ankylosing spondylitis: results of surgical treatment and prospective outcome analysis. Eur Spine J. 2010;19:57–64.

14. Van Royen BJ, De Gast A, Smit TH. Deformity planning for sagittal plane corrective osteotomies of the spine in ankylosing spondylitis. Eur Spine J. 2000;9:492–8.
15. von Royen BJ, Slot GM. Closing-wedge posterior osteotomy for ankylosing spondylitis. J Bone Joint Surg Br. 1995;77:117–21.
16. Tokala DP, Lam KS, Freeman BJ, et al. C7 decancellisation closing wedge osteotomy for the correction of fixed cervico-thoracic kyphosis. Eur Spine J. 2007;16:1471–8.
17. Khoueir P, Hoh DJ, Wang MY. Use of hinged rods for controlled osteoclastic correction of a fixed cervical kyphotic deformity in ankylosing spondylitis. J Neurosurg Spine. 2008;8(6):579–83.
18. Hoh DJ, Khoueir P, Wang MY, et al. Management of cervical deformity in ankylosing spondylitis. Neurosurg Focus. 2008;24(1):E9.
19. McMaster MJ. Osteotomy of the cervical spine in ankylosing spondylitis. J Bone Joint Surg Br. 1997;79(2):197–203.
20. Simmons EH. The surgical correction of flexion deformity of the cervical spine in ankylosing spondylitis. Clin Orthop Relat Res. 1972;86:132–43.
21. Mehdian SM, Freeman BJ, Licina P. Cervical osteotomy for ankylosing spondylitis: an innovative variation on an existing technique. Eur Spine J. 1999;8:505–9.

Surgery Planning in AS Thoracolumbar Kyphosis

6

Kai Song, Zheng Wang, Xuesong Zhang, Bing Wu, and Yan Wang

Ankylosing spondylitis (AS) is a chronic inflammatory disease, generally involving the sacroiliac joints, spinal column, and hip joints as pathogenesis develops [1]. A thoracolumbar kyphosis is the most common deformity which causes difficulty in standing, walking, looking horizontally, and so on. When the kyphosis occurs with cervical ankylosing and hip involvement, the health-related quality of life (HRQOL) would be even worse [2–14]. How do spine surgeons make surgery planning bring better HRQOL to the kyphosis? In this chapter, we would like to introduce our strategy in three aspects which determine the activity of daily living.

Restore Sagittal Balance in AS Thoracolumbar Kyphosis
With lumbar hypolordosis and thoracolumbar kyphosis, AS kyphotic patients have a positive sagittal imbalance which leads to patients' difficulty in standing and walking. Therefore, to restore sagittal balance is the first thing to be considered, and it is the most important in patients without cervical ankylosing and hip involvement [3–5, 7–12, 14]. What is the optimal radiographic parameter to assessing sagittal balance for AS kyphosis, and how do we achieve the optimal sagittal balance? In the first part, we introduce our understanding and the corresponding method.

K. Song · Z. Wang (✉) · X. Zhang · B. Wu · Y. Wang
Chinese PLA General Hospital (301 Hospital),
Beijing, China

Restore Chin-Brow Vertical Angle (CBVA)
For AS kyphotic patients without cervical ankylosing, we can easily deal with the CBVA, because when restoring the sagittal balance, optimal CBVA commonly is obtained at the same time depending on good cervical flexion-extension [6, 13]. However, if the cervical spine is ankylosing, surgeon must pay more attention. Sometimes, restoring good sagittal balance may lead to bad CBVA. CBVA determines patients' visual fields, and it is even more important for HRQOL than sagittal balance [13]. In the second part, we talk about the optimal CBVA for patients with cervical ankylosing and the method to achieve best CBVA.

Match with the Range of Motion (ROM) of the Hip Joints
The hips are the most commonly affected diarthrodial joint in patients with AS. For such cases, the range of motion (ROM) of the hip joints always decreases to various degrees [15–18]. In this case, if we merely pursue reconstructing the ideal sagittal balance and CBVA, poor clinical outcomes might occur. For example, some patients will lose sitting ability if they primitively had hip flexing limitation when they regain good sagittal balance [12]. In this case, optimal surgery should match patients' new trunk axis with the hip ROM. In the third part, we will discuss it in details and introduce the surgery design.

Y. Wang (ed.), *Surgical Treatment of Ankylosing Spondylitis Deformity*,
https://doi.org/10.1007/978-981-13-6427-3_6

1 Restore Sagittal Balance in AS Thoracolumbar Kyphosis

1.1 Sagittal Imbalance and Compensation

The harmony of the spinopelvic alignment in the sagittal plane allows for stable balance and is economical in terms of mechanical effects and muscular energy [19–21]. Generally, the center of gravity (CG) of the trunk always falls on the hip axis (HA) in the erect position. Even with spinal deformity, automatic compensatory mechanisms will relocate the CG of the trunk onto the HA to provide a new balance with minimal muscular energy expenditure, regardless of whether this can be achieved completely [21–23].

For fixed thoracolumbar kyphosis due to ankylosing spondylitis (AS), the CG is considerably anterior compared to normal, which means that the CG falls in front of the HA. However, this situation will not occur, because the body rotates the pelvis backward to relocate the CG on the HA to the greatest degree by extension of the hips and flexion of the knees [4, 8, 24]. Yet, this automatic compensation still leads to muscle fatigue and erect posture disability. Therefore, a pelvic neutral position has been considered as the goal for sagittal reconstruction.

1.2 Center of Gravity (CG) and Pelvic Rotation

For most adults with a well-balanced spine, the CG of the trunk is over the hip axis (HA) and directly under the promontory of the sacrum when the pelvis is in a neutral position [25, 26]. In spinal deformity, compensatory mechanisms still tend to locate the CG onto the HA by pelvic rotation in order to maintain a balanced upright posture with a minimum of muscular energy expenditure. This leads to the promontory of the sacrum to move either behind or in front of the HA. Thus, on one hand, we can use the line connecting the HA and the sacrum promontory as the pelvic neutral positional line. On the other hand, we can consider the vertical angle of the line connecting the HA and the sacrum promontory as the pelvic rotation angle (PRA).

For fixed thoracolumbar kyphosis caused by AS, the CG is anterior to normal, which means that the CG will fall in front of the HA. However, this position does not occur, as it appears that the body rotates the pelvis backward to relocate the CG on the HA by extension of the hips and flexion of the knees for balance and less energy expenditure [4, 8, 24] (Fig. 6.1a). When an insufficient PSO angle was achieved, the CG was relocated, although the pelvis did not need to rotate backward to the same degree as before; it was still in a backward rotation (Fig. 6.1b). If an excessive PSO angle was achieved, then the pelvis would rotate forward to compensate for locating CG on the HA (Fig. 6.1c). Therefore, we could only obtain a pelvic neutral position when the CG was relocated on the line connecting the HA and the sacrum promontory or named pelvic neutral positional line (Fig. 6.1d). So, all left we should do was to find CG.

1.3 Finding a Marker for Center of Gravity (CG)

How do we find the CG? Usually, it is not feasible to determine the position of the CG because of the irregular shape of the trunk and the irregular distribution of bones, fats, muscles, and internal organs. However, we come up with a different way to deal with this complex problem. To our knowledge, the CG of an irregular object can be obtained by hanging or supporting it in different points and directions, and the CG will be on the point of intersection. According to this principle of mechanics, we can use the pre- and postoperative HA vertical lines (or CG line) to locate the CG of the trunk (Fig. 6.2a, b).

One issue should be noted: the pre- and postoperative shapes of the trunk are different. So, why can we still use HA vertical lines to find the CG? Actually, when we consider the entire trunk as two parts, separated by the PSO level line, we find that the mass of the distal part is far less than that of the proximal. More importantly, the distal arm of force is also far shorter than the proximal. Thus, the CG of the entire trunk is nearly at the

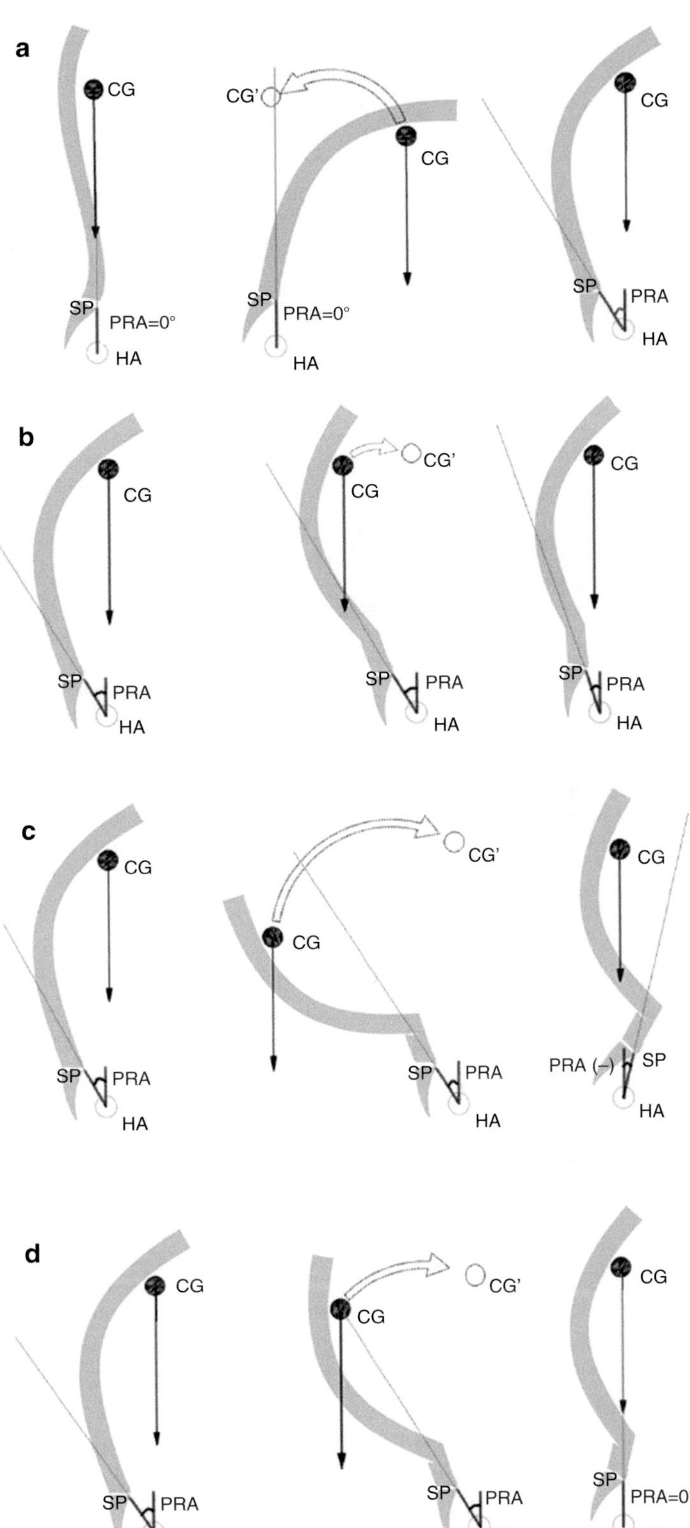

Fig. 6.1 (**a**) (1) For a healthy adult, CG and SP are on HA; (2) for AS kyphosis, CG is anterior compared to normal in the pelvic neutral position and is not a stable state; (3) the pelvis is rotated backward, and then CG fell on HA again, while SP was behind HA. (**b**) Insufficient PSO angle. (1) Preoperatively, CG is on HA, while SP is behind HA, so the pelvis is rotated backward; (2) after PSO, CG was behind HA, and this was not a stable state; (3) postoperatively, CG was on HA, while SP was still behind HA in spite of moving forward. (**c**) Excess PSO angle. (1) Preoperatively, CG was on HA, while SP was behind HA, so the pelvis was in backward rotation; (2) after PSO, CG was behind HA and was not a stable state; (3) postoperatively, CG was on HA, while SP was in front of HA because of rotating forward too much. (**d**) Adequate PSO angle. (1) Preoperatively, CG is on HA, while SP was behind HA, so the pelvis was in backward rotation; (2) after PSO, CG was behind HA and was not a stable state; (3) postoperatively, CG was on HA, and likewise SP was on HA as a result of rotating forward properly. Abbreviations: CG, center of gravity of the trunk; SP, sacrum promontory; HA, hip axis; PRA, pelvic rotation angle (Reprinted, with permission, from: Song K, Zheng G, Zhang Y, et al. Hilus pulmonis as the center of gravity for AS thoracolumbar kyphosis. Eur Spine J. 2014 Dec;23(12):2743–50. https://doi.org/10.1007/s00586-013-3134-5)

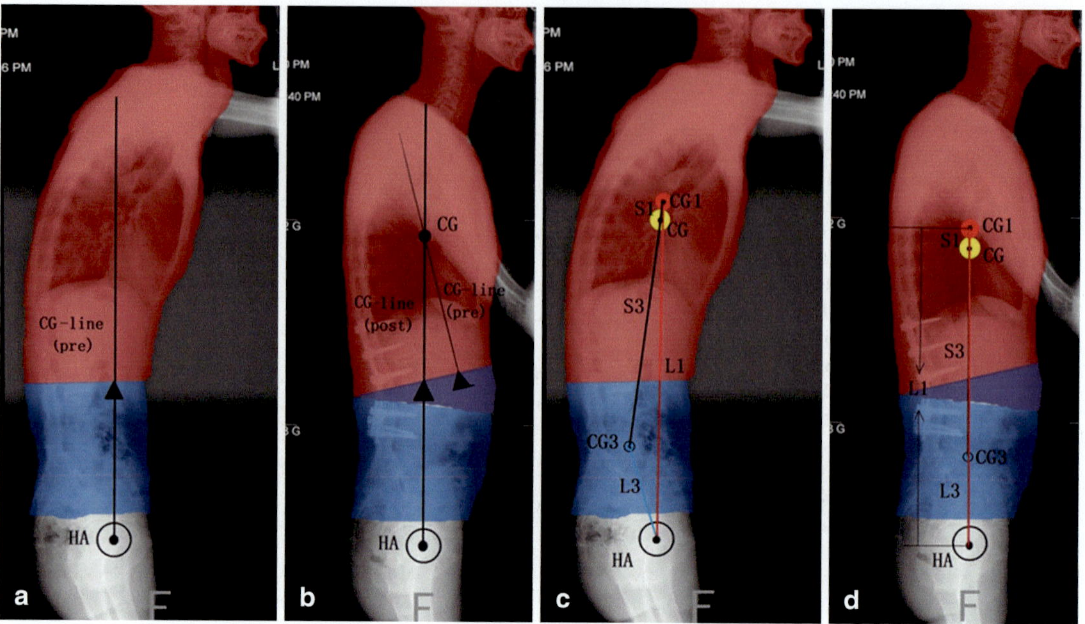

Fig. 6.2 (**a**) Pre-surgery and (**b**) post-surgery. CG, center of gravity, is on the crossing point of the preoperative CG-line and the postoperative CG-line. The shorter the distance is between the markers with the two lines, the better marker it is as the center of gravity. (**c**) Pre-surgery and (**d**) post-surgery. *CG* center of gravity of the entire trunk, *CG1* center of gravity of the proximal part of the trunk, *CG3* center of gravity of the distal part of the trunk. Mass of proximal part > mass of distal part; arm L1 > arm L3; mass CG1 * arm L1 >> mass CG3 * arm L3; S3/S1 = (mass CG1 * arm L1)/(mass CG3 * arm L3), so S3 >> S1. Thus, CG is next to CG1 (Reprinted, with permission, from: Song K, Zheng G, Zhang Y, et al. Hilus pulmonis as the center of gravity for AS thoracolumbar kyphosis. Eur Spine J. 2014 Dec;23(12):2743–50. https://doi.org/10.1007/s00586-013-3134-5)

center of the proximal trunk due to the hip axis fulcrum (Fig. 6.2c, d).

In previous study, Song found that pre- and postoperative horizontal distance between hip axis and hilus pulmonis was so small that we considered the hilus pulmonis (HP) to be located on the HA. This means that the HP could be thought of as approximating the CG of the trunk [11].

Where is the hilus pulmonis (HP)? The hilus pulmonis (HP) includes several principal structures: left main bronchus, right pulmonary artery, left pulmonary artery, and bronchus intermedius. The major components of the hilum are relatively clearly visible on a lateral view, especially the distal end of the left bronchus, which is a round lucency and typically located at or near the apparent center of the lungs on the lateral film. This is true even when the lungs are abnormally shaped. In addition, we defined the round lucency (left main bronchus) as the center of the hilus pulmonis [27–29] (Fig. 6.3).

1.4 Deformity Planning

Because we can use the hilus pulmonis (HP) as a marker for the CG, then placing the HP, the sacrum promontory, and the hip axis on one line can insure a postoperative pelvic neutral position [11] (Fig. 6.4).

However, there are certain types (with large PI) of spine-pelvis where the sacrum promontory does not lie in line with the hip axis, like Type 4 according to Roussouly [30]. Fortunately, more and more studies have demonstrated strong corrections between PT and SS and PI, so we can predict one's individual pelvic neutral position by calculating the theoretic PT or SS according to PI [31–33].

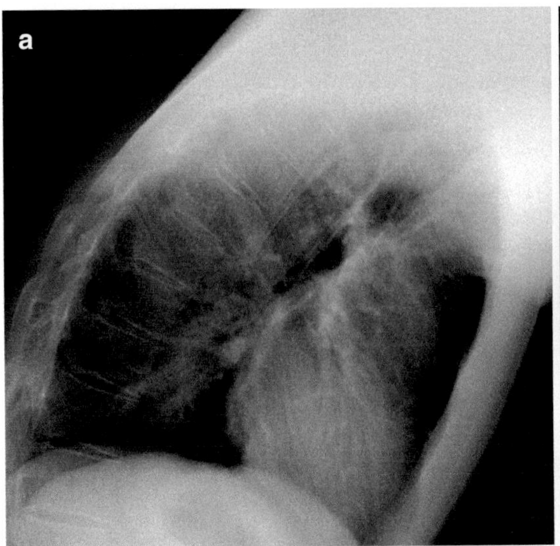

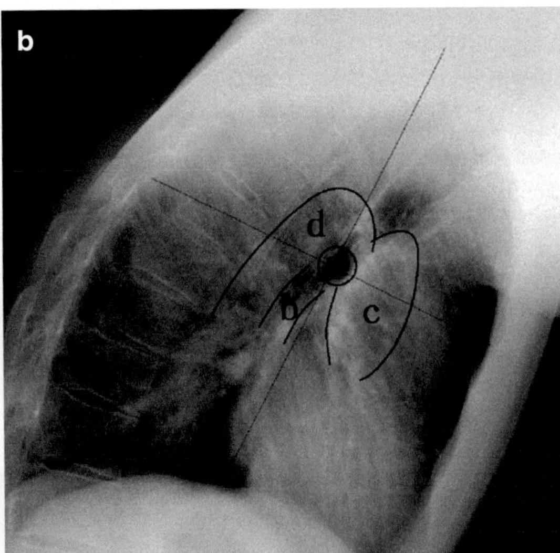

Fig. 6.3 (**a**) Close-up view of lateral hilum. (**b**) (*a*) Left main bronchus; (*b*) bronchus intermedius; (*c*) right pulmonary artery and interlobar artery; (*d*) left pulmonary artery. Draw a line connecting the apex pulmonis and midpoint of the diaphragm and another line segment dividing the antetheca and paries posterior of the lung; then the point of intersection of the two lines is mostly on or next to (*a*) (Reprinted, with permission, from: Song K, Su X, Zhang Y, et al. Optimal Chin-Brow Vertical Angle for Sagittal Visual Fields in Ankylosing Spondylitis Kyphosis. Eur Spine J. 2016;25 (8):1–9. https://doi.org/10.1007/s00586-016-4588-z)

Here the formula, PT = 0.37*PI − 7°, could be used for us to locate the pelvic neutral position exactly and individually [33].

So what is the procedure to make a deformity planning? First, we measure preoperative PI, and then the theoretic PT (ideal postoperative PT) could be calculated. Second, use the theoretic PT to locate exact pelvic neutral positional line rather than the line through hip axis and sacrum promontory. Third, shift hilus pulmonis to the line. Then, the deformity planning becomes individual and more adequate [10, 11, 14] (Figs. 6.5 and 6.6).

As shown in previous study, different osteotomy levels contribute different abilities to restore sagittal balance. It depends on the different arm of force of the trunk [14]. If the same degree is obtained, osteotomy in distal vertebrae can do more for sagittal balance than in proximal vertebrae. In other words, to restore a same sagittal balance, osteotomy angle in distal vertebrae needed might be smaller than in the proximal. A two-level PSO involve not only a proximal vertebra but also a distal one, and it is not the simple thing to choose a middle vertebrae to instead. It is a complicated calculation. As we can see in Fig. 6.7a, different angles were required at different levels (T12 = 85°, L1 = 72°, and L2 = 60°) for sagittal balance, and it is not an exact angle when we used middle level to replace the total angle of two-level osteotomy as in Fig. 6.7a, b (L1 = 72° ≠ 65° = L2 + T12). In addition, different contributed angles in levels resulted in different total angles for osteotomy as shown in Fig. 6.7b, c (L2 + T12 = 45° + 20° = 65° and L2 + T12 = 30° + 40° = 70°).

1.5 Supplement

In most papers, sagittal vertical axis was considered as a design standard for surgery. However, recent research indicates that the C7 plumb line is actually not the CG line. Actually, it is impossible

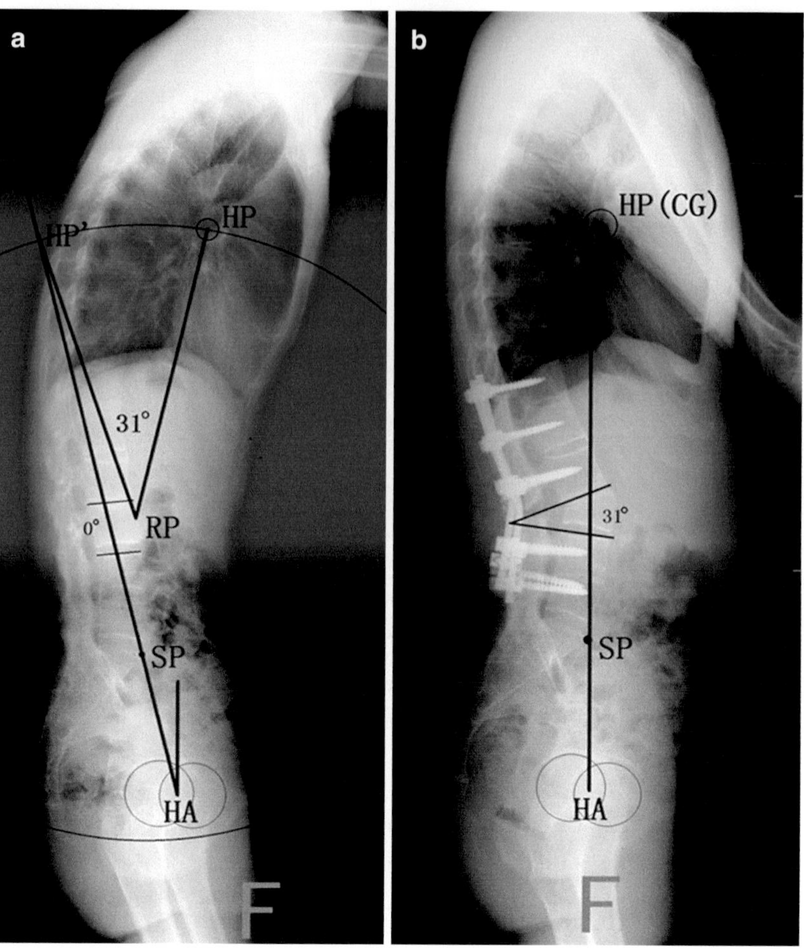

Fig. 6.4 Osteotomy design. (**a**) Draw a straight line through HA and SP, and make a circle with RP (rotation point: the middle point at the front edge of PSO vertebra) as the center and RP-HP as the radius; then, HP' is the intersection with SP-HA. Theoretical osteotomy angle = ∠HP'-RP-HP = 31°. (**b**) After achieving a PSO = 31°, CG and SP were on HA (Reprinted, with permission, from: Song K, Zheng G, Zhang Y, et al. Hilus pulmonis as the center of gravity for AS thoracolumbar kyphosis. Eur Spine J. 2014 Dec;23(12):2743–50. https://doi.org/10.1007/s00586-013-3134-5)

to restore a pelvic neutral position exactly when using C7. Moreover, it is also impossible to restore SVA to be normal in AS kyphosis.

The cases we introduced in the paper are perfect, however, it is hard to obtain so exact angles in clinical practice. Actually, we just want to present a reasonable method to calculate exact angles to restore the sagittal balance. All that remains is to get the exact angle as possible as we can in intra-operation.

In addition, considering that it has been a long time for AS patients with the kyphosis, their bodies might have already adapt to the kyphotic situation to some degree, and all the corresponding muscles have changed, so there is no need to restore a normal theoretical PT, and a little larger PT may be better.

2 Restore Chin-Brow Vertical Angle (CBVA)

Chin-brow vertical angle (CBVA) is very important in correction of thoracolumbar kyphotic deformity in ankylosing spondylitis (AS), especially for the patients with cervical ankylosis [13]. For AS kyphotic patients without cervical ankylosing, we can easily deal with the CBVA, because when restoring the sagittal balance, optimal CBVA commonly is obtained at the same time depending on good cervical flexion-extension. However, if the cervical spine is ankylosing, surgeon must pay more attention. Sometimes, restoring good sagittal balance may lead to bad CBVA. CBVA determines patients' visual fields, and it is even more important for

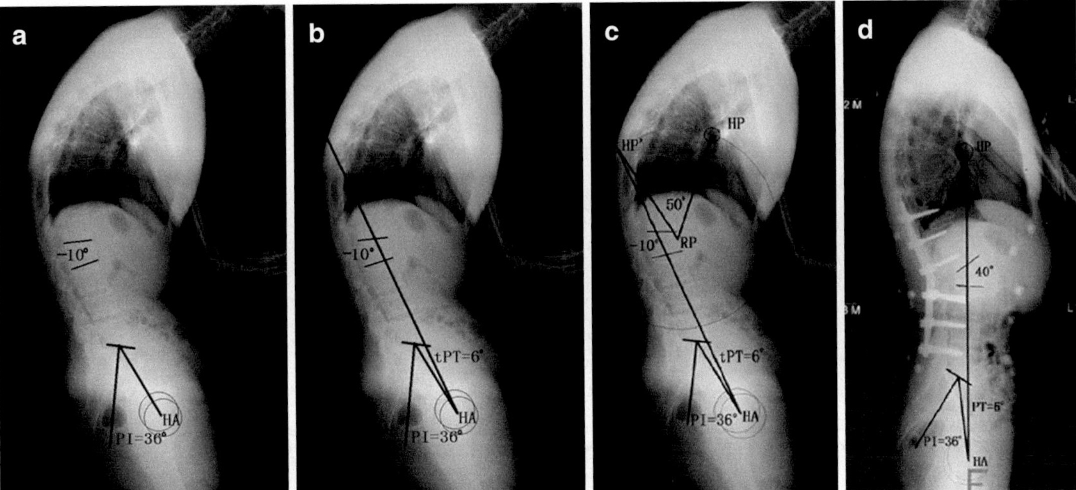

Fig. 6.5 Personalized single-level osteotomy design. A 26-year-old female with AS. (**a**) The preoperative PI was 36°, and the kyphosis of the osteotomy site was 10°. (**b**) Thus, PT = 0.37*36–7 = 6°. The postoperative plumb line (or named pelvic neutral positional line) was drawn according to the theoretic PT (tPT). (**c**) A circle was drawn by taking the anterior column of the second vertebra (rotation point, RP) as the center and the distance between these points to the *hilus pulmonis* as the radius. The included angle was 50°; thus the exact required osteotomy angle was 50°. (**d**) Postoperative lordosis of the osteotomy site was 40°, the real osteotomy angle was 40° + 10° = 50°, and PT was 6° (equal to tPT). Good sagittal balance was achieved (Reprinted, with permission, from: Song K, Zheng G, Zhang Y, et al. A new method for calculating the exact angle required for spinal osteotomy. Spine (Phila Pa 1976). 2013;38(10):E616–620. https://doi.org/10.1097/BRS.0b013e31828b3299)

HRQOL than sagittal balance. In previous study, Suk et al. stated that the patients with CBVA between −10° and 10° had better horizontal gaze [13]. Unfortunately, in clinical practice, we found the patients with CBVA between −10° and 10° after surgery usually complained of difficulty in cooking, cleaning, desk working, and the like, although they had excellent horizontal gaze. In other words, for the patients with cervical ankylosis, good horizontal gaze existed together with poor downward gaze.

2.1 CBVA and Life Quality

It is easy to image that a variety of CBVA is suitable for various tasks. Song notes that, when −10 < CBVA < 10°, the patients indeed had better horizontal gaze and outdoor activities (walking on road, taking public vehicles, shopping, standing communication, looking at the sky and tall building, climbing upstairs). However, the CBVA lead to inability of seeing downward which is the basis of most indoor activities (maintaining personal hygiene, dressing, eating, cooking, cleaning the house, desk working, and sitting communication). When CBVA was between 10° and 20°, both outdoor activities and indoor activities are satisfactory. When 20° ≤ CBVA ≤ 30°, the patients are satisfied with most indoor and outdoor activities, almost as that when 10° ≤ CBV A <20°. Some indoor activities like desk working and cooking are even better, but the subject head-neck appearance does not meet the patients' demand. The patients may prefer to tilt their head backward a little just because of good appearance. When CBVA was 30–40°, the patients are satisfied with neither outdoor or indoor activities nor the subjective head-neck appearance. When CBVA was >40°, the patients are extremely dissatisfied, and the life quality is very low. So, most AS thoracolumbar kyphotic patients with cervical ankylosis have the best satisfaction when 10° ≤ CBVA < 20° [13].

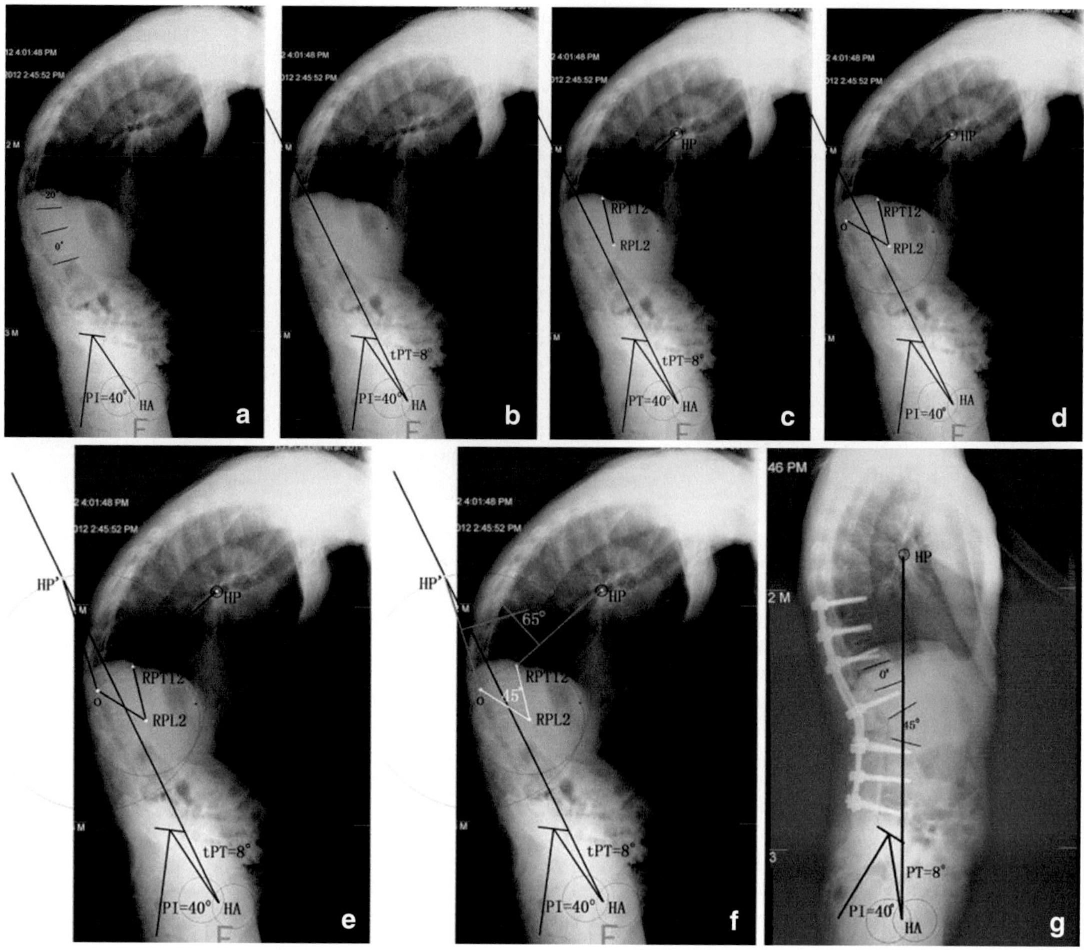

Fig. 6.6 Personalized bi-level osteotomy design. (**a**) Measure preoperative PI (40°), and then the theoretic PT (tPT = 0.37 * PI − 7 = 0.37 * 40 − 7 = 8°) could be calculated. (**b**) Use the tPT to locate the exact pelvic neutral positional line (HA-HP'). (**c**) Mark RPL2 (rotation point at L2, the middle point at the front edge of PSO vertebra) and RPT12 (rotation point at T12, the middle point at the front edge of PSO vertebra). (**d**) Make a circle with RPL2 as the center and RPL2-RPT12 as the radius, make a little on the circle and mark it O, which decided the osteotomy angle for L2. (**e**) Make another circle with O as the center and RPT12-HP as the radius; HP' is the intersection with HP'-HA. (**f**) Theoretical osteotomy angle for L2 = ∠O-RPL2-RPT12 = 45°. Theoretical osteotomy angle for T12 = ∠HP'-O − RPT12-HP − ∠O-RPL2-RPT12 = 65° − 45° = 20°. (**g**) After achieving a PSO angle in L2 of 45° (45° postoperative lordosis + 0° preoperative kyphosis), and a PSO angle in T12 of 20° (20°postoperative lordosis + 0°preoperative kyphosis), for a total of 65°, the postoperative PT = 8°, individual pelvic neutral positon was reconstructed successfully. (Reprinted, with permission, from: Song K, Zheng G, Zhang Y, et al. Hilus pulmonis as the center of gravity for AS thoracolumbar kyphosis. Eur Spine J. 2014 Dec;23(12):2743–50. https://doi.org/10.1007/s00586-013-3134-5)

Actually, due to the compensation of the lower extremities, the trunk of the patients could tilt forward and backward, which may contribute to some change of CBVA. Hence, most of the daily activities could be finished even at a bad CBVA. Nevertheless, the compensation for CBVA would cause instant sagittal imbalance and body fatigue as well. The CBVA of a patient with free-standing position was the most comfortable one. Therefore, the measurement of CBVA should be a free-standing posture CBVA [13].

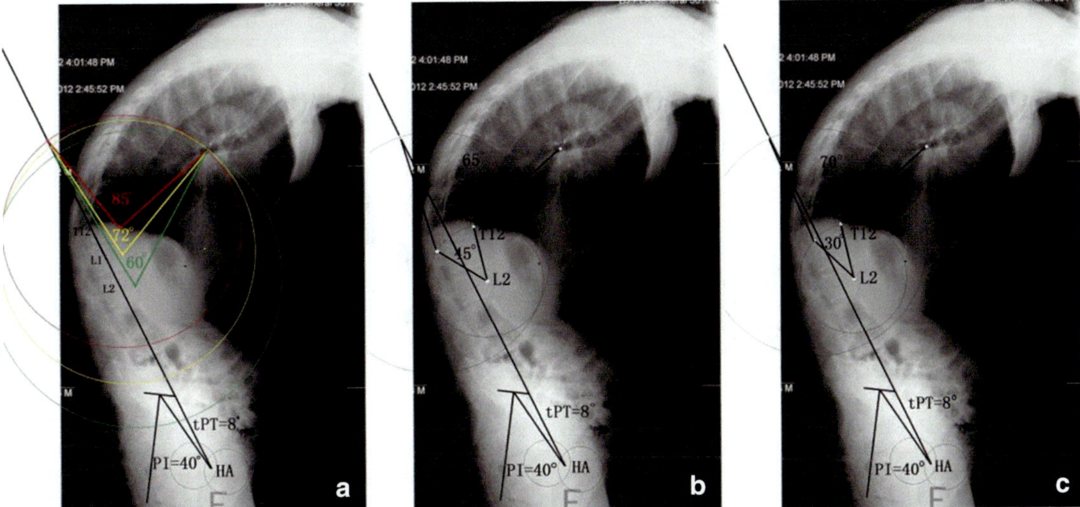

Fig. 6.7 Different osteotomy levels contribute differences to restore sagittal balance

2.2 Prediction of Postoperative CBVA

The harmony of sagittal spinopelvic alignment allows for stable balance and is economical in terms of mechanical effects and muscular energy. In general, the center of gravity (CG) of the trunk always falls on the hip axis (HA) when one stands freely. Even for the spinal deformities, automatic compensatory mechanisms relocate the CG of the trunk onto the HA, because it can provide a new balance with minimal muscular energy expenditure, no matter whether or not this can be achieved completely [21, 23, 34].

For fixed thoracolumbar kyphotic deformity secondary to AS, the CG (center of gravity) should be considerably anterior compared to normal conditions, and it means that the CG is anterior to the hip axis (HA) (Fig. 6.8a); however, it does not occur, because the pelvis is rotated posteriorly to relocate the CG on the HA to the greatest degree by "flexion of the knees" and "extension of the hips" for a new balance and minimal muscular energy expenditure [4, 8, 11] (Fig. 6.8b).

When osteotomies are performed to reconstruct spinopelvic alignment, the CBVA (50°) will change to CBVA' (−10°) theoretically, and the difference is equal to the osteotomy angle, α (60°). This situation does not occur either, because at the same time CG will be shifted to CG' and falls posteriorly behind the HA (Fig. 6.8c).

In fact, the patient will rotate the pelvis anteriorly ($\beta = 35°$) to obtain a new balance by "extension of the knees" and "flexion of the hips," just in contrast with the way before [4, 8, 11]. Thus, CG' will be relocated on HA, and the patient will obtain a new balance. In this situation, CBVA' (−10°) changes to CBVA" (25°), with the difference equal to β (35°; Fig. 6.8d). Therefore, CBVA" (25°) rather than CBVA' (−10°) is the actual postoperative CBVA (Fig. 6.8e).

As we have seen in Fig. 6.8, the preoperative CBVA (CBVA) is decreased by osteotomy (α) and is increased by pelvic rotation (β). Thereafter, the postoperative CBVA (CBVA") is obtained. Thus, we can derive the equation CBVA" = CBVA-α + β, which is the key to predict the postoperative CBVA.

2.3 Make Surgery Planning

As previously mentioned, we introduced that we could consider hilus pulmonis (HP) as the CG of the trunk for AS kyphotic deformity [11]. Then, in the lateral X-ray, HP can be used to

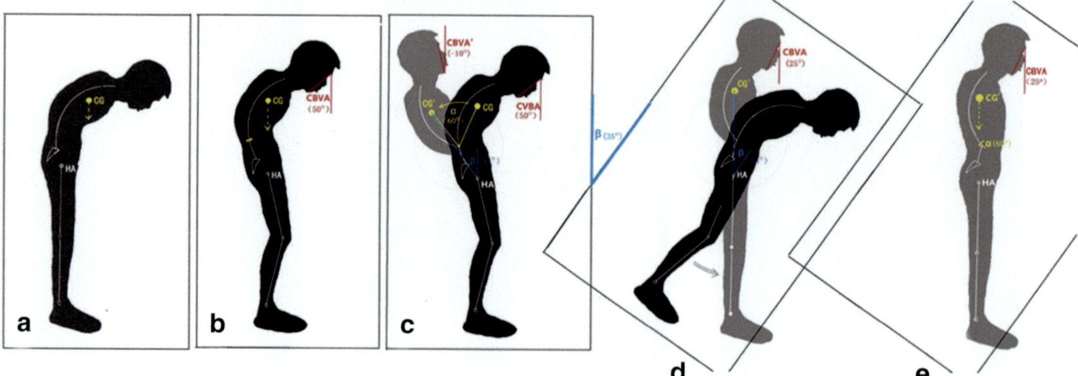

Fig. 6.8 CBVA of the AS and the change before and after surgery. *α* osteotomy angle, *β* pelvic rotation angles, *CG* center of gravity, *CBVA* chin-brow vertical angle, *RP* rotation point, the middle point at the front edge of osteotomy vertebra, *HA* hip axis. (**a**) For AS thoracolumbar kyphotic deformity, without extremity compensation, the CG is anterior to the HA; however, it does not occur. (**b**) In the free-standing position, the pelvis is rotated posteriorly to relocate the CG on the HA to the greatest degree by "flexion of the knees" and "extension of the hips" for a new balance. The preoperative CBVA can be measured (CBVA = 50°). (**c**) It is a simulation of osteotomy. First, make a circle with RP as the center and RP-CG as the radius; then, make a little on the circle as CG' with ∠CG'-RP-CG = *α* = 60°; in this situation, the CBVA (50°) will change to CBVA' (−10°), and the difference is just equal to *α* (60°); however, it does not occur, because CG' falls behind the HA. Second, draw a straight line through CG' and HA; then, the CG'-HA vertical angle (*β* = 35°) can be measured, and the pelvis will be rotated clockwise by *β* (35°). (**d**) After clockwise rotation (*β* = 35°), CG' falls onto the HA, by "extending the knees" and "flexing the hips" compensatory; in this situation, CBVA' (−10°) changes to CBVA" (25°) with deviation equal to *β* (35°). (**e**) CG' falls onto the HA, and CBVA"(25°) is the real postoperative CBVA. (Reprinted, with permission, from: Song K, Su X, Zhang Y, et al. Optimal Chin-Brow Vertical Angle for Sagittal Visual Fields in Ankylosing Spondylitis Kyphosis. Eur Spine J. 2016;25(8):1–9. https://doi.org/10.1007/s00586-016-4588-z)

locate CG. It offered us a possibility for predicting the postoperative CBVA.

Figure 6.9 shows an AS thoracolumbar kyphosis with cervical ankylosis (preoperative CBVA = 37°). In the preoperative surgery design, we planned to perform an osteotomy with L3 as the hinge (PSO at L3 and SPO at L3/4 and L2/3) and a total angle of $\alpha = 60°$. Luckily, a 60° osteotomy was exactly achieved in intra-operation under our control. Thus, as in the surgery design, HP, which took place of CG, was shifted to HP', and the pelvic anterior rotation could be predicted by measuring β (HP'-HA vertical angle) = 23°. Then, the postoperative CBVA should be CBVA" = CBVA − α + β = 37–60 + 23 = 0°. After surgery, the CBVA was finally 0°, as it was expected. The CBVA was the same as the surgery planning.

2.4 Match CBVA with Sagittal Balance

Reconstruction of sagittal balance is also important for AS thoracolumbar kyphosis with cervical ankylosis. Generally, the distal (proximal) osteotomy level contributes to a smaller (greater) CBVA change compared to the proximal (distal) osteotomy level. In contrast, the proximal (distal) osteotomy level contributes to a smaller (greater) change in sagittal balance compared to distal (proximal) osteotomy. Thus, we could try different levels when the sagittal balance and CBVA were not well-matched. Figure 6.10 presents a case on how we match CBVA with sagittal balance by choosing different osteotomy levels.

2.5 Supplement

Sometimes, it is impossible to match CBVA and sagittal balance well. Our experience suggests that CBVA is more important for the patients with cervical ankylosing. In this situation, try various insufficient spinal osteotomy angles and then predict the postoperative CBVA by the method we introduced; when 10 < CBVA < 20, do it. However, sometimes, for the cases with severe cervical lordosis or severe kyphosis, the only way was to do cervical osteotomy. We introduce it in other chapter.

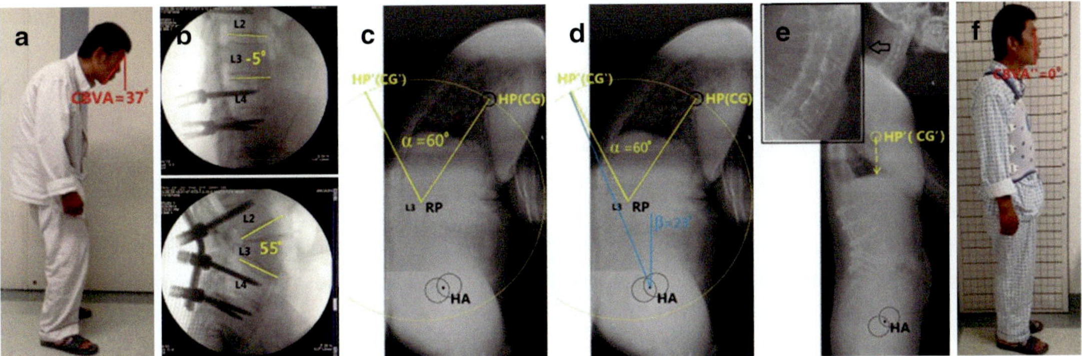

Fig. 6.9 Case. *α* osteotomy angle, *β* pelvic rotation angle, *CG* center of gravity, *RP* rotation point, the hinge at the front edge of osteotomy vertebra; *HA* hip axis, *HP* hilus pulmonis, *CBVA* chin-brow vertical angle. (**a**) CBVA was 37° in free-standing posture preoperatively. (**b**) Intraoperative X-ray in the prone position; Cobb angle from the upper end plate of L4 to the lower end plate of L2 was −5° before postural reduction and 55° after postural reduction; thus 60° osteotomy was obtained; it is the same as surgery design. (**c**) Lateral X-ray in free-standing posture in pre-operation, L3 was chosen as the center of osteotomy, and then RP would be the hinge of restoration, and HP would be on HP' after a planning osteotomy ($\alpha = 60°$). (**d**) Draw a straight line through HP' and HA, and the vertical angle of the line ($\beta = 23°$) is measured, which would be the angle the pelvis is rotated clockwise after surgery. Therefore, we predicted the postoperative CBVA = CBVA − α + β = 37–60 + 23 = 0°. (**e**) Lateral X-ray in free-standing posture in post-operation, HP' was relocated onto the HA by automatic compensatory mechanisms. In the magnified image, the fused cervical spine can be seen, especially in the laminae. (**f**) In free-standing posture in pre-operation, CBVA" is 0° which is equal to the predicted CBVA. The man is an orchard worker who always needs to pick the peaches, so CBVA=0° is optimal for him. (Reprinted, with permission, from: Song K, Su X, Zhang Y, et al. Optimal Chin-Brow Vertical Angle for Sagittal Visual Fields in Ankylosing Spondylitis Kyphosis. Eur Spine J. 2016;25(8):1–9. https://doi.org/10.1007/s00586-016-4588-z)

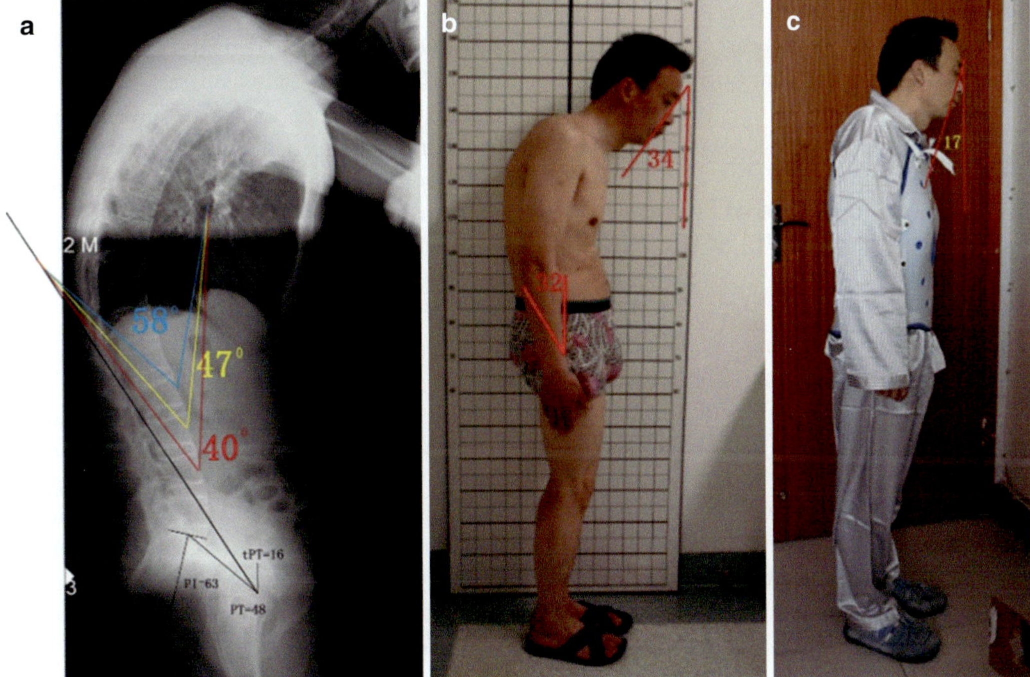

Fig. 6.10 (**a**) PI = 63°, PT = 48°, tPT = 16°. For the case, sagittal balance would be reconstructed well when we have different osteotomy angles (L2 = 58°, L3 = 47°, L4 = 40°). (**b**) The CBVA was 34°, and the pelvic rotation angle was 32° (β = PT − tPT = 48–16 = 32°). So, the CBVA' = CBVA + β = 34 + 32 = 66°. If we chose different osteotomy levels, different postoperative CBVA would occur (L2CBVA = 66–58 = 8°, L3CBVA = 66–47 = 15°, L4CBVA = 66–40 = 26°). Because 10 < CBVA < 20 was optimal, osteotomy at L2 was chosen (**c**) Postoperative CBVA = 17°, the patient had both optimal CBVA and sagittal balance

In addition, we would like to remind that it was approximate that hilus pulmonis is the center of gravity. Indeed, not every patient can be predicted exactly as in the case above. Therefore, it is important for us to leave adequate leeway during surgery planning. A bigger CBVA is better than a smaller CBVA. Even for patients without cervical ankylosis, measurement of the preoperative CBVA at the cervical flexion position is necessary to avoid careless correction of CBVA.

3 Match with the Range of Motion (ROM) of the Hip Joints

The hips are the most commonly effected diarthrodial joint in patients with AS. For such cases, the range of motion (ROM) of the hip joints always decreases to various degrees [15–18]. In this case, if we merely pursue reconstructing the ideal sagittal balance and CBVA, poor clinical outcomes might occur. For example, some patients will lose sitting ability if they primitively had hip flexing limitation when they regain good sagittal balance [12]. In this case, optimal surgery should match patients' new trunk axis with the hip ROM.

3.1 Changed Range of Flexion-Extension (ROFE) of the Hip Joint

For healthy adults, the range of flexion-extension (ROFE) of the hip joint is about 140° (−15° to 125° in flexion) [35, 36]. With normal joints and a flexible spine, all of the activities in daily living could be performed easily [37]; however, it is much more difficult for AS kyphotic patients. Because, the spinal kyphosis changed the normal trunk axis, and then with reference to the trunk axis, the ROFE of the hip joint changed as well and led to a decreased effective ROFE. For example, a patient had the trunk axis forward for 30° because of spinal kyphosis, and as a result the ROFE of the hip joint changed to 15–155° in flexion. Then, the patient had a redundant flexion and an insufficient extension in the hip joints (Fig. 6.11a–c). Most AS kyphotic patients need to flex knees to compensate for insufficient hip extension when standing [4, 11]. With spinal correction, the trunk axis of the patients changed back, and as a result, the ROFE changed back as well (Fig. 6.11d). Thus, the upright activities turned to be much improved postoperatively.

However, the patients with hip involvement were more complicated.

The patients had a limited range of flexion-extension (ROFE) of the hip joints, and for those patients, spinal correction should be performed with care. If the spinal correction was excessive, patients might lose the ability to forward bending, such as squatting and putting on socks, and even sitting on the toilet and chairs. In contrast, an insufficient spinal correction would lead to an inability to stand and walk. Only with adequate spinal correction, the forward bending and upright activities could compromise each other (Fig. 6.12).

In the previous clinical practice, we focused on sagittal balance in AS kyphosis and did not pay attention on the patients with hip involvement. It led to a failed operative effect. Some patients underwent excessive spinal correction and consequently had difficulties sitting on the toilet or chairs; some underwent insufficient spinal correction and consequently had difficulties in standing upright [12].

3.2 Make Surgery Planning

Based on the above theoretical explanation, Song investigated an easy way to make an evaluation for AS thoracolumbar kyphotic patients with hip involvement [12]. However, they also added that the examination depended on spinal stability; if there had been a pseudarthrosis or occult fracture, the examination should be made in other ways.

1. First, the patient is asked to sit on a chair of the right height to keep the thigh parallel to

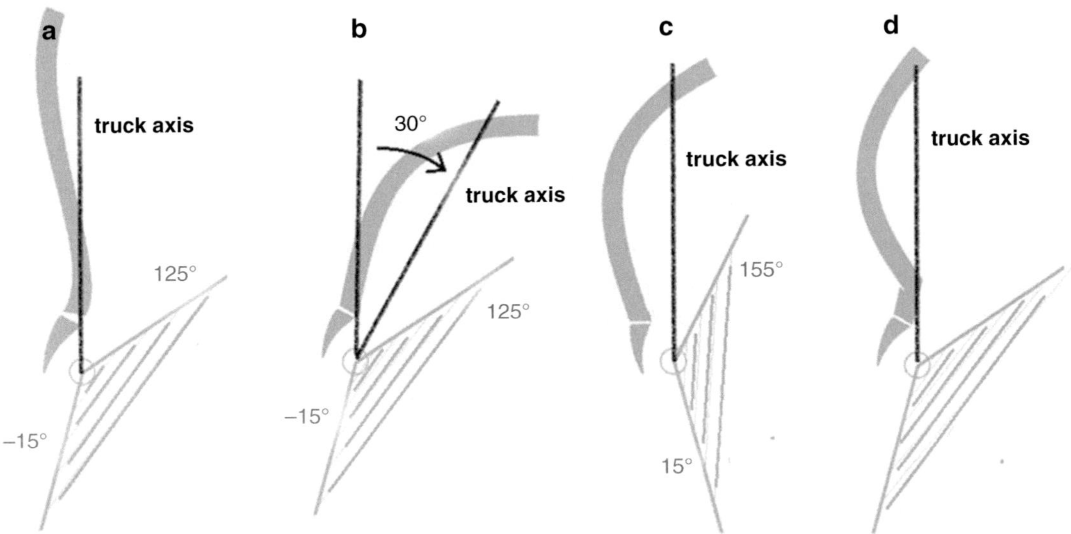

Fig. 6.11 Changes in range of flexion-extension (ROFE) of hips in AS kyphosis. (**a**) ROFE of hip joints in healthy adults. (**b**) ROFE in AS kyphosis. (**c**) ROFE in free-standing position. (**d**) ROFE in after spinal correction in free-standing position

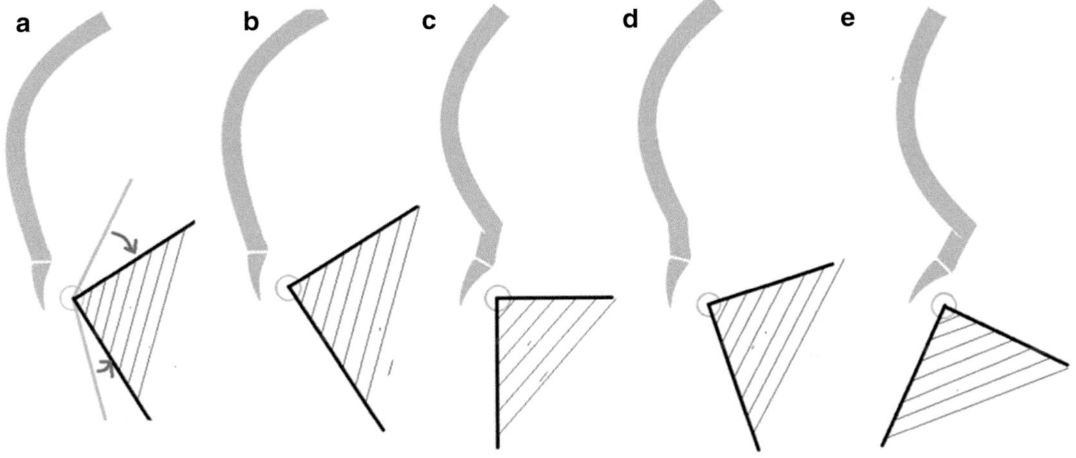

Fig. 6.12 Changes in range of flexion-extension (ROFE) of hip joints in AS kyphosis with hip involvement. (**a**) Smaller ROFE of hip joints in AS kyphosis with hip involvement. (In fact, AS kyphosis had hip joints hyperextension more often.) (**b**) ROFE in free-standing posture. (**c**) ROFE after proper spinal correction. (**d**) ROFE after insufficient spinal correction. (**e**) ROFE after excessive spinal correction

the floor and try to bend over, and then a lateral photograph was taken. Second, a vertical line through the surface topography of the hip axis was made on the photograph. Third, the surface topography of the planning osteotomy vertebra was represented and marked with an "O." Fourth, a circle with an "O" is made in the center with an "O"-shoulder as the radius and then the circle intersected with the vertical line. Finally, the sector angle, designated as "*a*," was the "max osteotomy angle for sitting." Only when the osteotomy angle was smaller than "a" could the patient sit freely (Fig. 6.13a).

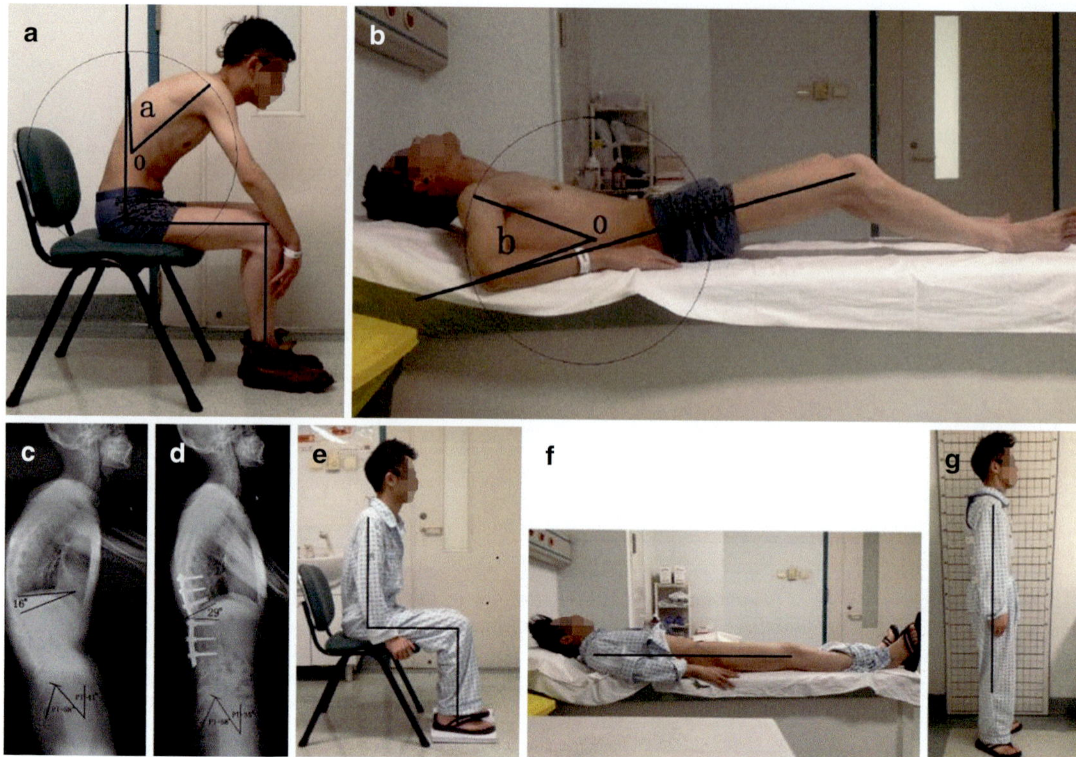

Fig. 6.13 Deformity planning for AS kyphosis with hip involvement. (**a**) "*a*" was "max osteotomy angle for sitting." (**b**) "*b*" was "min osteotomy angle for straightening." The patient had obvious thoracolumbar kyphosis and mild lumbar lordosis loss, so the osteotomy was selected in the thoracolumbar level; $a = 50°$ and $b = 40°$, and the optimal deformity planning was "b (40°) < osteotomy angle < a (50°)." (**c**) Preoperatively, CobbT12 = 16°; (**d**) Postoperatively, CobbT12 = −29°; the osteotomy angle was totally 45°. (**e**) Good sitting postoperatively. (**f**) Good lying. (**g**) Good standing

2. First, the patient lies down on the back and tried to straighten the body (if there was a spinal instability, the patient tried the best to stand upright instead) and then took a lateral photograph. Second, on the photograph a thigh line was made through the surface topography of the hip axis. Third, the surface topography of the planning osteotomy vertebra was represented and marked with an "O." Fourth, a circle was made with an "O" as the center with an "O"-shoulder as the radius and then the circle intersected with the thigh line. Finally, the sector angle, designated as "*b*," was the "min osteotomy angle for straightening." Only the osteotomy angle was greater than "*b*," and the patient could stand upright and lie flat (Fig. 6.13b).

Therefore, when $b <$ osteotomy angle $< a$, the patient could sit, stand, and lie freely (Fig. 6.13). When the osteotomy angle $>b$ and $>a$, the patient could stand upright, but could not sit freely (Fig. 6.14). When the osteotomy angle $<a$ and $<b$, the patient could sit freely, but could not stand upright and lie flat (Fig. 6.15).

A different osteotomy level contributes differently to sagittal balance and CBVA, and the principle is equally applicable to the deformity planning. Generally, a distal osteotomy level is more beneficial for body straightening, while the

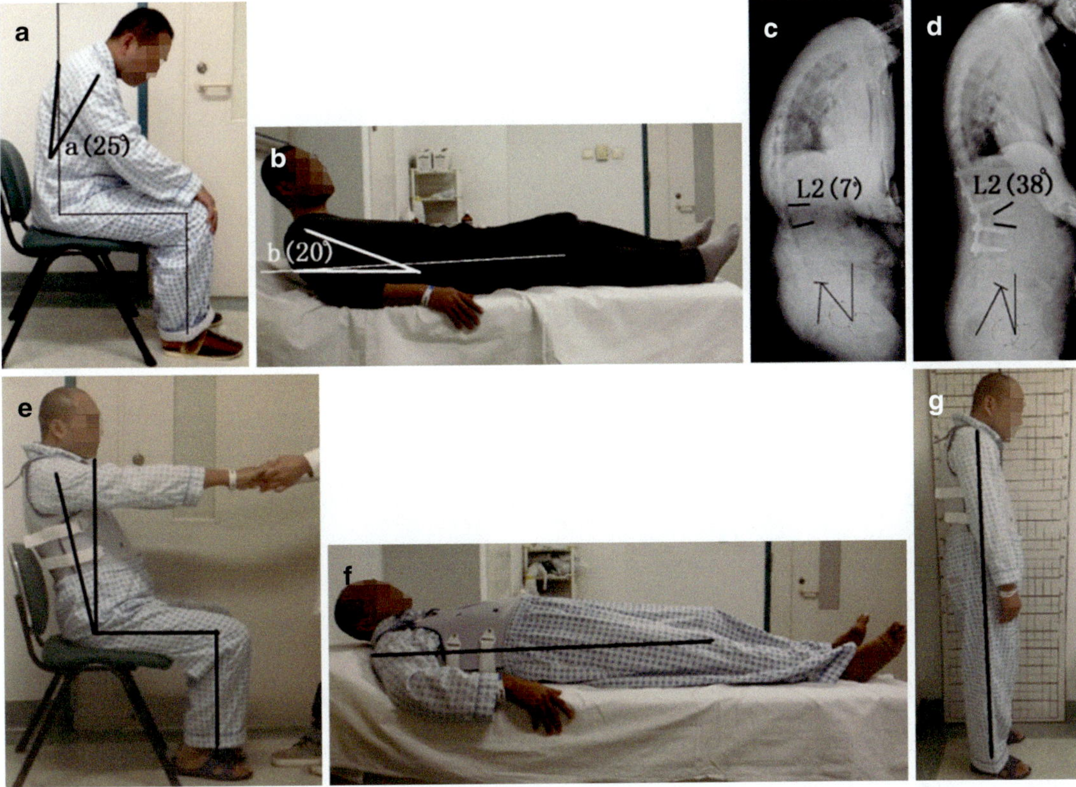

Fig. 6.14 Excessive osteotomy in AS kyphosis with hip involvement. (**a**) "*a*" = 25°. (**b**) "*b*" = 20°; the optimal deformity planning was "*b* (20°) < osteotomy angle < *a* (25°)." (**c**) Pre-operatively, CobbL2 = 7°. (**d**) Postoperatively, CobbL2 = −38°; the osteotomy angle was totally 45°. (**e**) Bad sitting postoperatively. (**f**) Good lying. (**g**) Good standing. The patient had good ability to lie flat and stand upright; however, he lost part of the ability to sit, and he complained of difficulties in sitting for defecation and driving a car at the follow-up

proximal osteotomy level is more beneficial for the body bending. Thus, in clinical practice, we could try different osteotomy levels to make the planning more feasible. Unfortunately, it is sometimes impossible to meet the requirement "*b* < osteotomy angle < a" because the range of flexion-extension (ROFE) of the hip joints is not large enough (<90°). That means the patient could not sit freely and stand upright at the same time. In this case, we should think more about patients' careers and habits and make it clear that which capacity is more important for the patient. In addition, whether or not the patient had received total hip replacement (THR) and would receive THR after the spinal correction should also be considered.

Generally, ROFE of 60° is enough for most patients. For the patients with total ankylosing hip joints, THR is needed.

3.3 THR and Spinal Correction

THR or spinal correction? Which should be performed first for a AS kyphosis with ankylosing hip? It is a controversial issue, even in our own department.

Before we discuss the issue, one thing must be known. Change of spinal alignments could lead to change of pelvic orientation, so does the acetabular component [12, 38–40]. Thus, when THR was performed first, how to determine a correct

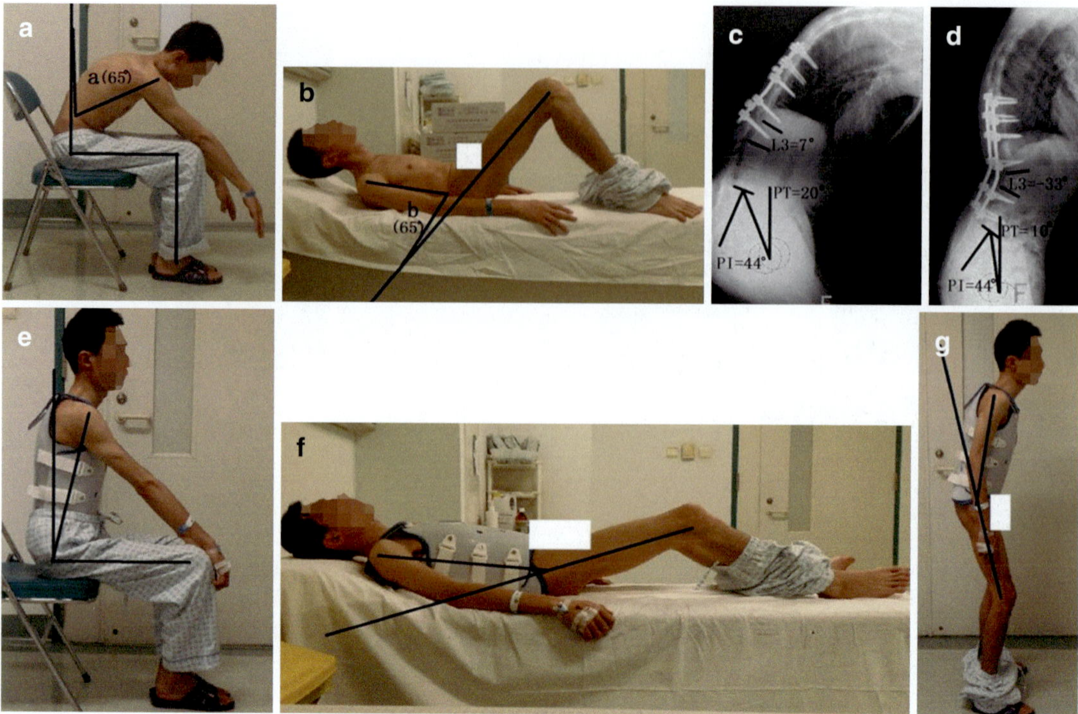

Fig. 6.15 Insufficient osteotomy in AS kyphosis with hip involvement. (**a**) "*a*" = 65°. (**b**). "*b*" = 65°; the optimal deformity planning was "*b* (65°) < osteotomy angle < *a* (65°)." (**c**) Preoperatively, CobbL2 = 7°. (**d**). Postoperatively, CobbL2 = −33°; the osteotomy angle was totally 40°. (**e**) Good sitting postoperatively. (**f**) Bad lying. (**g**) Bad standing. The revision patient had a good ability to sit; however, he lost part of the ability to lie flat and stand upright. If a larger osteotomy angle had been performed, or a distal osteotomy level had been selected, better results could be achieved.

orientation of the cup? How do we define the anteversion angle and abduction angle? Tang [39] described two ways of defining the cup alignment in THR: the cup anatomical position (CAP) and the cup functional position (CFP). CAP was the cup alignment with reference to anterior pelvic plane (APP) (the two anterior superior iliac spines (ASISs) and the pubic symphysis (PS) of the pelvis). CFP was the cup alignment with reference to the level ground with the patient assuming a standing posture. In addition, sagittal anterior pelvic plane angle (SAPPA) was defined to describe the pelvic sagittal plane angle. So, for a kyphotic patient, if we perform THR according to the CFP, after spinal osteotomy, because the patients' pelvis and cup would rotate anteriorly, cup anteversion angle and abduction angle would decrease. It may cause impingement of superior lip of the cup and impair hip flexion. Some patients could not sit well as a result to some degree (Fig. 6.16). If we perform THR according to the CAP, before spinal osteotomy, because the patients' pelvis and cup rotate backward to compensate the sagittal imbalance, cup anteversion angle and abduction angle would increase. It may cause anterior dislocation of femoral head prosthesis, theoretically (Song [12] did not think so). Until after the spinal osteotomy, the cup anteversion angle and abduction angle would restore to normal (Fig. 6.17). Therefore, Tang [39] recommends referring to CAP and improved CFP when determine a cup orientation if we perform THR first.

Some professors like Zheng [41] and Tang [39] recommended that spinal correction should be performed before THR. They had the idea that when the spinal alignment was restored by osteotomy, hip surgeons could perform the THR

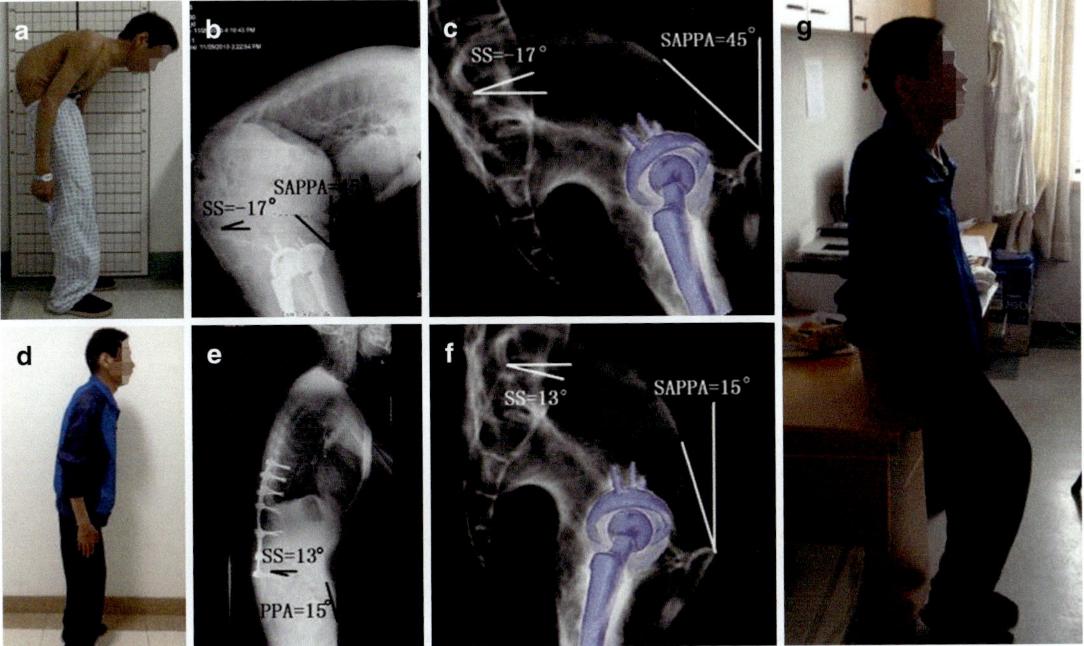

Fig. 6.16 AS kyphosis with THR referring to CFP. (**a**) The patient in free-standing posture, after THR and before spinal osteotomy. (**b**) Exceeding pelvic retroversion (SAPPA = 45°, SS = −17°). (**c**) Acceptable cup anteversion in CT image reconstruction (SAPPA = 45°, SS = −17°). (**d**) The patient in free-standing posture, after spinal osteotomy. (**e**) Moderate pelvic retroversion (SAPPA = 15°, SS = 13°). (**f**) Insufficient cup retroversion in CT image reconstruction (SAPPA = 15°, SS = 13°). (**g**) Bad sitting

easily without considering the cup orientation changing. In addition, the patients could make a goal-oriented functional exercise (sit well and stand uprightly). However, there was also a problem [12]. When the patients had already underwent spinal correction before THR, they usually acted as “a straight stick” and therefore had a much lower health quality of life (HQOL). With no bending joint, the patients could not walk and sit, and they could not take care of themselves in daily life, and they required special care to keep. The only thing they could do is lying down on the bed or standing immovably with assistance. Until the THR were performed, their low HQOL could not be improved [12]. In previous years, we sometimes performed THR in a short time (1 or 2 weeks) after spinal correction to avoid the problem. However, it led to other problems. First, patients could not tolerate the two major operations (spinal osteotomy and THR) in a short period. Second, postoperative recovery for the two operations contradicts to each other. Spinal osteotomy needed immobilization postoperatively, while THR needed early functional exercise. If the patient followed the spine surgeons’ advice, ROFE of hip prostheses might lose. If the patient followed the hip surgeons’ advice, failure of spinal internal fixation might occur (Fig. 6.18).

Song [12] recommended a planning on the premise that the spine surgeon and hip surgeon both had thorough comprehension of the compensatory mechanism in sagittal balance of the spine and lower extremities.

Firstly, make a co-planning. The spine surgeon should be clear about the range of the future body trunk axis by spinal osteotomy, and the hip surgeon should be clear about the future range of flexion-extension (ROFE) of the hip joints by THR according to the bone and soft tissue. Then, the spine surgeon and hip surgeon compromise to achieve a common goal that the future body axis matches with the future ROFE well (Fig. 6.19).

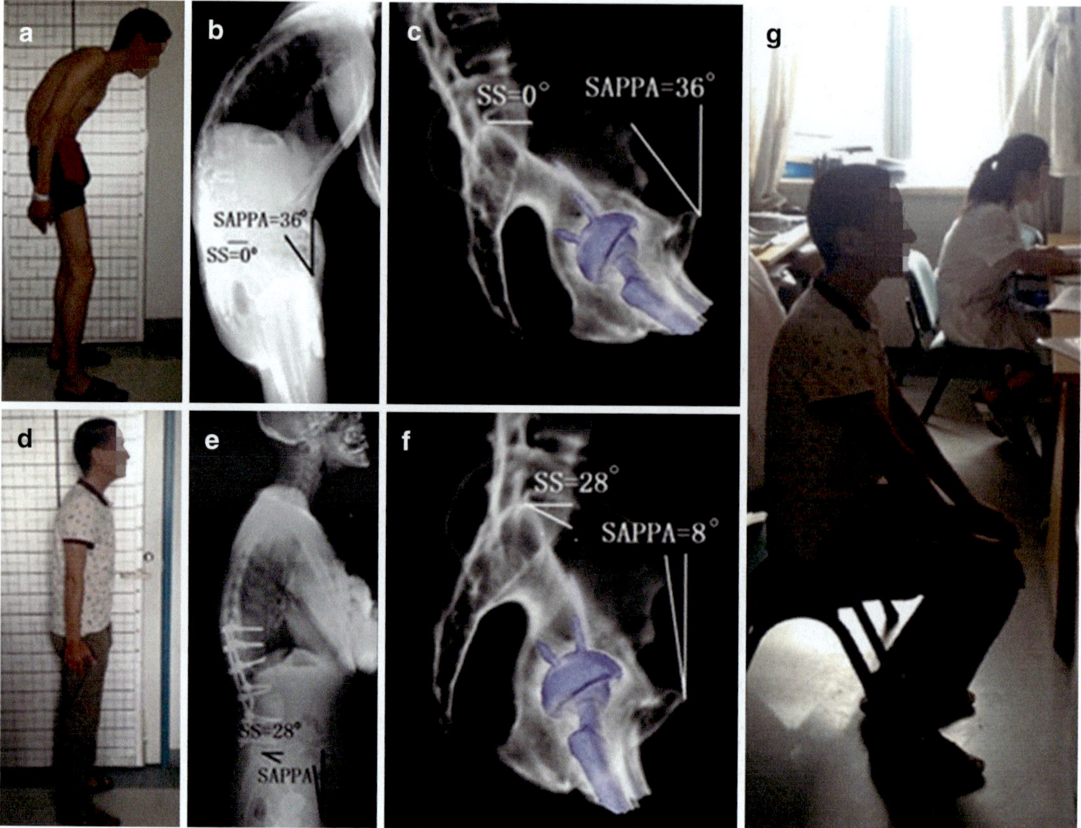

Fig. 6.17 AS kyphosis with THR referring to CAP. (**a**) The patient in free-standing posture, after THR and before spinal osteotomy. (**b**) Exceeding pelvic retroversion (SAPPA = 36°, SS = 0°). (**c**) Exceeding cup anteversion in CT image reconstruction (SAPPA = 36°, SS = 0°). (**d**) The patient in free-standing posture, after spinal osteotomy. (**e**) Mild pelvic retroversion (SAPPA = 8°, SS = 28°). (**f**) Acceptable cup retroversion in CT image reconstruction (SAPPA = 8°, SS = 28°). (**g**) Good sitting

Secondly, do THR first. When performing THR, the cup should be placed with reference to the future body axis, but not cup anatomical position (CAP) or the cup functional position (CFP). The intraoperative ROFE may be different as expected. No need to release the anterior soft tissue of hips overly and no need to worry about anterior dislocation.

Thirdly, do proper hip functional exercise for at least 3–6 months. Lots of patients and even surgeons misunderstand the real hip flexion because of the compensation of kyphotic body trunk. The patient appears to sit well, and actually it relies on spinal kyphosis but not good hip flexion function. So, after the spinal correction, no more good sitting function remains (Fig. 6.20).

Fourthly, after at least 3–6 months, the ROFE would be stable, and then do spinal correction. Before performing the surgery, make the evaluation for the patients with hip involvement as we mentioned before, and try to meet the requirement "b < osteotomy angle < a" (Fig. 6.13a, b). If the ROFE is smaller than 90°, do some simple release of hips before or after spinal osteotomy with general anesthesia.

3.4 Supplement

This part could be considered as a supplement of the surgery design for AS kyphosis. Thus, we first make the surgery planning to restore sagittal balance and CBVA; if the planning meet

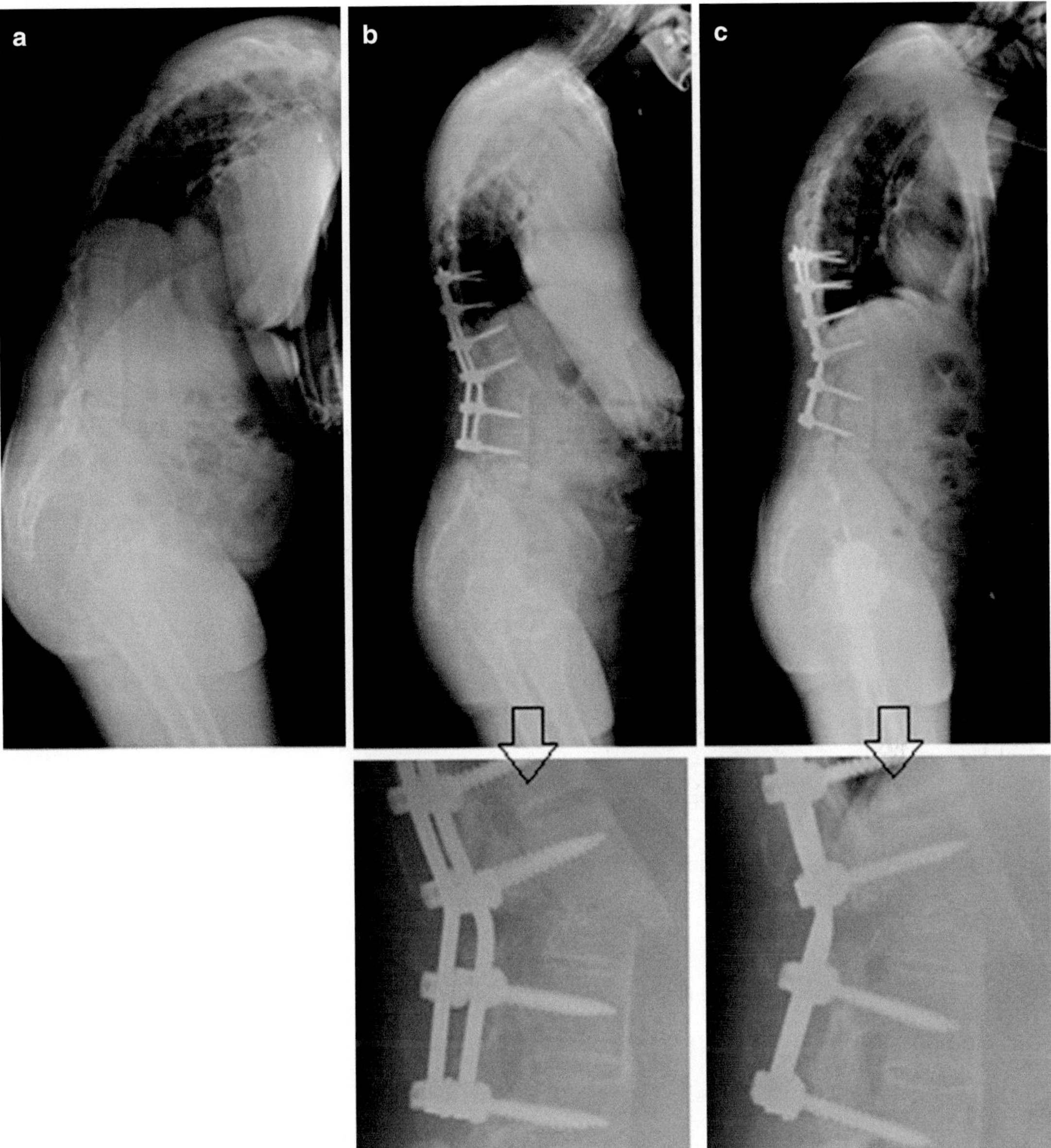

Fig. 6.18 The AS kyphotic patient was with ankylosing hips (**a**), and he underwent spinal osteotomy first (**b**). Because he could not stand the complete inactivity like "a straight stick," we performed THR only 7 days after the spinal osteotomy. After THR, the hip doctor told him to do early functional exercise to avoid hip prosthesis ankylosing, and it led to a pedicle-screw cutting in the lowest two levels and a larger ST (**b**, **c**). Luckily, no neural symptom occurred except back pain; after 3 months with conservative treatment, the spinal fusion was achieved. However, the ROFE was not as good as expected without early functional exercise which was restricted by the spine surgeon after the failure of the spinal internal fixation

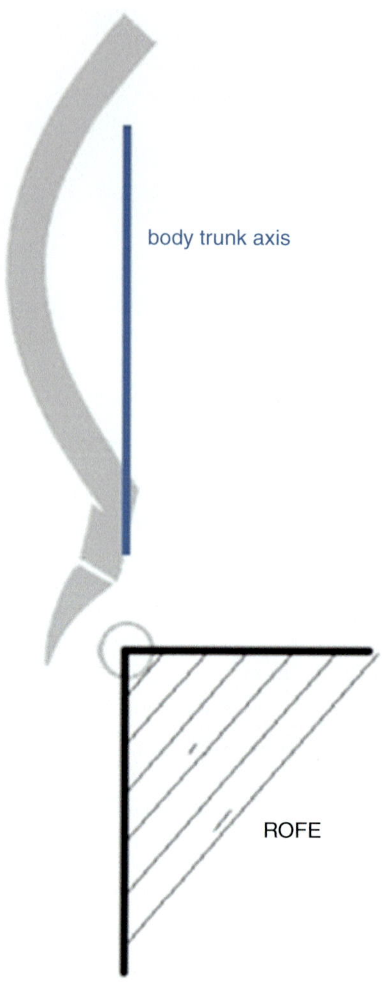

Fig. 6.19 Body trunk axis and hip ROFE

"b < osteotomy angle < a," then do it; if it does not meet it, try different osteotomy levels and angles. In addition, whether or not the patient had received THR and would receive THR after the spinal correction should also be considered.

Acknowledgement To memorize our respectful Professor Yonggang Zhang who made the most outstanding contributions to the study.

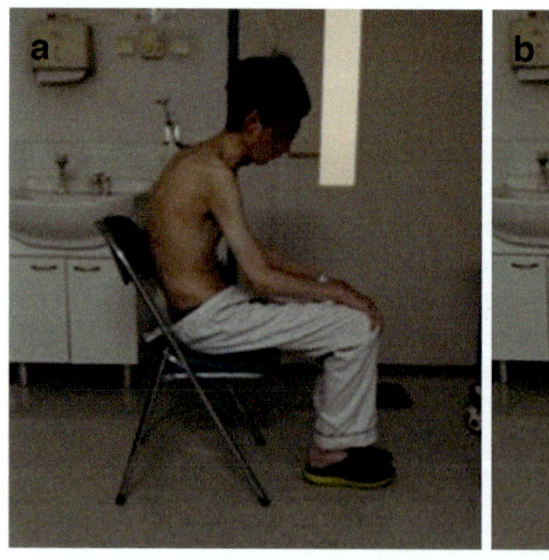

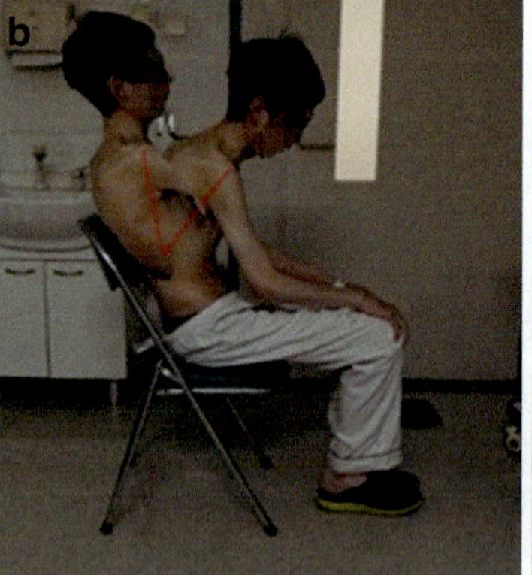

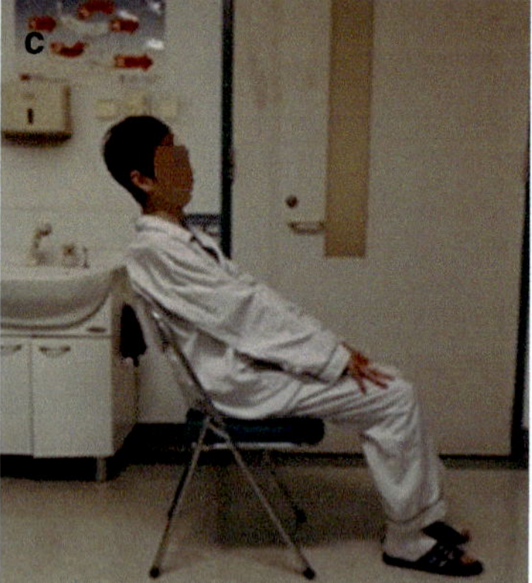

Fig. 6.20 The patient who had underwent THR appeared to sit well (**a**), so he did not do more exercises to flex his hips. However, spinal correction would improve the kyphotic body trunk (**b**), so after the spinal correction, he could not sit well (**c**). Unfortunately, he missed the best time to do hip exercise, and as a result limited flexion function could be obtained further

References

1. Braun J, Sieper J. Ankylosing spondylitis. Lancet. 2007;369:1379–90.
2. Smith-Petersen MN, Larson CB, Aufranc OE. Osteotomy of the spine for correction of flexion deformity in rheumatoid arthritis. J Bone Joint Surg. 1945;27:1–11.
3. Van Royen BJ, De Gast A. Lumbar osteotomy for correction of thoracolumbar kyphotic deformity in ankylosing spondylitis: a structured review of three methods of treatment. Ann Rheum Dis. 1999;58:399–406.
4. Van Royen BJ, Gast AD, Smit TH. Deformity planning for sagittal plane corrective osteotomies of the spine in ankylosing spondylitis. Eur Spine J. 2000;9:492–8.
5. Kim KT, Suk KS, Cho YJ, et al. Clinical outcome results of pedicle subtraction osteotomy in ankylosing spondylitis with kyphotic deformity. Spine. 2002;27:612–8.
6. Suk KS, Kim KT, Lee SH, et al. Significance of chin brow vertical angle in correction of kyphotic deformity of ankylosing spondylitis patients. Spine. 2003;28:2001–5.
7. Bridwell KH, Lewis SJ, Lenke LG, et al. Pedicle subtraction osteotomy for the treatment of fixed sagittal imbalance. J Bone Joint Surg Am. 2003;85-A:454–63.
8. Debarge R, Demey G, Roussouly P. Radiological analysis of ankylosing spondylitis patients with severe kyphosis before and after pedicle subtraction osteotomy. Eur Spine J. 2010;19:65–70.
9. Kim KT, Lee SH, Suk KS, et al. Outcome of pedicle subtraction osteotomies for fixed sagittal imbalance of multiple etiologies: a retrospective review of 140 patients. Spine. 2012;37(19):1667–75.
10. Song K, Zheng G, Zhang Y, et al. A new method for calculating the exact angle required for spinal osteotomy. Spine (Phila Pa 1976). 2013;38(10):E616–20.
11. Song K, Zheng G, Zhang Y, et al. Hilus pulmonis as the center of gravity for AS thoracolumbar kyphosis. Eur Spine J. 2014;23(12):2743–50.
12. Song K, Zhang Y, Fu J, et al. Changes of activities and qualities of life related to hip joints after spinal correction of thoracolumbar kyphosis in ankylosing spondylitis. Chin J Spine Spinal Cord. 2015;10: 871–82.
13. Song K, Su X, Zhang Y, et al. Optimal chin-brow vertical angle for sagittal visual fields in ankylosing spondylitis kyphosis. Eur Spine J. 2016;25(8):1–9.
14. Zheng G, Song K, Yao Z, et al. How to calculate the exact angle for two-level osteotomy in ankylosing spondylitis? Spine. 2016;41(17):E1046.
15. Bisla RS, Ranawat CS, Inglis AE. Total hip replacement in patients with ankylosing spondylitis with involvement of the hip. J Bone Joint Surg Am. 1976;58:233.
16. Williams E, Taylor AR, Arden GP, et al. Arthroplasty of the hip in ankylosing spondylitis. J Bone Joint Surg Br. 1977;59:393.
17. Walker LG, Sledge CB. Total hip arthroplasty in ankylosing spondylitis. Clin Orthop. 1991;262:198–204.
18. Sochart DH, Porter ML. Long-term results of total hip replacement in young patients who had ankylosing spondylitis: eighteen to thirty-year results with survivorship analysis. J Bone Joint Surg Am. 1997;79(8):1181–9.
19. Duval-Beaupère G, Robain G. Visualization on full spine radiographs of the anatomical connections of the centre of the segmental body mass supported by each vertebra and measured in vivo. Int Orthop. 1987;11:261–9.
20. Jackson RP, Hales C, Cert CH. Congruent spinopelvic alignment on standing lateral radiographs of adult volunteers. Spine. 2000;25:2808–15.
21. Legaye J, Duval-Beaupère G. Gravitational forces and sagittal shape of the spine. Clinical estimation of their relations. Int Orthop. 2008;32:809–16.
22. Le Huec JC, Saddiki R, Franke J, et al. Equilibrium of the human body and the gravity line: the basics. Eur Spine J. 2011;20:S558–63.
23. Schwab F, Lafage V, Boyce R, et al. Gravity line analysis in adult volunteers age-related correlation with spinal parameters, pelvic parameters, and foot position. Spine. 2006;31:E959–67.
24. El Fegoun AB, Schwab F, Gamez L, et al. Center of gravity and radiographic posture analysis: a preliminary review of adult volunteers and adult patients affected by scoliosis. Spine. 2005;30:1535–40.
25. Takemitsu Y, Harada Y, Iwahava T, et al. Lumbar degenerative kyphosis. Clinical, radiological and epidemiological studies. Spine. 1988;13:1317–26.
26. Chang KW. Quality control of reconstructed sagittal balance for sagittal imbalance. Spine. 2011;36:E186–97.
27. McComb BL. The chest in profile. J Thorac Imaging. 2002;17:58–69.
28. Feigin DS. Lateral chest radiograph a systematic approach. Acad Radiol. 2010;17:1560–6.
29. Raoof S, Feigin D, Sung A, et al. Interpretation of plain chest roentgenogram. Chest. 2012;141(2):545–58.
30. Roussouly P, Gollogly S, Berthonnaud E, et al. Classification of the normal variation in the sagittal alignment of the human lumbar spine and pelvis in the standing position. Spine (Phila Pa 1976). 2005;30(3):346–53.
31. Duval-Beaupère G, Schmidt C, Cosson PH. A barycentremetric study of the sagittal shape of spine and pelvis: the conditions required for an economic standing position. Ann Biomed Eng. 1992;20:451–62.
32. Legaye J, Duval-Beaupère G, Hecquet J, et al. Pelvic incidence: a fundamental pelvic parameter for three-dimensional regulation of spinal sagittal curves. Eur Spine J. 1998;7:99–103.
33. Vialle R, Levassor N, Rillardon L, et al. Radiographic analysis of the sagittal alignment and balance of the spine in asymptomatic subjects. J Bone Joint Surg Am. 2005;87:260–7.
34. Roussouly P, Gollogly S, Noseda O, et al. The vertical projection of the sum of the ground reactive forces of a standing patient is not the same as the C7 plumb line:

a radiographic study of the sagittal alignment of 153 asymptomatic volunteers. Spine. 2006;31:E320–5.

35. Roach KE, Miles TP. Normal hip and knee active range of motion: the relationship to age. Phys Ther. 1991;71:656–65.
36. Boone D, Azen S. Normal range of motion in male subjects. J Bone Joint Surg. 1979;16:756–9.
37. Tully EA, Wagh P, Galea MP. Lumbofemoral rhythm during hip flexion in young adults and children. Spine. 2002;27(20):E432–40.
38. Tang WM, Chiu KY. Primary total hip arthroplasty in patients with ankylosing spondylitis. J Arthroplast. 2000;15:52–8.
39. Tang WM, Chiu KY, Kwan MF, et al. Sagittal pelvic malrotation and positioning of the acetabular component in total hip arthroplasty: three-dimensional computer model analysis. J Orthop Res. 2007;25(6):766–71.
40. Legaye J. Influence of the sagittal balance of the spine on the anterior pelvic plane and on the acetabular orientation. Int Orthop. 2009;33(6):1695–700.
41. Zheng GQ, Zhang YG, Chen JY, et al. Decision making regarding spinal osteotomy and total hip replacement for ankylosing spondylitis: experience with 28 patients. Bone Joint J. 2014;96-B(3):360–5.

7 Basic Surgical Technique for Management of AS Kyphosis

Guoquan Zheng, Zhijun Xin, and Yan Wang

1 Introduction

Ankylosing spondylitis (AS) results in typical spinal deformities, for example, flattening of lumbar lordosis or lumbar kyphosis, as well as worsening of smooth thoracic hyperkyphosis. These fixed kyphosis and synthetic positive sagittal deformities not only damage the walking ability but also lead to significant pain, which may limit many patients' mental activity and physiological functions, such as interpersonal communication, walking, driving, and the like. Surgery may be the appropriate option for managing these patients [1]. Of course, dysfunction's degree is a vital factor when considering surgery [2], because most patients require spinal osteotomy to obtain adequate correction, so patients are a huge challenge for spine surgeons during surgery.

In theory, the apical vertebrae osteotomy has a better correction effect. The root tip of most AS patients is located at the junction of the thoracolumbar vertebrae and the lumbar vertebrae. Therefore, the overall correction effect is best under lumbar intervention. The kyphosis is best treated with lumbar lordosis osteotomy, because thoracic correction is restricted by the ankylosis of the costovertebral joints [3–5], and the thoracic spinal canal is narrower, so that the midthoracic spinal cord has more chance to get perioperative injury than the cauda equina. The spinal canal is more susceptible to damage when it is wider. A lower horizontal osteotomy allows for a better sagittal alignment due to the long arm length though the correction has the same angle.

G. Zheng · Z. Xin · Y. Wang (✉)
Chinese PLA General Hospital, Beijing, China

In addition to the choice of osteotomy site, the selection of osteotomy type is also important. There are several potential spinal osteotomies for the treatment of kyphosis, including the opening wedge osteotomy (OWO), also known as Smith-Petersen osteotomy (SPO); closing wedge osteotomy (CWO), also named as pedicle subtraction osteotomy (PSO) [6, 7]; and closing-opening wedge osteotomy and/or spinal dislocation (vertebral column decancellation, VCD) [1].

2 Smith-Petersen Osteotomy (SPO)

Smith-Petersen osteotomy (SPO) [1, 8] is the first spine osteotomy technique proposed in 1945 to treat kyphosis caused by AS. It is intended to be a 30–40° correction with one-level osteotomy at L1, L2, and L3 initially. However, due to the large elongation of the anterior column, this technique is associated with some serious complications, such as aortic rupture. Subsequently, the concept of multiple SPO osteotomy was

Y. Wang (ed.), *Surgical Treatment of Ankylosing Spondylitis Deformity*,
https://doi.org/10.1007/978-981-13-6427-3_7

used in AS, which was to create a harmonious lordosis by multilevel resection of the posterior joint between the facet joints to achieve a sufficient and satisfactory correction [5, 9].

3 Indication

Smith-Petersen osteotomy (SPO) is an anterior opening wedge osteotomy (OWO) technique [10] which needs a complete resection of the posterior elements at the level of the osteotomized region, including the lamina, ligamentum flavum, and facets, and then the anterior column is extended by strong stretching of the disc spaces at osteotomized level [11, 12] (Fig. 7.1). Hence, for SPO, a minor, long, rounded, smooth flexible, thoracolumbar kyphosis secondary to AS is the most common indication. Clinically, SPO offers unique merits, especially for those spinal kyphotic deformities with anterior column that are not fused and ossified.

4 Operative Technique

The technique involves the removal of a single segment or multiple segments of the posterior column structures between the facets, compressing the posterior column spacing, and cutting through the intervertebral disc to lengthen the anterior column through a powerful artificial extension. During the operation, the spinous process was removed by an osteotome at first, and the edges of laminae and the synovial joints were resected using high-speed bur or piezosurgery and machined into a V-shaped fashion region. Then, use the Krissen forceps to remove the ligamentum flavum. After the spinal rod is prebended and implanted, the pedicle screw or interspinous cantilever operation is combined with compression forceps, especially in the case of osteoporosis, which can shorten the posterior column. Under normal circumstances, there is no need to interrupt the disc in SPOs (Fig. 7.2). Discectomy helps to destroy the anterior longitudinal ligament,

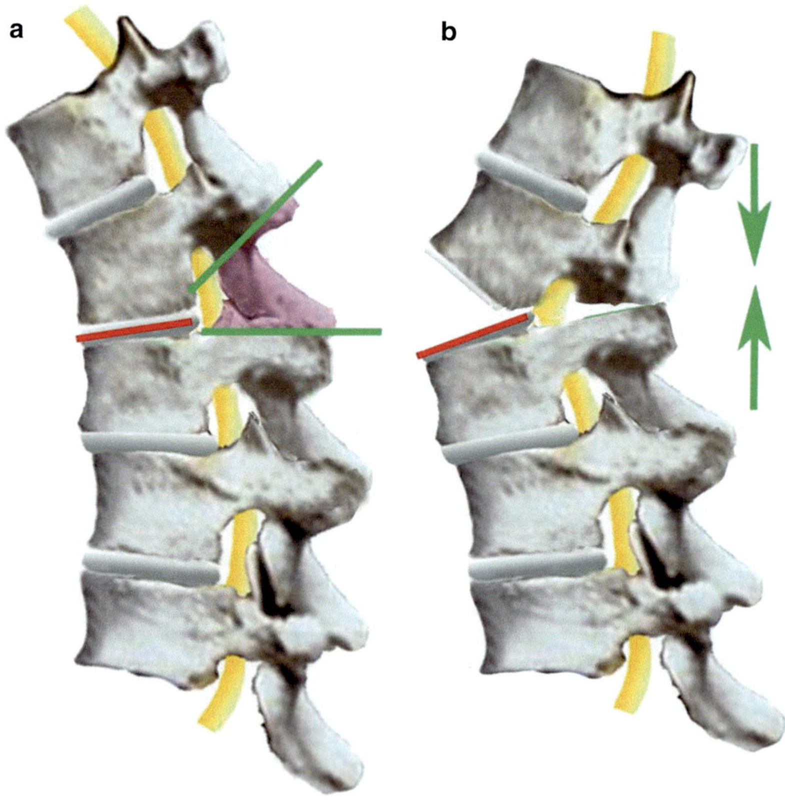

Fig. 7.1 Sketch map of single-level SPO. (**a**) The posterior structures were removed before correction; (**b**) the correction can be achieved by manufacturing a single segmental intervertebral opening wedge

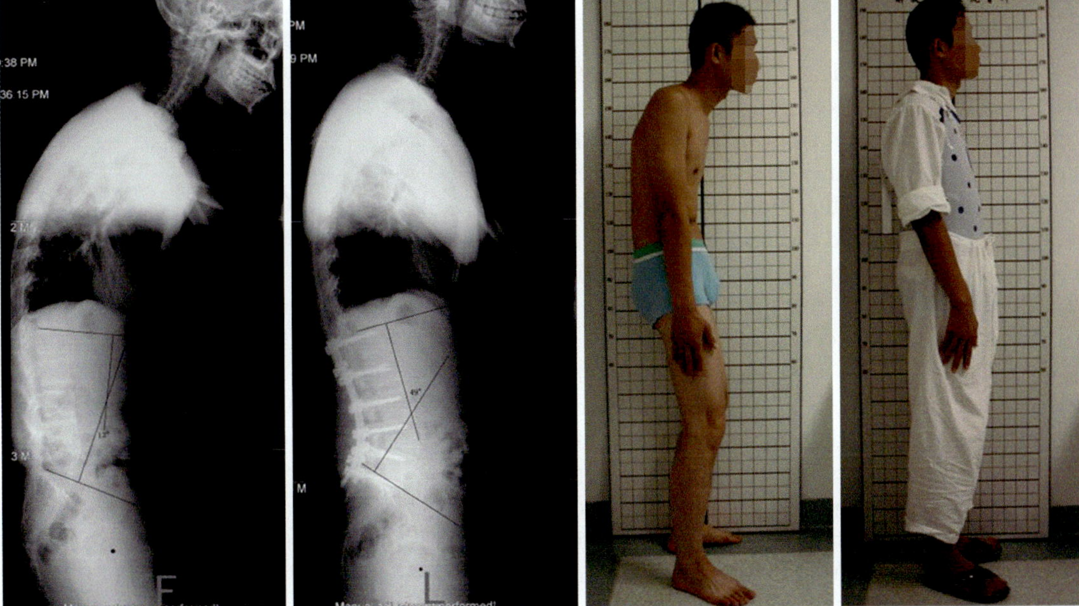

Fig. 7.2 Illustration of mutilevel SPO (SPOs) for AS. A 26-year-old man with AS with thoracolumbar kyphosis underwent five-level SPOs performed at L1~L2, L2~L3, L3~L4, L4~L5, and L5~S1. Preoperative and postoperative clinical appearances and lateral radiographs were as shown. A 7° correction was obtained for each layer, resulting in a total correction of 36°. The round and smooth curve was stabilized. (Reprint with permission from: Zhang YG. et al. (2015) The Management of Thoracolumbar Kyphotic Deformity in Ankylosing Spondylitis. In: Wang Y., Boachie-Adjei O., Lenke L. (eds) Spinal Osteotomy. Springer, Dordrecht)

which facilitates anterior column opening and creates a monosegmental intervertebral open wedge (Fig. 7.1). While, this technique requires extending the anterior column, which may increase the risk of abdominal vessels damage, intestinal paralysis, delayed healing and rod breakage.

5 Pedicle Subtraction Osteotomy

Under the comparison with SPO, pedicle subtraction osteotomies (PSO) are more complicated, and the operation time and blood loss are significantly increased. However, because of its closed osteoclasis rather than an open wedge, this technique avoids the use of sudden force in correcting the spine. Therefore, this technique can reduce neurological complications and blood vessels (aortic rupture). The two methods have good clinical results, not only to perfect the quality of life of patients but also have high patient satisfaction.

6 Indications

Pedicle subtraction osteotomies (PSO) are more suitable for fixed sagittal deformities with sharp or angular kyphosis in patients with severe global positive sagittal imbalance >8 cm [1]. However, PSO technique, as a closing-wedging osteotomy to produce a shortening of the posterior and middle columns, may result in buckling of the dura and spinal cord, which is very dangerous, and authors have recommended usually using at non-spinal cord area and limiting the correction to 30–40° [13–15]. von Royen and Slot [16] recommended that corrective osteotomy should be performed in the lower lumbar spine to maximize correction and safety.

7 Operative Technique

PSO techniques include posterior column resection and pedicle wedge incision, as well as a hinge located in the anterior cortex of the vertebral body [17]. After exposure, the pedicle screw is placed into the cephalad and caudad vertebral body avoided the intended site of the osteotomy. Osteotomy maneuver was begun with removing all of the posterior structures (ligament, spinous process, lamina, and facet joints). The transverse process is removed at the base. After the pedicle is separated, the cancellous bone is taken, and holes were made via the pedicles into the vertebral body with curette. Then, the cancellous bone of the vertebral body can be removed (or decancellation) using a bone spur or curette through the hole of pedicles, and a "V"-shaped bony defect cavity was made. It is important to ensure that the bone is taken evenly, which will result in an asymmetrical closure of the osteotomy site. After appropriate cancellous bone removal, the lateral cortex of the vertebral body walls, the inferior wall of pedicle adjacent to the exiting nerve root, and finally the posterior cortex of the vertebral body were removed. The dura mater and nerve roots above and below the resected pedicle should be freed. The posterior and middle column osteotomy gap can be closed with a bent spinal rod cantilever which supports stability of the spine, or it can be closed with the operating table stretching. Then the middle and posterior column bone defects are closed without extending the front column. In the case of asymmetric osteotomy or cantilever maneuvers, sagittal translation sometimes occurs, which can lead to catastrophic dural impact. Therefore, the center of the lamina should be enlarged to check the thecal sac and nerve roots to ensure that nothing hits them (Figs. 7.3 and 7.4).

Regarding the potential risks of PSO, it requires resecting and removing the multiple elements circumferentially around the neural structures and thus creates potential risk of neurological injuries and temporary instability. In addition, due to the limitations of the technical principle, when the same angle needs to be corrected, anterior column fixation will inevitably require greater posterior column shortening, which will increase the risk of nerve injury.

8 Vertebral Column Decancellation

We named the vertebral column decancellation (VCD) osteotomy technique as a modified VCR for the first time in a series of 13 patients with severe adult congenital kyphosis [18]. This technique is used to integrate the multiple advantages of eggshell technology, SPO, PSO, and VCR [19].

VCD technology is based on the following understandings: (1) Rational treatment of sagittal spinal deformity can be achieved by anterior extension, posterior shortening, or a combination of the two. In theory, the more the hinge position is pulled back, the shorter the shortening is required for the spinal cord, and the safer the correction. (2) In order to reduce the complications of spinal cord or other neural structure shortening, the middle column of the osteotomized vertebra must be removed as little as possible. (3) The rearrangement process of the spinal sagittal profile is also the decompression process of the spinal cord. Spinal shortening during the correction process may lead to the backward movement of the spinal cord, so it is necessary to remove enough posterior elements to adapt to the spinal cord and avoid new compression. (4) Limited and precise selective decancellation of the deformed vertebral body may facilitate rearrangement of spinal deformity. (5) Osteoporosis of the anterior cortex of the osteotomized vertebra helps the opening and elongation of the anterior column, which reduces the shortening required for the posterior column, thereby reducing the risk of neurological deficits. (6) The residual vertebral bone can replace the metal mesh described in the VCR technique as a "bone cage"; it can bring better immediate stability and better fusion in the foreseeable future. (7) The order of operation is

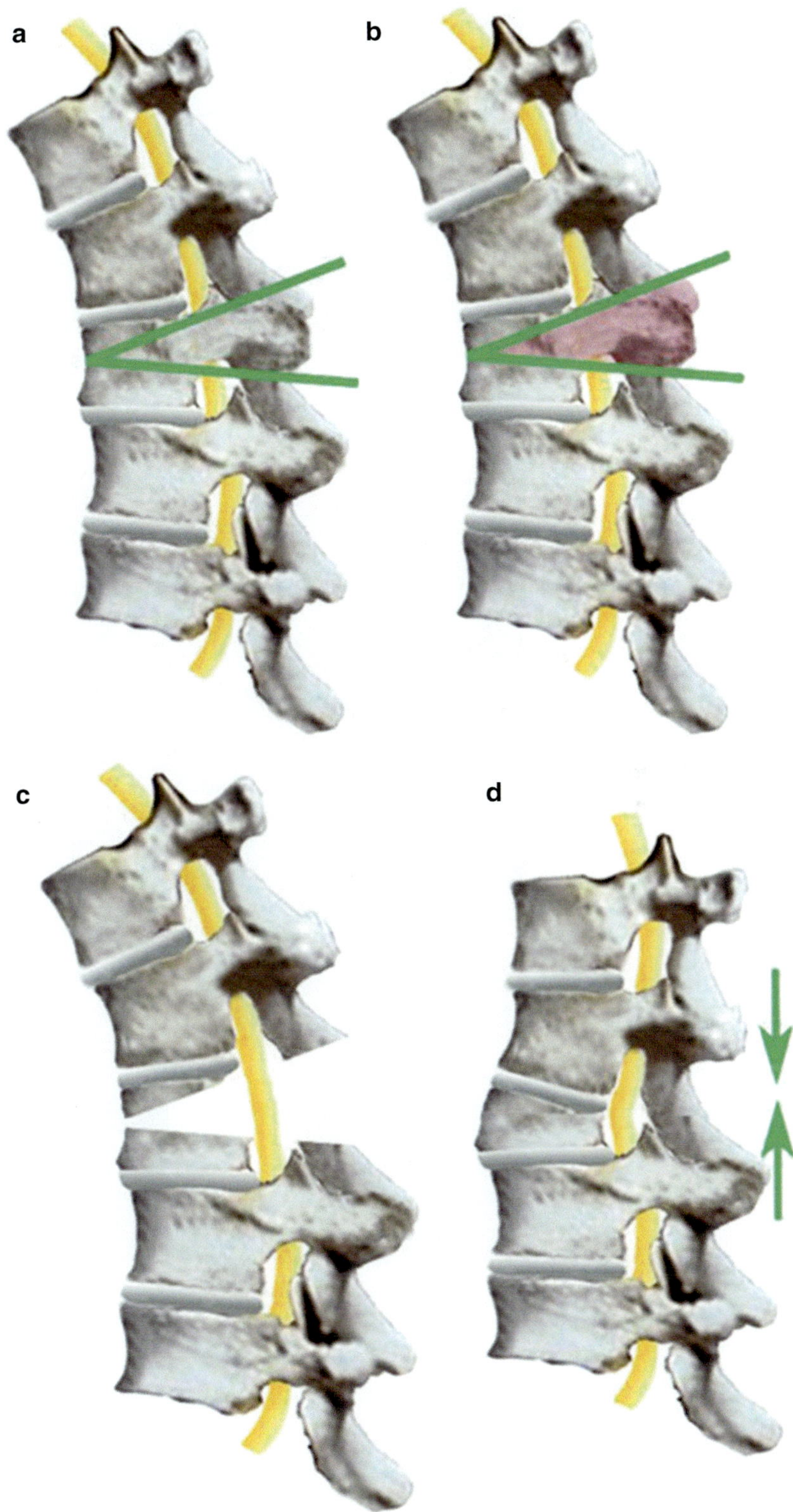

Fig. 7.3 Sketch map of PSO. (**a**–**c**) PSO includes posterior column resection and transpedicular wedge osteotomy; (**d**) hinge at the anterior cortex of the vertebral body

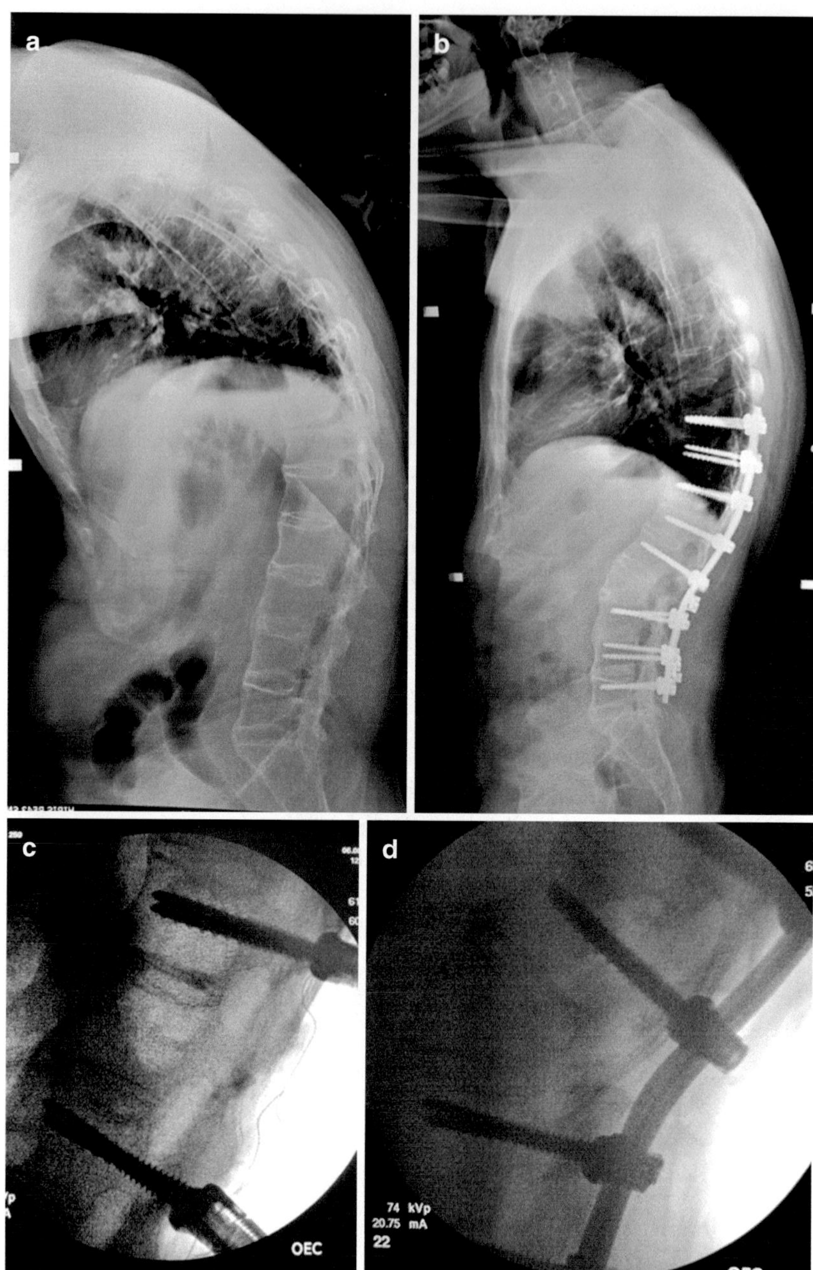

Fig. 7.4 Illustration of PSO for AS kyphosis. (**a**, **b**) Preoperative and postoperative X-ray; (**c**–**d**) intraoperative confirmation of the correction; (**e**–**f**) appearance before and after the surgery

Fig. 7.4 (continued)

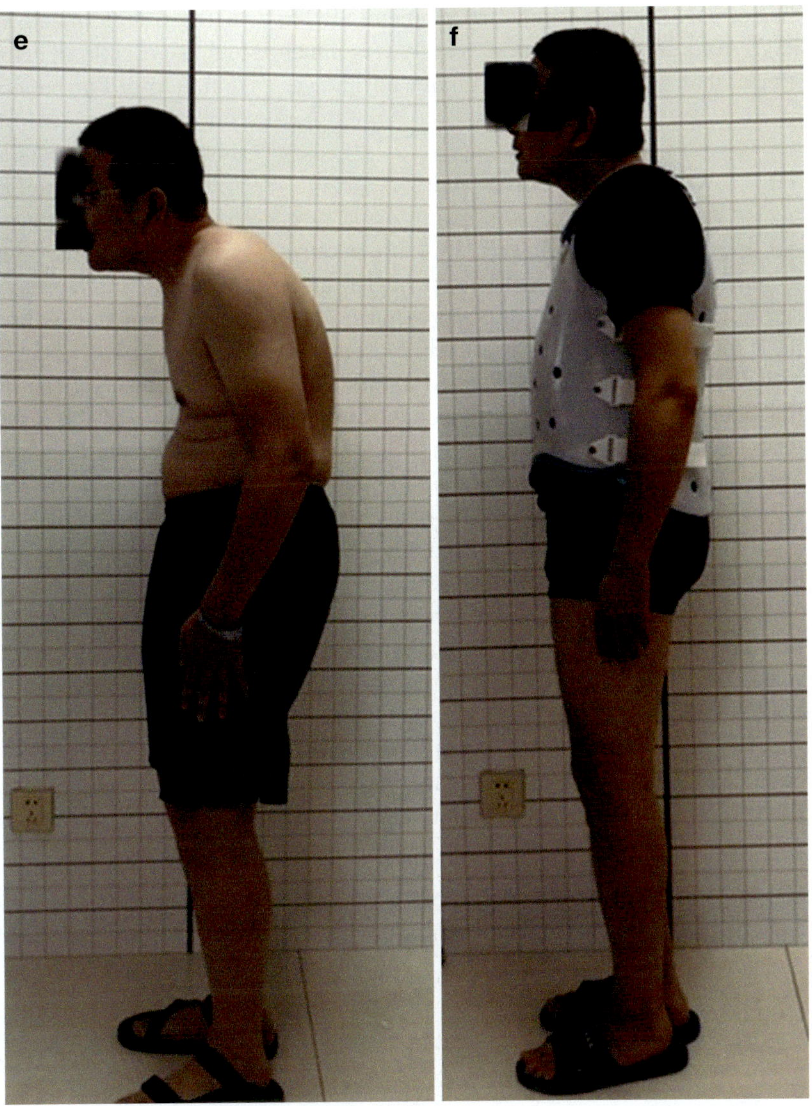

from inside to outside (eggshell technique), rather than from outside to inside, which means that in most cases, there is no need to manage segmental blood vessels, and that can reduce the occurrence of vascular complications. (8) The hinge in the PSO technique is located at the anterior longitudinal ligament of the osteotomy site. The excessive shrinkage of the osteotomy area during correction may lead to spinal cord curved or kinked or potentially damaged. VCD is a close-opening technique in which the corrective hinge is adjustable according to the need, which is consistent with previous closing-opening wedge osteotomy (COWO).

9 Indications

The indications for the first phase of VCD are restricted to severe angular spine deformities [19]. The main consideration is the balancing operation itself and the potential achievements and complication. Severe patients with long rounded smooth kyphoscoliosis also face the same conditions, and spinal osteotomy is also an option to ensure alignment intervention, because adequate recovery not only allows for better fusion but also decompression. Therefore, if the exact correction angle required for AS-related kyphosis is less than 40° and the height of the previous column is close to the normal vertebrae, then we recommend SPO or PSO. And if the correction required is much greater than 40°, VCD offers a unique advantage.

10 Operative Technique

All operations were monitored by intraoperative somatosensory evoked potential system. The anterior column of the vertebral body is normal and has a rounded angular deformity, and most decancellation manipulation is performed in one vertebral body. Vertebral column decancellation (VCD) was initiated with the probe action of the osteotomy vertebrae. The pedicle hole is then enlarged with a high-speed drill bit or a "V"-shaped spacer until the corresponding wall becomes soft and easily collapses under a lateral pressure.

The middle column cancellous bone is pressed into a "V"-shaped bony defect cavity with special spacer, and then the anterior column cancellous bone is removed in a line gap with a small curette. In VCD, the entire osteotomy gap before orthopedic surgery is Y-shape rather than V-shape in PSO (Fig. 7.5). The anterior and middle column of the osteotomized vertebrae was removed as less as possible to decrease the shortening of the spinal cord. For patients with sagittal combined coronal plane deformity, asymmetric VCD should be recommended.

After the vertebral bodies were decancellated, the posterior column structures such as spinous processes, laminae, facet joints, and transverse processes are resected. Two prebending spinal rods were fixed with cranial and caudal pedicle screws, respectively. Then, the upper, middle, and lower walls of the pedicle are clamped and removed, and the posterior wall of the vertebral body is pushed forward into the osteotomy gap. Intraoperative application of two clamps grasping the spinal rod, one clamp fixed at the cranial of the osteotomy site, another clamp fixed at the caudal of the osteotomy site, and fracturing the anterior cortex of the osteotomy vertebral body through forceful strength, then extending the lumbar anterior column and closing posterior column wedge osteotomy gap, and to disrupt the anterior longitudinal ligament, and then, an anterior monosegmental opening wedge created by the stretch of the anterior column in the end (Fig. 7.6).

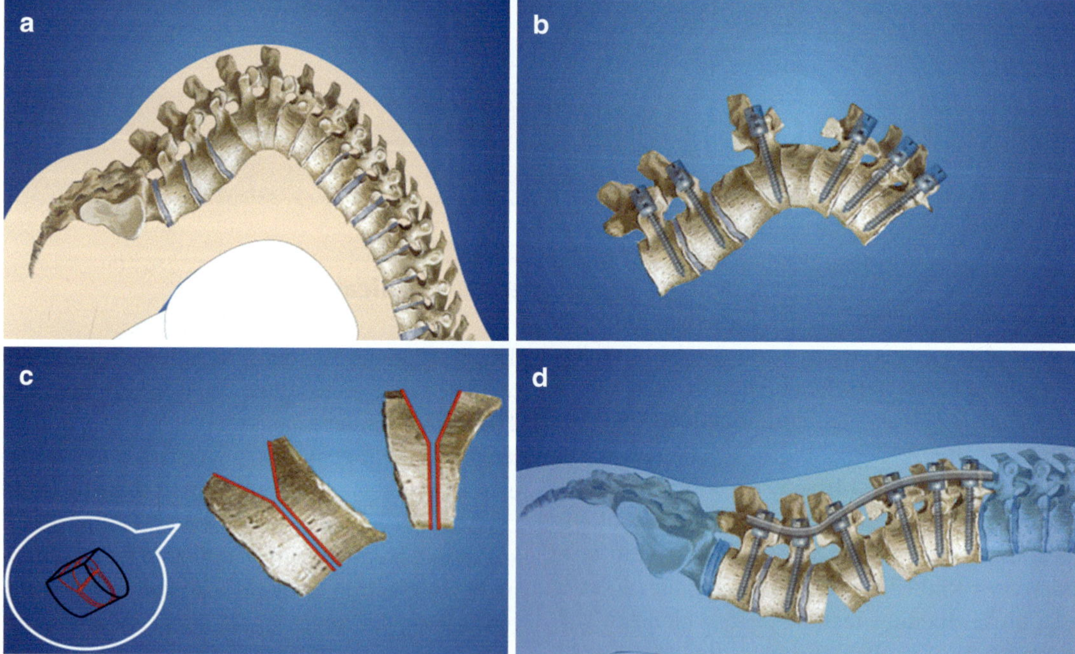

Fig. 7.5 Sketch map of VCD. (**a**) AS deformity is a typical round angular spine deformity; (**b**) pedicle screws were inserted before the osteotomy was performed; (**c**) decancellation of the osteotomized vertebrae into a Y-shape rather than V-shape using the high-speed drill and curette; (**d**) postoperative lateral view shows that correction is achieved by elongating or opening the anterior column and shortening the posterior column

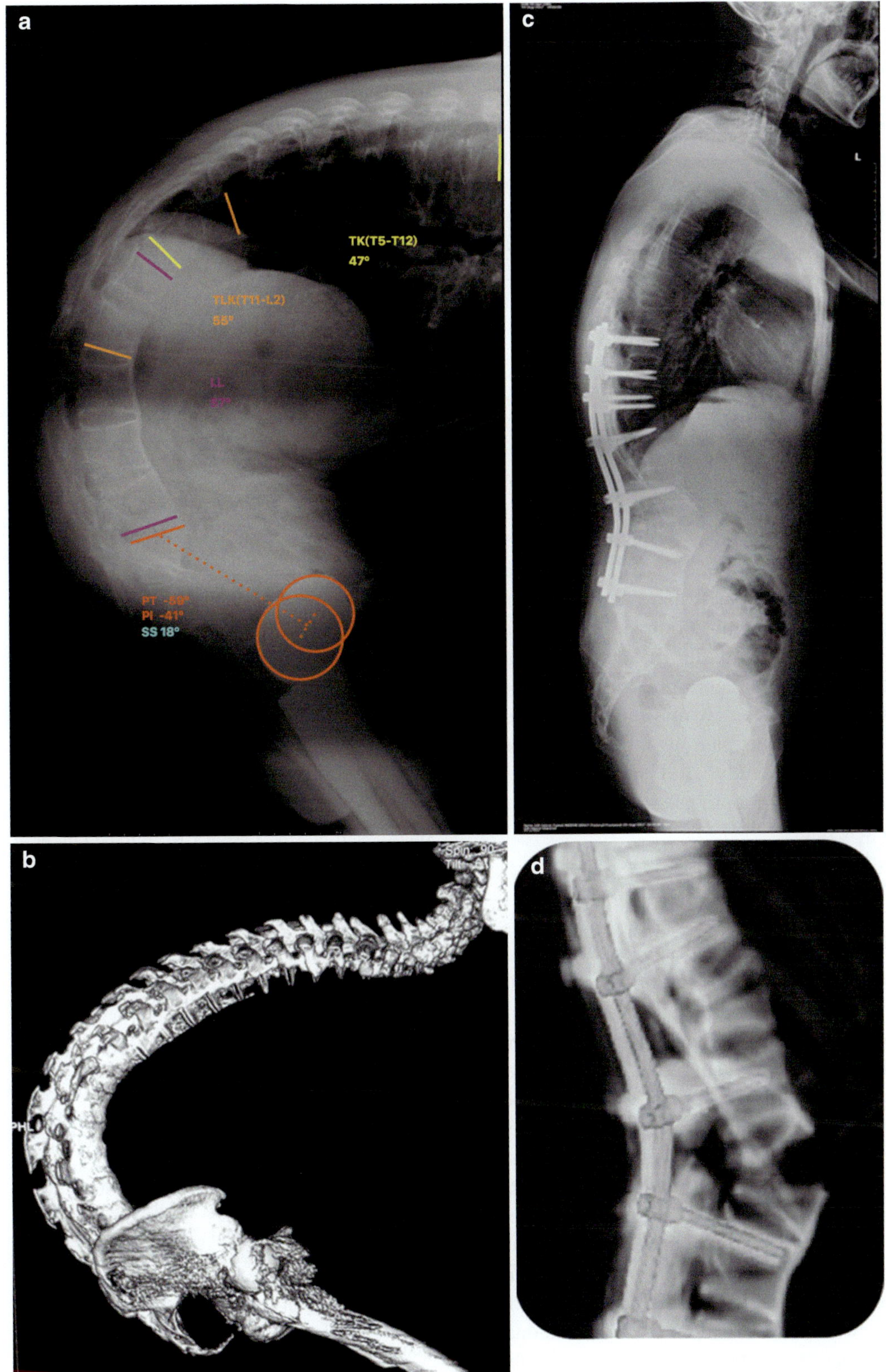

Fig. 7.6 Illustration of a two-level VCD for severe AS kyphosis. (**a**, **b**) Preoperative X-ray and CT three-dimensional reconstruction; (**c**, **d**) postoperative X-ray and CT scan showed that the osteotomy gap was opened in the "Y"-shape with total correction of 105°

The corrective hinge was located at the anterior column when the middle column was closed and located at the middle column when the anterior column was elongated. After confirming the free of the exiting nerve roots and the intraoperative fluoroscopy confirmed that the degree of correction was consistent with the preoperative design, the pedicle screw was locked and fixed. Hemostatic agents, such as gelatin sponge or liquid gelatin, can reduce bleeding in the vertebral body and spinal canal and help to control blood loss.

11 Postoperative Management

Closed suction drains were inserted at the surgical sites in all patients. All drains of the patients who underwent VCD were extubated after the output decreased to <50 ml/24 h, which was usually 3–5 days after surgery. Patients were allowed to ambulate with a thoracolumbosacral orthosis within 48–72 h after the drain tube was pulled out. The thoracolumbosacral orthosis was worn thereafter with ambulation for 3 months. All patients were evaluated by X-ray before and immediately after surgery, on the 3rd, 6th, and 12th month postoperatively, and then once a year.

12 Conclusion

Vertebral column decancellation (VCD) technology is a combination of multiple spinal surgery techniques and is a technically demanding method. In experienced surgeons, the incidence of complications of this procedure is acceptable compared to other similar procedures. Compared with PSO, the VCD osteotomy gap is more like a Y-shape than a V-shape. The elongation of the anterior column reduces the shortening required of the posterior column, reduces the risks of new compressions such as dura bulking, and improves the corrective capacity as well. VCD is a selective local excision, and the residual bone replaces the metal mesh described in the VCR technique and acts as a "bone cage," which may bring better immediate stability and better fusion in the future.

References

1. Bridwell KH. Decision making regarding Smith-Petersen vs. pedicle subtraction osteotomy vs. vertebral column resection for spinal deformity. Spine. 2006;31:S171–8.
2. Simmons EH. Kyphotic deformity of the spine in ankylosing spondylitis. Clin Orthop. 1977;128:65–77.
3. Gerscovich EO, Greenspan A, Montesano PX. Treatment of kyphotic deformity in ankylosing spondylitis. Orthopedics. 1994;17:335–42.
4. McMaster MJ. A technique for lumbar spinal osteotomy in ankylosing spondylitis. J Bone Joint Surg Br. 1985;67:204–10.
5. Hehne HJ, Zielke K, Bohm H. Polysegmental lumbar osteotomies and transpedicled fixation for correction of long-curved kyphotic deformity in ankylosing spondylitis: report on 177 cases. Clin Orthop. 1990;258:49–55.
6. Bridwell K, Lewis S, Rinella A, et al. Pedicle subtraction osteotomy for the treatment of fixed sagittal imbalance. Surgical technique. J Bone Joint Surg Am. 2004;86:44–9.
7. Thiranont N, Netrawichien P. Transpedicular decancellation closed wedge vertebral osteotomy for treatment of fixed flexion deformity of spine in ankylosing spondylitis. Spine. 1993;18:2517–22.
8. Smith-Petersen MN, Larson CB, Aufranc OE, et al. Osteotomy of the spine for correction of flexion deformity in rheumatoid arthritis. J Bone Joint Surg Am. 1945;27:1–11.
9. Chen IH, Chien JT, Yu TC. Transpedicular wedge osteotomy for correction of thoracolumbar kyphosis in ankylosing spondylitis: experience with 78 patients. Spine (Phila Pa 1976). 2001;26:E354–60.
10. Styblo K, Bossers GT, Slot GH. Osteotomy for kyphosis in ankylosing spondylitis. Acta Orthop Scand. 1985;4:294–7.
11. Zheng G-Q, Song K, Zhang Y-G, Wang Y, Huang P, Zhang X-S, et al. Two-level spinal osteotomy for severe thoracolumbar kyphosis in ankylosing spondylitis; Wang Y, Lenke LG. Vertebral column decancellation for the management of sharp angular spinal deformity. Eur Spine J. 2011;20:1703–10.
12. Liu H, Yang C, Zheng Z, Ding W, Wang J, Wang H, et al. Comparison of Smith-Petersen osteotomy and pedicle subtraction osteotomy for the correction of thoracolumbar kyphotic deformity in ankylosing spondylitis. Spine. 2015;40:570–9.

13. Kawaharu H, Tomita K. Influence of acute shortening on the spinal cord: an experimental study. Spine. 2005;30:613–20.
14. Lehmer SM, Keppler L, Buscup RS, et al. Posterior transvertebral osteotomy for adult thoracolumbar kyphosis. Spine. 1994;19:2060–7.
15. Gertzbein SD, Harris MB. Wedge osteotomy for the correction of posttraumatic kyphosis. Spine. 1992;17:374–9.
16. von Royen BJ, Slot GM. Closing-wedge posterior osteotomy for ankylosing spondylitis. J Bone Joint Surg Br. 1995;77:117–21.
17. Boachie-Adjei O, Ferguson JI, Pigeon RG, et al. Transpedicular lumbar wedge resection osteotomy for fixed sagittal imbalance: surgical technique and farly results. Spine. 2006;31:485–92.
18. Wang Y, Zhang Y, Zhang X, et al. A single posterior approach for multilevel modified vertebral column resection in adults with severe rigid congenital kyphoscoliosis: a retrospective study of 13 cases. Eur Spine J. 2008;17(3):361–72.
19. Wang Y, Lenke LG. Vertebral column decancellation for the management of sharp angular spinal deformity. Eur Spine J. 2011;20(10):1703–10.

8 Vertebral Column Decancellation Technique for Thoracolumbar Kyphosis in Ankylosing Spondylitis

Yan Wang, Xuesong Zhang, Yonggang Zhang, Zheng Wang, Guoquan Zheng, and Zhifa Zhang

1 Thoracolumbar Kyphosis in Ankylosing Spondylitis

Ankylosing spondylitis (AS) is a chronic inflammatory disease, primarily involving the sacroiliac joints and spinal column from caudal to cranial.

Kyphosis in ankylosing spondylitis may affect the cervical and thoracolumbar spine.

According to the classification of kyphotic deformity of AS in Table 8.1, kyphotic deformity was divided into four types according to the location of apex of kyphosis: lumbar (type I), thoracolumbar (type II), thoracic (type III), and cervical or cervicothoracic junction (type IV) [1]. This chapter only discusses kyphosis affecting thoracolumbar spine (type II). Thoracolumbar kyphosis is the most common deformity of AS, which is classified as type II kyphosis according to classification of AS kyphosis based on the database of our institution [2, 3].

Table 8.1 The classification of kyphotic deformity of AS

Type	Description
Type I	Lumbar kyphosis
Type II	Thoracolumbar hyper-kyphosis
	A. With relative normal lumbar lordosis – Thoracolumbar kyphosis (20–35°) + Thoracolumbar kyphosis >35°
	B. With lumbar kyphosis – Thoracolumbar kyphosis (20–35°) + Thoracolumbar kyphosis >35°
Type III	Thoracic hyper-kyphosis
	A. With relative normal lumbar lordosis – Thoracic kyphosis (50–65°) + Thoracic kyphosis >65°
	B. With lumbar kyphosis – Thoracic kyphosis (50–65°) + Thoracic kyphosis >65°
Type IV	Cervical or cervicothoracic kyphosis

2 Several Spinal Osteotomy Techniques

Several spinal osteotomy techniques are available for treating AS spinal deformities, including Smith-Petersen osteotomy (SPO) and pedicle subtraction osteotomy (PSO) [4]. SPO was originally described in 1969 by Smith-Peterson for the treatment of ankylosing spondylitis [5]. Classical SPO involves resection of posterior elements including the bilateral facet joints and the lamina and removal of the posterior ligaments at the osteotomy level. In the correction of mechanism, SPO is opening wedge osteotomy (OWO), which is closed with the hinge at the posterior aspect of the disc space by manual extension with the widening of the anterior disc space and disruption of the anterior longitudinal ligament. Performing multiple SPO to achieve the desired correction angle requires a mobile anterior column, which may not be applied to entirely fused and severe AS kyphosis [6, 7].

Y. Wang (✉) · X. Zhang · Y. Zhang
Z. Wang · G. Zheng · Z. Zhang
Chinese PLA General Hospital, Beijing, China

Y. Wang (ed.), *Surgical Treatment of Ankylosing Spondylitis Deformity*,
https://doi.org/10.1007/978-981-13-6427-3_8

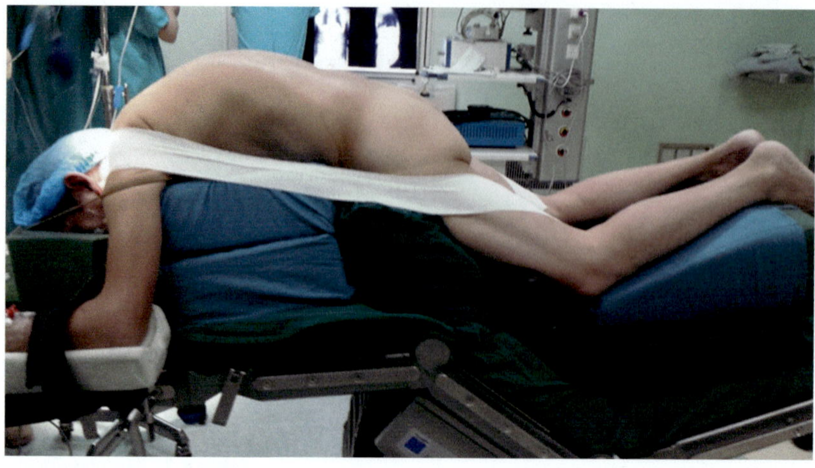

Fig. 8.1 After anesthesia by intubation with fiber-optic laryngoscopes, the patient was in a prone position on the operation table with the sponge pads under the abdomen fitting the fold body

PSO is a posterior-based three-column osteotomy performed for a fixed sagittal or coronal deformity [8]. It is characterized with the hinge located at anterior column of vertebral body by the resection of posterior column and transpedicle wedging osteotomy [9]. Considering the correction of mechanism, PSO belongs to closing wedging osteotomy (CWO) which is described as shortened posterior and middle column without opening of the anterior column. PSO is confirmed and accepted as the effective treatment for spine deformity [10].

As the most powerful osteotomy for correction of spinal deformity, VCR is generally reserved for severe fixed sagittal and coronal imbalance for substantial neurologic risks and complications. And due to its technical difficulty and potential for complications, Suk et al. called this procedure a "formidable last resort technique for the most tenacious spinal deformities" [11, 12].

3 Vertebral Column Decancellation

Vertebral column decancellation (VCD), a new spinal osteotomy, is firstly introduced in series studies for 13 adult patients with severe rigid congenital kyphoscoliosis and nine patients with severe Pott's kyphosis [13, 14]. The technique of VCD is conceived and designed on the basis of combination of advantages of eggshell technique, SPO, PSO, and VCR [2, 14–16]. VCD osteotomy technique is characterized by the programmed management, repeatable operation, and effective and safe correction for the treatment of AS kyphosis. Considering the opening of the anterior part and bilateral part of the osteotomy vertebrae, VCD is an entire three-column osteotomy compared with PSO [8, 17, 18]. This chapter is to introduce and report VCD technique as a new, effective, and safe option for correction of AS patients with rigid thoracolumbar kyphosis.

4 Surgical Technique of VCD

4.1 Preparation Before Osteotomy

All surgeries were monitored by intraoperative somatosensory-evoked potential (SEP) and motor-evoked potential (MEP) system. A special operation position is carefully designed for every patient before surgery according to kyphotic degree, which will be particularly described in relevant chapter (Fig. 8.1). C-arm fluoroscopy was used to confirm the correction angle of the osteotomy segment as planned (Fig. 8.2). Ultrasonic bone scalpel is an important tool and is fully applied in the whole process of osteotomy [19–21] (Fig. 8.3). A standard skin incision was made in the midline, and the spine was exposed by dissection lateral to the

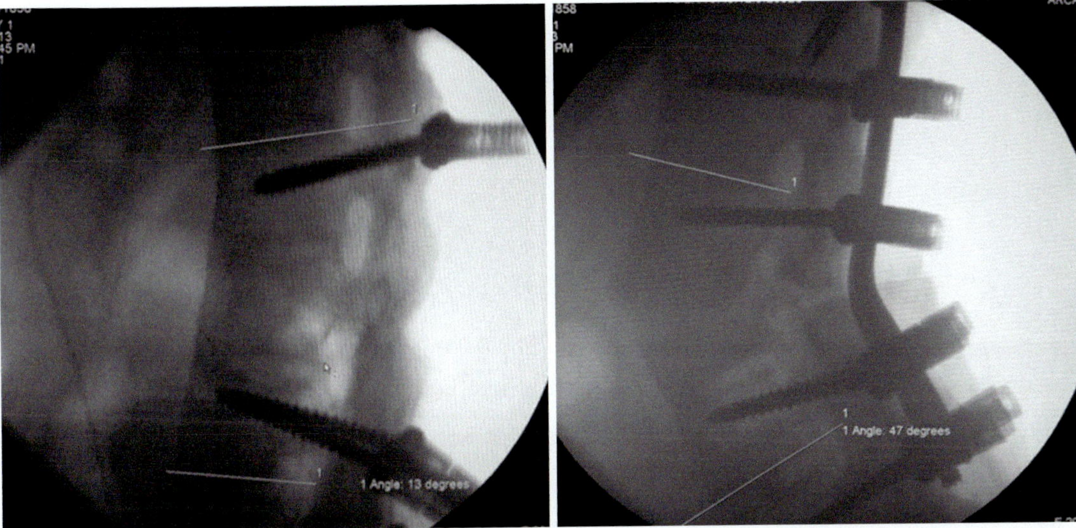

Fig. 8.2 The adequate correction angle of the osteotomy segment was obtained under control of instrument rod by cantilever during the monitoring of C-arm as planned

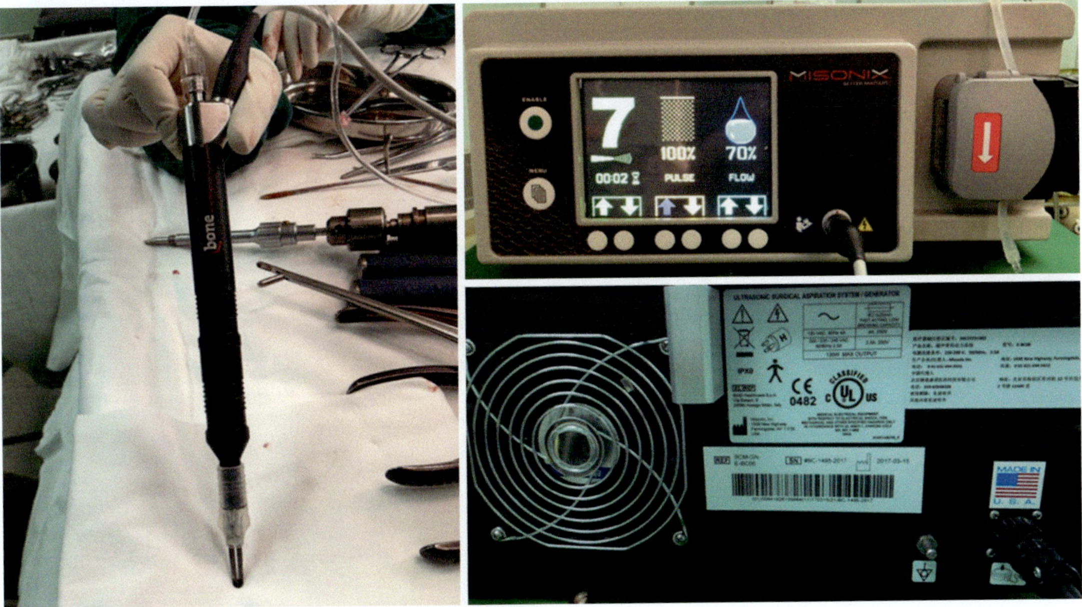

Fig. 8.3 Ultrasonic surgical bone scalpel and generator system

costotransverse joint at the thoracic level and the lumbar transverse process. Pedicle screws were usually placed extending three levels above and three levels below the osteotomy site. Bleeding was controlled by electric cauterization and hemostatic gauze. Then the posterior spinous processes of corresponding osteotomy zone were removed.

4.2 Remove Posterior Elements of the Osteotomy Vertebrae Via Ultrasonic Bone Scalpel

- *Step 1*
- Transverse processes were clearly visualized and resected by ultrasonic bone scalpel (Fig. 8.4a).

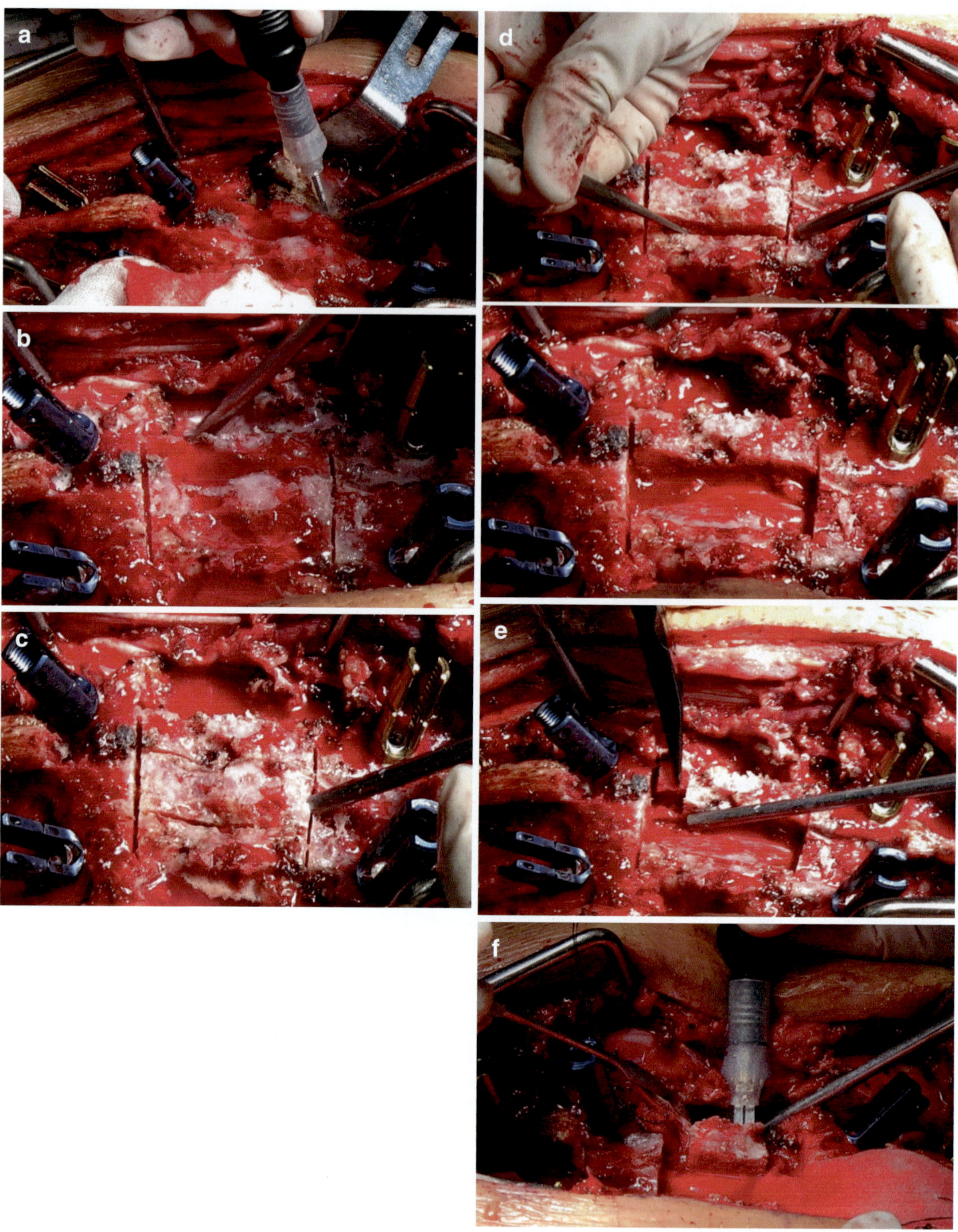

Fig. 8.4 (**a**) Transverse processes were clearly visualized and resected by ultrasonic bone scalpel. (**b**) Transverse incision was performed through the lamina in the below the above pedicles and above the below pedicles. (**c**) Longitudinal incision was performed inside the pedicles of the osteotomy vertebrae. (**d**) The bone resected was removed and the duras were clearly seen. (**e**) The fused facets and lamina were incised around the osteotomy vertebrae like Ponte osteotomy and pedicles were isolated. (**f**) The two pedicles of the osteotomy vertebrae were resected via ultrasonic bone scalpel

- *Step 2*
- Transverse incision was performed through the lamina in the below the above pedicles and above the below pedicles (Fig. 8.4b).
- *Step 3*
- Longitudinal incision was performed inside the pedicles of the osteotomy vertebrae. The bone resected was removed and the dura were clearly seen (Fig. 8.4c, d).
- *Step 4*
- The fused facets and lamina were incised around the osteotomy vertebrae like Ponte osteotomy, and pedicles were isolated (Fig. 8.4e).
- *Step 5*
- The two pedicles of the osteotomy vertebrae were resected via ultrasonic bone scalpel (Fig. 8.4f).

4.3 The Core of VCD: Osteotomy of Vertebral Body (Fig. 8.5)

- *Step 1*
- The sites of the pedicles (resected) in the osteotomy were dilated by the drill (Fig. 8.6a).

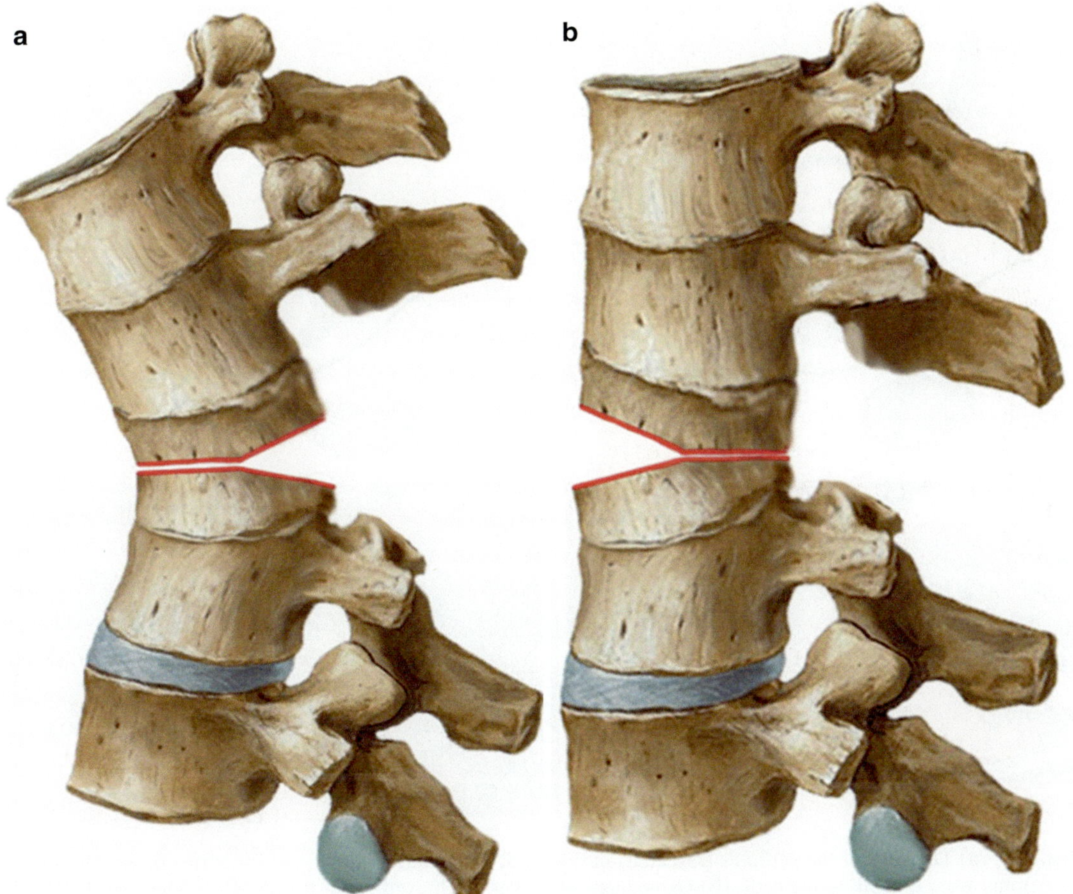

Fig. 8.5 (**a**) After corresponding spinous processes, lamina and facet joints were removed, posterior cancellous bone of the osteotomy vertebrae were removed partly by a drill or a curette through pedicles, and the posterior wall cortex of vertebral body was removed. (**b**) Linear osteoclasis of anterior cortex and lateral walls were achieved by ultrasonic bone scalpel. VCD osteotomy was well illustrated when osteoclasis of anterior and bilateral cortex and closing of posterior wedge osteotomy were completed

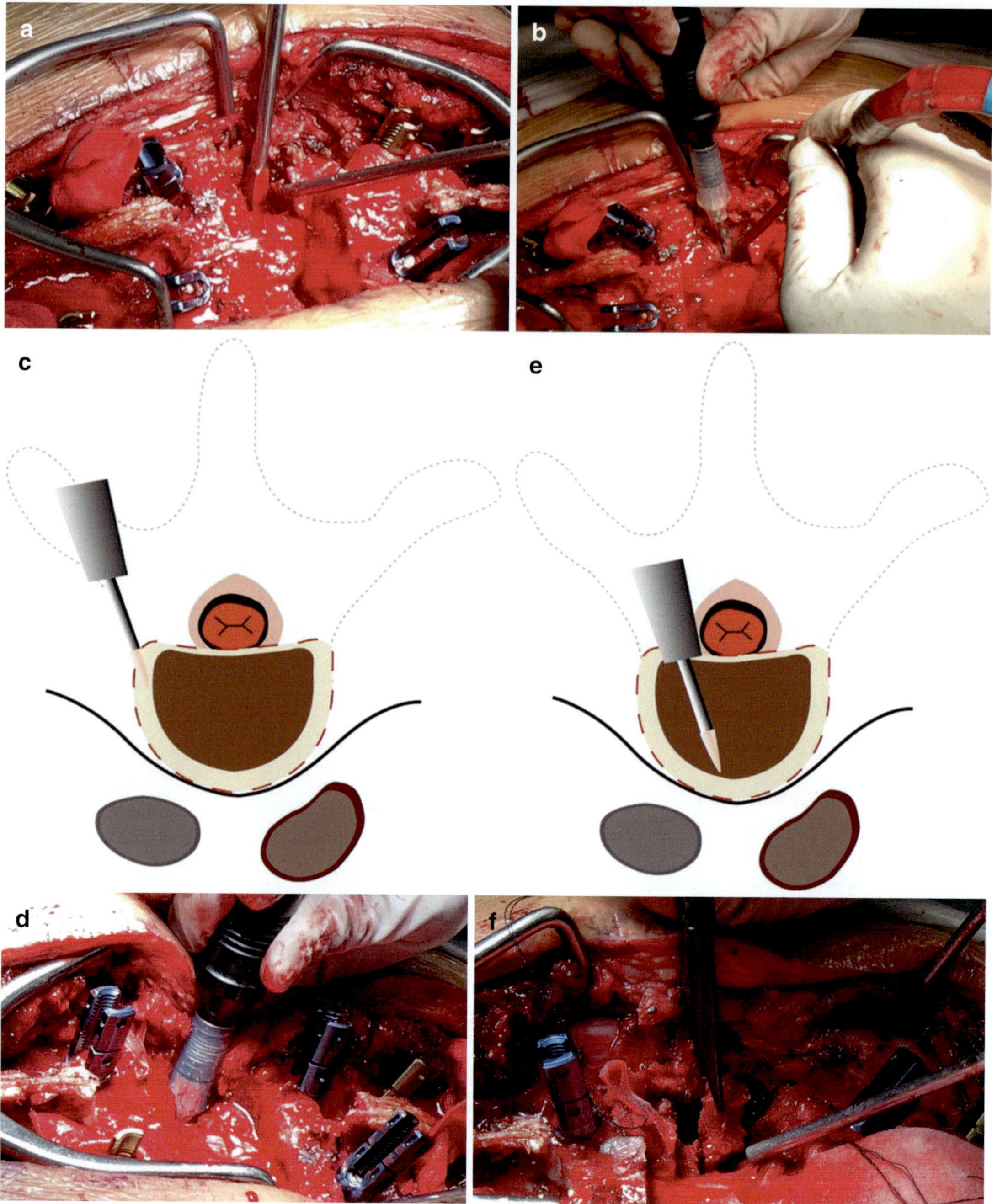

Fig. 8.6 (**a**) The sites of the pedicles (resected) in the osteotomy were dilated by the drill. (**b**) Osteoclasis of the bilateral cortex of vertebral body was achieved by via ultrasonic bone scalpel. (**c**) Illustration of osteoclasis of the bilateral cortex of vertebral body. (**d**) Osteoclasis of the anterior cortex of vertebral body was achieved via ultrasonic bone scalpel. (**e**) Illustration of osteoclasis of the anterior cortex of vertebral body. (**f**) The posterior wall cortex of the osteotomy vertebrae was removed

- *Step 2*
- Osteoclasis of the bilateral cortex of vertebral body was achieved via ultrasonic bone scalpel (Fig. 8.6b, c).

- *Step 3*
- Osteoclasis of the anterior cortex of vertebral body was achieved via ultrasonic bone scalpel (Fig. 8.6d, e).

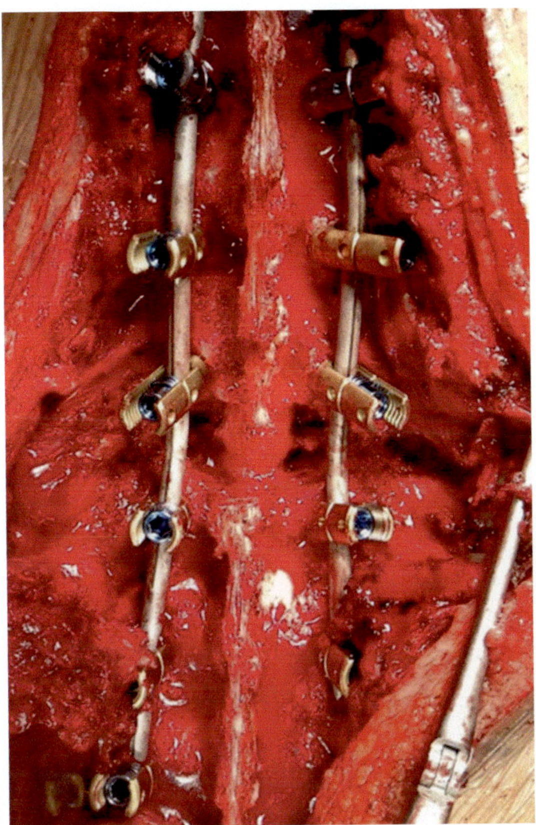

Fig. 8.7 The final internal fixation was applied after the confirmation of correction on fluoroscopy

- *Step 4*
- The posterior wall cortex of the osteotomy vertebrae was removed (Fig. 8.6f).

4.4 Restore the Sagittal Balance

A temporary stabilizing rod is needed to be attached to, at a minimum, two to three pedicle screws both above and below the resection area. Before correction of the kyphosis deformity, the angle of adjacent tails of the pedicle screw beside the osteotomy was obtained as planned. The final internal fixation was applied after the confirmation of correction on fluoroscopy (Figs. 8.2 and 8.7).

5 Discussion

5.1 Principles of VCD

Due to osteoclasis of the anterior cortex wall, an anterior mono-segmental vertebral opening wedge was created as designed and was observed in CT scan postoperative immediately (Figs. 8.9 and 8.10). Obviously, VCD is a close-open osteotomy rather than close wedge osteotomy [8] (Fig. 8.8a, b). The anterior half cancellous bone of the osteotomy column should be reserved as much as possible. The hinge of the correction was located at the posterior half of the column, which was well illustrated in Fig. 8.5a, b.

Intraoperatively, the degree of correction was adjusted by the hinge, according to the preoperative surgery planning, through opening the anterior column and closing the posterior wedge in assistance of operation table and spinal rod until the adequate degree of correction was accomplished. After the confirmation of proper correction on fluoroscopy, final internal fixation was completed (Fig. 8.2).

5.2 Key Points of VCD

The main procedures of VCD osteotomy include removal of the posterior elements, transpedicular decancellation of the posterior half cancellous bone of the osteotomy vertebral column, osteoclasis of anterior column and bilateral cortex, and the correction by the hinge or leverage.

The key points of VCD technique are (1) preserving as much as possible the posterior half of the osteotomy column as the hinge, which also serves as "leverage" or "bony cage" [22], (2) a Y-type osteotomy rather than V-type osteotomy properly makes the reasonable shortage of posterior column, (3) and appropriate opening of anterior column, for adequate correction of rigid deformity in AS patients, is of great importance and essential [23] (Fig. 8.5).

For AS patients with thoracolumbar sagittal kyphotic deformities, considering muscles around the pelvic, hip, and knee joints consistently contracting to maintain the erect position, surgery planning for adequate correction degree should be prepared for every case to achieve an optimal sagittal balance [24, 25].

VCD osteotomy is a unique technique, which is entirely three-column osteotomy in terms of removal of posterior elements and opening of the middle column and anterior column, compared with SPO and PSO [2].

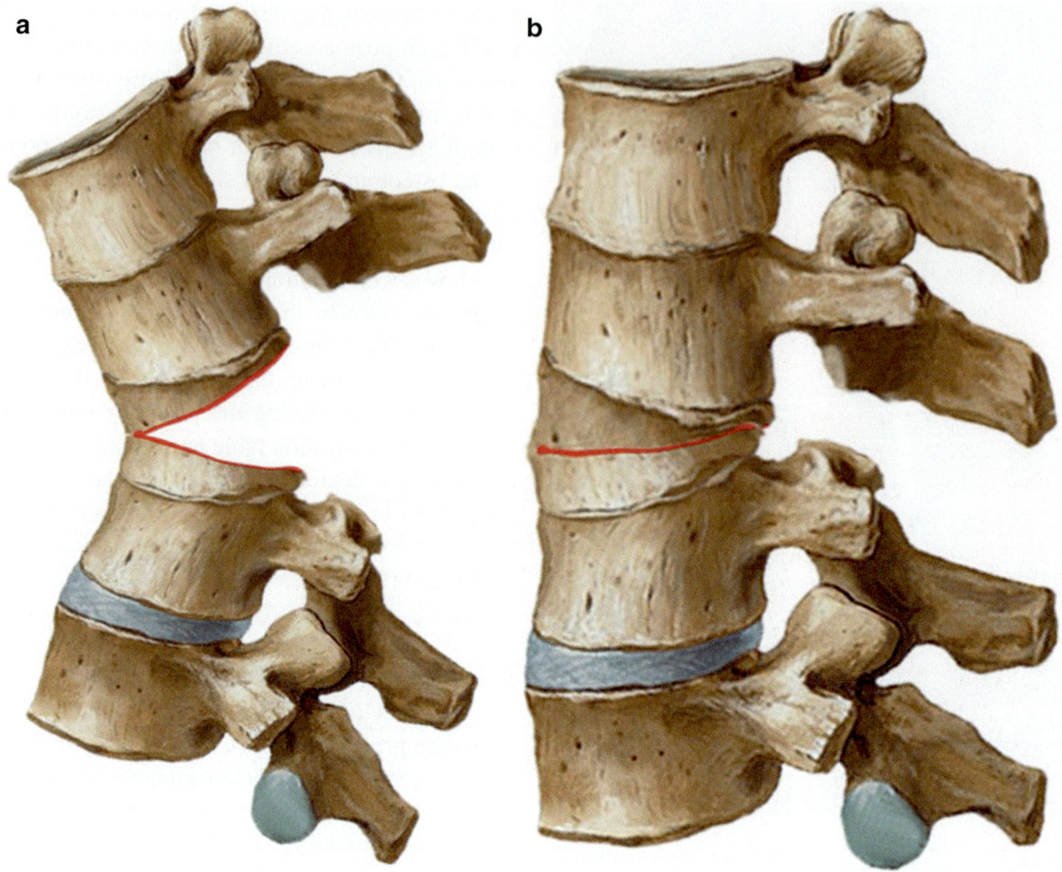

Fig. 8.8 (**a**) The classic PSO osteotomy mechanism, V-shaped osteotomy. (**b**) The completion status of PSO osteotomy

5.3 Correction Mechanism of VCD

In the correction mechanism, SPO is characterized by opening wedge osteotomy (OWO) through a mobile disc space opened, and PSO is described as closing wedge osteotomy (CWO) with the hinge located at an anterior cortex of vertebral body (Fig. 8.5) [10, 26, 27].

VCD is a new spinal osteotomy which preserves the middle column as the hinge, thus achieving the satisfying correction angle by reasonable anterior opening and rational posterior closing and avoiding the occurrence of sagittal translation. This obvious difference between COWO and VCD is well illustrated in Fig. 8.5a, b [15, 18, 28].

5.4 The Advantages of VCD

The advantages of VCD were assessed and recognized as follows: (1) lengthening the anterior column and shortening the posterior column can be achieved both by VCD for reasonable management of rigid thoracolumbar kyphosis [2]. (2) The osteoclasis of anterior and bilateral cortex of the osteotomy vertebrae helps to appropriately open and elongate the anterior column, which may decrease the need for shortening of the posterior column, decreasing the risk of neurological deficits. Theoretically, the more the hinge is posteriorly located, the smaller the need for shortening of the spinal cord, thus for safer correction [13]. (3) Preservation of the middle of the

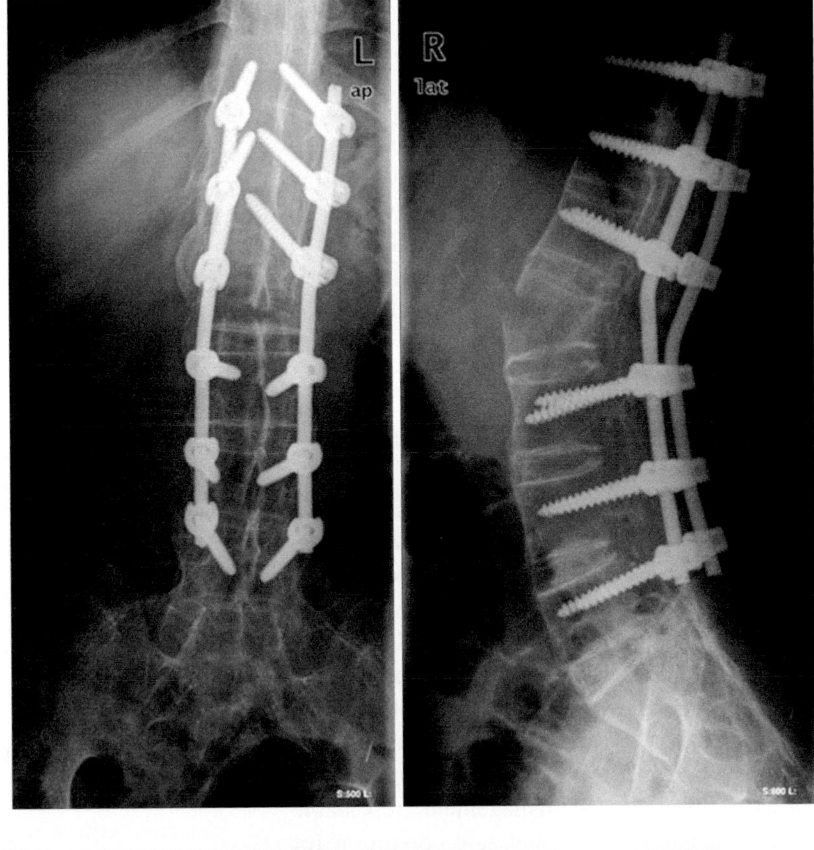

Fig. 8.9 In an ideal condition, the almost Y-shaped osteotomy could be exactly observed in the X-ray after the surgery of VCD immediately

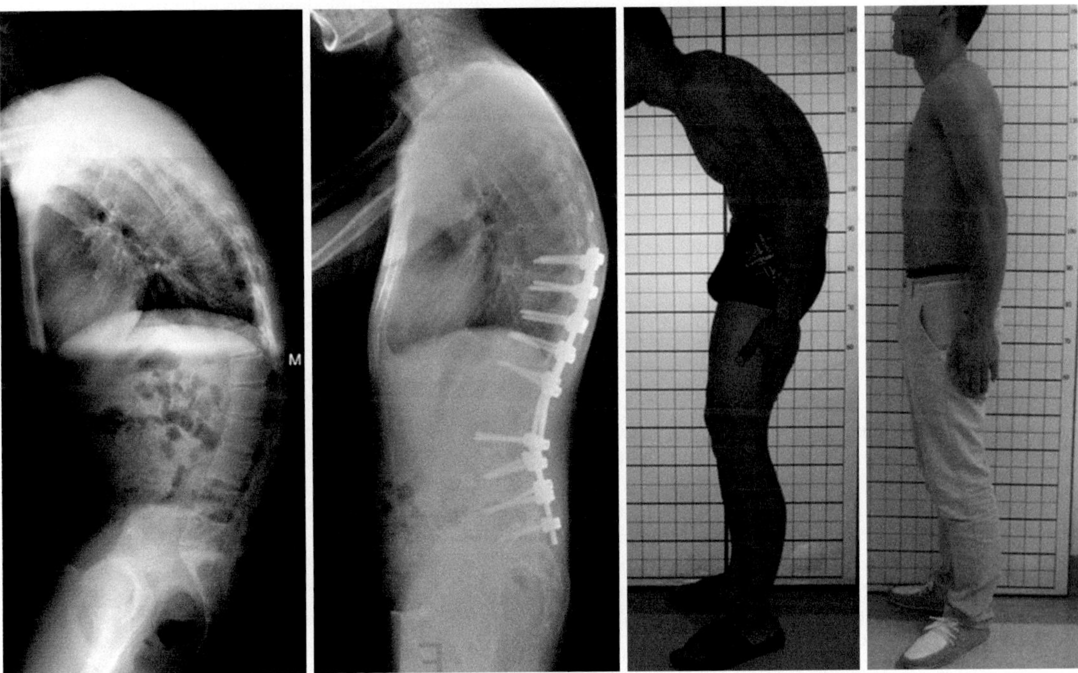

Fig. 8.10 The photograph showed a pre- and postoperative full-length spine X-ray and appearance picture of 36-year-old man with thoracolumbar kyphosis secondary to ankylosing spondylitis. After the osteotomy of VCD, the thoracolumbar kyphosis was almost corrected by about 50°. The osteotomy site was clearly observed and the sagittal balance was almost restored. In the follow-up of 2 years, no obvious sagittal translation and great correction loss was observed

osteotomy vertebrae as the hinge increases the adjustability of the correction [22]. (4) The reserved spongy bone of osteotomy vertebrae serves as a "bony cage" [1, 22, 23], which may bring better stability instantly and better fusion in the future; (5) the vertebral body osteotomy order was from inside to outside (eggshell technique) rather than from outside to inside, which means it is not necessary to expose the segmental vessels in most cases, with less vascular complication expected [16, 29].

6 Conclusions

Vertebral column decancellation (VCD) technique is a combination of several spinal surgery techniques, which is newly developed spinal three-column osteotomy. For cases with rigid sagittal thoracolumbar deformity, VCD offers a safe and reliable way to achieve good results, including realignment of the kyphotic spine, decompression of neurological elements, and then improvement in neurologic function. In terms of programmed management, repeatable operation, and effective and safe correction for the treatment of AS kyphosis, VCD can be accepted as a new, effective, and safe option for correction of AS patients with rigid thoracolumbar kyphosis.

Ethical Approval The consent for publication of this study was obtained from all the patients involved. And the study was approved by the ethical committee of PLA General Hospital.

References

1. Zhang Y, et al. The management of thoracolumbar kyphotic deformity in ankylosing spondylitis. In: Wang Y, Boachie-Adjei O, Lenke LG, editors. Spinal osteotomy. Dordrecht: Springer; 2014. p. 149–62.
2. Zhang X, Zhang Z, Wang J, et al. Vertebral column decancellation: a new spinal osteotomy technique for correcting rigid thoracolumbar kyphosis in patients with ankylosing spondylitis. Bone Joint J. 2016;98-B(5):672–8.
3. Song K, Zheng G, Zhang Y, et al. Hilus pulmonis as the center of gravity for AS thoracolumbar kyphosis. Eur Spine J. 2014;23(12):2743–50.
4. Thiranont N, Netrawichien P. Transpedicular decancellation closed wedge vertebral osteotomy for treatment of fixed flexion deformity of spine in ankylosing spondylitis. Spine (Phila Pa 1976). 1993;18(16):2517–22.
5. Smith-Petersen MN, Larson CB, Aufranc OE. Osteotomy of the spine for correction of flexion deformity in rheumatoid arthritis. Clin Orthop Relat Res. 1969;66:6–9.
6. Trent G, Armstrong GW, O'Neil J. Thoracolumbar fractures in ankylosing spondylitis. High-risk injuries. Clin Orthop Relat Res. 1988;227:61–6.
7. Van Royen BJ, De Gast A, Smit TH. Deformity planning for sagittal plane corrective osteotomies of the spine in ankylosing spondylitis. Eur Spine J. 2000;9(6):492–8.
8. Chang KW, Chen YY, Lin CC, Hsu HL, Pai KC. Closing wedge osteotomy versus opening wedge osteotomy in ankylosing spondylitis with thoracolumbar kyphotic deformity. Spine (Phila Pa 1976). 2005;30(14):1584–93.
9. Chang KW, Chen HC, Chen YY, Lin CC, Hsu HL, Cai YH. Sagittal translation in opening wedge osteotomy for the correction of thoracolumbar kyphotic deformity in ankylosing spondylitis. Spine. 2006;31(10):1137–42.
10. Kim KT, Park DH, Lee SH, Lee JH. Results of corrective osteotomy and treatment strategy for ankylosing spondylitis with kyphotic deformity. Clin Orthop Surg. 2015;7(3):330–6.
11. Suk KS, Kim KT, Lee SH, Kim JM. Significance of chin-brow vertical angle in correction of kyphotic deformity of ankylosing spondylitis patients. Spine (Phila Pa 1976). 2003;28(17):2001–5.
12. Suk SI, Chung ER, Lee SM, Lee JH, Kim SS, Kim JH. Posterior vertebral column resection in fixed lumbosacral deformity. Spine. 2005;30(23):E703–10.
13. Wang Y, Zhang Y, Zhang X, et al. A single posterior approach for multilevel modified vertebral column resection in adults with severe rigid congenital kyphoscoliosis: a retrospective study of 13 cases. Eur Spine J. 2008;17(3):361–72.
14. Wang Y, Zhang Y, Zhang X, et al. Posterior-only multilevel modified vertebral column resection for extremely severe Pott's kyphotic deformity. Eur Spine J. 2009;18(10):1436–41.
15. Lenke LG, Sides BA, Koester LA, Hensley M, Blanke KM. Vertebral column resection for the treatment of severe spinal deformity. Clin Orthop Relat Res. 2010;468(3):687–99.
16. Boachie-Adjei O. Role and technique of eggshell osteotomies and vertebral column resections in the treatment of fixed sagittal imbalance. Instr Course Lect. 2006;55:583–9.
17. Thomasen E. Vertebral osteotomy for correction of kyphosis in ankylosing spondylitis. Clin Orthop Relat Res. 1985;194:142–52.
18. Arun R, Dabke HV, Mehdian H. Comparison of three types of lumbar osteotomy for ankylosing spondylitis: a case series and evolution of a safe

technique for instrumented reduction. Eur Spine J. 2011;20(12):2252–60.

19. Nakagawa H, Kim SD, Mizuno J, Ohara Y, Ito K. Technical advantages of an ultrasonic bone curette in spinal surgery. J Neurosurg Spine. 2005;2(4):431–5.
20. Nakase H, Matsuda R, Shin Y, Park YS, Sakaki T. The use of ultrasonic bone curettes in spinal surgery. Acta Neurochir. 2006;148(2):207–12; discussion 12–3.
21. Kim K, Isu T, Matsumoto R, Isobe M, Kogure K. Surgical pitfalls of an ultrasonic bone curette (SONOPET) in spinal surgery. Neurosurgery. 2006;59(4 Suppl 2):ONS390–3; discussion ONS3.
22. Wang Y, et al. History of spine osteotomy. In: Wang Y, Boachie-Adjei O, Lenke LG, editors. Spinal osteotomy. Dordrecht: Springer; 2014. p. 1–10.
23. Wang Y, et al. Posterior vertebral column decancellation (VCD) for severe rigid spinal deformities. In: Wang Y, Boachie-Adjei O, Lenke LG, editors. Spinal Osteotomy. Dordrecht: Springer; 2014. p. 1–10.
24. Zhao Y, Wang Y, Wang Z, Zhang X, Mao K, Zhang Y. Effect and strategy of 1-stage interrupted 2-level transpedicular wedge osteotomy for correcting severe kyphotic deformities in ankylosing spondylitis. Clin Spine Surg. 2017;30(4):E454–e9.
25. Yao Z, Zheng G, Zhang Y, et al. Selection of lowest instrumented vertebra for thoracolumbar kyphosis in ankylosing spondylitis. Spine (Phila Pa 1976). 2016;41(7):591–7.
26. Zhang G, Fu J, Zhang Y, et al. Lung volume change after pedicle subtraction osteotomy in patients with ankylosing spondylitis with thoracolumbar kyphosis. Spine. 2015;40(4):233–7.
27. Xu H, Zhang Y, Zhao Y, Zhang X, Xiao S, Wang Y. Radiologic and clinical outcomes comparison between single- and two-level pedicle subtraction osteotomies in correcting ankylosing spondylitis kyphosis. Spine J. 2015;15(2):290–7.
28. Wang Y, Zheng G, Zhang X, Zhang Y, Xiao S, Wang Z. Temporary use of shape memory spinal rod in the treatment of scoliosis. Eur Spine J. 2011;20(1):118–22.
29. Danisa OA, Turner D, Richardson WJ. Surgical correction of lumbar kyphotic deformity: posterior reduction "eggshell" osteotomy. J Neurosurg. 2000;92(1 Suppl):50–6.

Selection of the Fusion Level in AS Kyphosis

9

Ziming Yao, Keya Mao, and Zheng Wang

Ankylosing spondylitis (AS) is a chronic inflammatory disease, generally involving the sacroiliac joints and spinal column and advancing from caudal to cranial vertebrae [1, 2]. A fixed thoracolumbar kyphosis is the most common deformity that causes difficulty standing, walking, looking horizontally, and lying flat on one's back. In severe cases, visceral compression may also cause intra-abdominal complications or impair respiratory function [3]. Surgical correction of the kyphosis is necessary for many AS kyphosis patients. Recently, pedicle subtraction osteotomy (PSO) or verteverte-bral column decancellation (VCD) has been applied to correct thoracolumbar kyphosis secondary to AS [4–7]. Selection of the upper instrumented vertebra (UIV) and lowest instrumented vertebra (LIV) determines the proximal and distal fusion level. In other patients with spinal deformity, reducing fusion level can preserve more spinal motion [8, 9]. However, in AS patients whose spine is fixed, reduction of fusion level still contributes to the operation and could be economical. We conducted studies to investigate the optimal selection of LIV and UIV relative to the osteotomied vertebra (OV) for common kyphosis caused by AS.

In the first study, we reviewed continuous AS cases surgically treated in our institution from January 2010 to May 2013. Collection and analysis of radiographic and clinical data were performed by individuals not directly involved in the patients' surgery. The inclusion criteria were as follows: (1) AS patients with thoracolumbar kyphosis who were treated by single or interrupted two-level PSO, (2) with minimum 2-year follow-up, and (3) having distal OV at L2, L3, or L4 with the LIV from L4 to S1. The exclusive criteria were as follows: (1) having a preoperative coronal curve of more than 10°, (2) with a previous spinal surgery, and (3) with pathological spinal fractures or pseudarthrosis. This study, therefore, consisted of a group of 123 patients with AS (110 males and 13 females) with a mean age of 36.1 years (range, 21–56 years). The mean follow-up was 29.3 months (range, 24–60 months).

We checked and calculated the relative location of OV and LIV and recorded the time used for implanting per pedicle screw at each vertebra, with the averaged time of right and left screw taken as the final result. All the included patients were divided into three groups based on the relative position of LIV and distal OV. Group OV+2 (n = 68) had LIV at the second vertebra below OV, Group OV+3 (n = 53) had LIV at the third vertebra below OV, and Group OV+4 (n = 2) had LIV at the fourth vertebra below OV. Since there were only two patients in Group OV+4, the former two groups were compared for preoperative and 2-year postoperative radiographic parameters and clinical data.

Z. Yao
Beijing Children's Hospital, Capital Medical University, National Center for Children's Health, Beijing, China

K. Mao · Z. Wang (✉)
Chinese PLA General Hospital, Beijing, China

Y. Wang (ed.), *Surgical Treatment of Ankylosing Spondylitis Deformity*,
https://doi.org/10.1007/978-981-13-6427-3_9

Additionally, according to whether LIV was S1, all patients were divided into Group S1 (n = 18) and Group Non-S1 (the LIV was L5 or above, n = 105). Preoperative and 2-year postoperative radiographic and clinical data of these two groups were compared again.

The radiographic data include global kyphosis (GK, the angle between the superior endplate of the maximally tilted upper end vertebra and the inferior endplate of the maximally tilted lower end vertebra), thoracolumbar kyphosis (TLK, the angle between the upper endplate of the T11 vertebra and the lower endplate of the L2 vertebra), lumbar lordosis (LL, the angle between the superior endplate of L1 and S1, positive value indicates lumbar kyphosis, and negative value indicates lumbar lordosis), and sagittal vertical axis (SVA, the distance measured between the C7 plumb line and the posterosuperior corner of S1 vertebra). All of these parameters were measured on the lateral X-ray plain of the full spine. The clinical data including age, sex, number of fused vertebra, intraoperative blood loss, operation duration, Oswestry disability index (ODI), visual analogue scale (VAS) of lumbosacral pain and incidence of pressure sores at the sacral area, proximal junctional kyphosis (PJK), and fixation failure at the last follow-up were reviewed. PJK was identified when the junctional kyphotic angle worsened more than 10° compared to the preoperative value.

Of the 123 patients, 69 underwent single-level PSO and 54 underwent two-level PSO. The single-level PSO or the lower PSO of two-level PSO was at L2 in 56 patients, L3 in 63, and L4 in the remaining 4. The LIV was L4 in 13 patients, L5 in 92, and S1 in the remaining 18.

The mean time spent to implant per screw was counted from locating the screw entrance point to finishing the screw insertion. The time of checking the screw position by C-arm was equally shared per screw. Compared with that used by implanting a screw at L1–L5, the time used by implanting a S1 screw was significantly longer.

Sixty-eight patients in Group OV+2 and 53 patients in Group OV+3 (Fig. 9.1) were equivalent with regard to the average age, sex distribution, preoperative ODI, and preoperative sagittal parameters (GK, TLK, LL, and SVA). Both groups obtained similar kyphosis and SVA corrections at the last follow-up. There was no significant difference for the improvement of ODI and incidence of PJK at the last follow-up. However, Group OV+3 had more fused vertebra than Group OV+2.

There were 18 patients in Group S1 and 105 patients in Group Non-S1. These two groups were equivalent with regard to the average age, intraoperative blood loss, and operation duration. Preoperative ODI and preoperative sagittal parameters (GK, TLK, LL, and SVA) had no significant difference in two groups. Both groups obtained similar kyphosis and SVA corrections at the last follow-up. There was no significant difference for the improvement of ODI and incidence of PJK at the last follow-up. However, Group S1 had more fused vertebra, lower ODI score, higher VAS score, and higher incidence of pressure sores at the last follow-up than Group Non-S1.

No instrumentation failure occurred by the last follow-up. No deformity progression or spinal fracture occurred at the distal junctional region by the last follow-up.

In AS patients, unlike in other patients with spinal disease, the whole spine was fused, and shorter fusion might not preserve more spinal mobility and growth potential. The main role of instrumentation is to maintain the correction after the surgery. However, minimizing the instrumented level is still beneficial to AS patients not only for the economic reason but also for surgical safety.

The distal anchor points should be chosen according to the location of the spinal osteotomy. Our study shows that two pairs of pedicle screws below the OV are enough to maintain the stability and correction. No patients with OV+2 suffered from fixation failure and deformity progression. Thus fixing three or more vertebrae below the OV is unnecessary. So, we suggest that OV+2 is an optimal LIV in AS thoracolumbar kyphosis treated by PSO. The reasons are as follows:

1. After the lordosis was reconstructed, the interface between the vertebra and pedicle is compressive and shear stressed rather than tensile stressed. Figure 9.2 shows the force component imposed on pedicle screw.

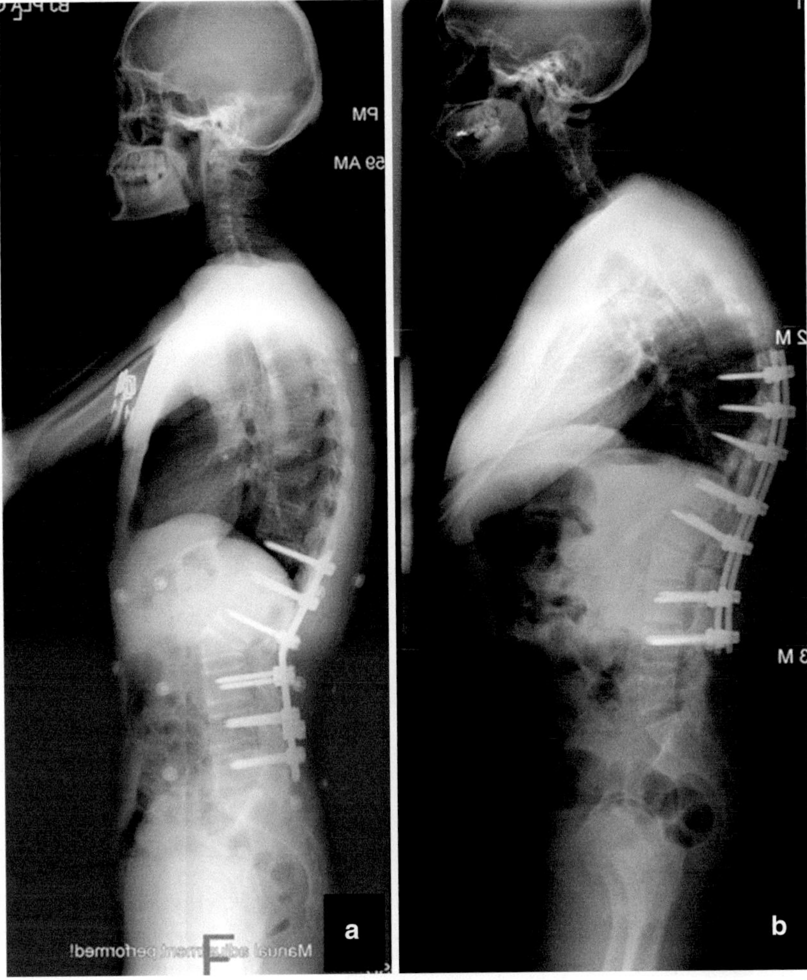

Fig. 9.1 Radiographs of two patients with distal PSO at L2. (**a**) Patient has a LIV at L5 (OV+3); (**b**) Patient has a LIV at L4 (OV+2)

2. Fusion between LIV and the vertebra below LIV is firm, and no junctional deformity or fracture happened.
3. Although the vertebra body has osteoporosis, ossification of ligament and excessive bone formation lead to a hard and thick cortex [10], which contributes to the force holding of a screw.

Our results show that the effect of correction and fusion is satisfactory whether S1 be instrumented or not. However, during the follow-up, the patients with S1 instrumentation had more pressure sores, and their lumbosacral pain was more serious. Thus, we suggest that don't take S1 as LIV in most AS thoracolumbar kyphosis treated by PSO. The reasons are as follows:

1. S1 screw was closer to the skin, which more likely leads to pressure sores, lumbosacral pain, and feeling of protrusion (Fig. 9.3).
2. Fusion between L5 and S1 is firm, and no junctional deformity or fracture happened.
3. Implanting a S1 screw takes a longer time than implanting another screw.

To our experience, it's more difficult to expose S1 entrance point and implant S1 screw because of iliac cover caused by fusion of the sacroiliac joint.

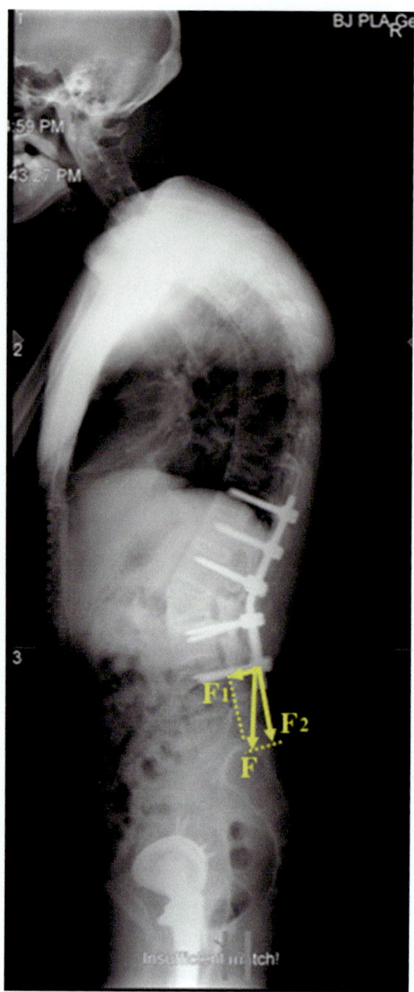

Fig. 9.2 The total force (F) suffered from the upper trunk can be divided into two parts: the compressive stress (F1, along the screw) and shear stress (F2, perpendicular to screw)

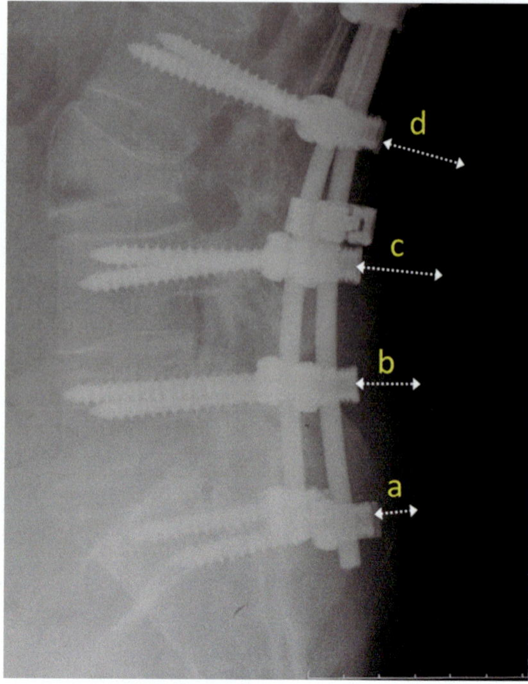

Fig. 9.3 The different distances between the skin and screw end. *a*, *b*, *c*, and *d* indicate the different distances between the screw of S1, L5, L4, and L2 and the skin

Instrumentation of S1 is necessary only in some specific conditions, such as the screw above S1 becomes loose or there is occult fracture on L4 level. Otherwise, we don't suggest to instrument S1.

Another issue is how to choose the OV, since hip axis plays the role of the hinge center of the upper trunk in a fixed spine like AS patients. Theoretically, the shorter the distance between the OV and hip joint, the larger the influence of the whole sagittal imbalance. To maximize correction and safety, von Royen recommended that the corrective osteotomy should be performed in the lower lumbar spine [11]. However, according to our study, performing a PSO at L4 needs to fix S1 (OV+2), which could bring a lot of problems to the patients. Therefore, from the perspective of instrumentation, performing a PSO at L3 or above is optimal.

In addition, thoracolumbar and lumbar regions are usually the most kyphotic regions in AS patients. We suggest choosing L2 as the osteotomy site at the thoracolumbar region and L3 as the osteotomy site at the lumbar region, considering this level is a non-cord region and the vertebral canal is relatively spacious, which is an advantage factor to prevent cord injury [3]. When the magnitude of kyphosis is severe and two-level PSO is needed, we recommend carrying out the first PSO at L3 and the second PSO at T12 or L1, according to the characteristics of the patients' deformities [12].

In brief, for the correction of thoracolumbar or lumbar kyphosis caused by AS, we recommend to take OV+2 as LIV instead of OV+3 and restrict the instrumentation of S1. That means, when L2 was the distal PSO vertebra, L4 should be chosen as the LIV; when L3 was the distal PSO vertebra, L5 should be chosen as the LIV; and L4 was not suitable to be taken as the OV [13]. And to our experience, this selection was also appropriate for patients undergoing VCD osteotomy.

To determine the optimal selection of UIV in AS thoracolumbar kyphosis, we did the second research with the same cases in the first study. We reviewed AS thoracolumbar kyphosis cases treated with PSO or VCD. According to the relationship between UIV and proximal OV, all cases were divided into Group A, UIV was the third vertebra cranial to the proximal OV, and Group B, UIV was the fourth vertebra or more cranial to the proximal OV (Fig. 9.4). The two groups were

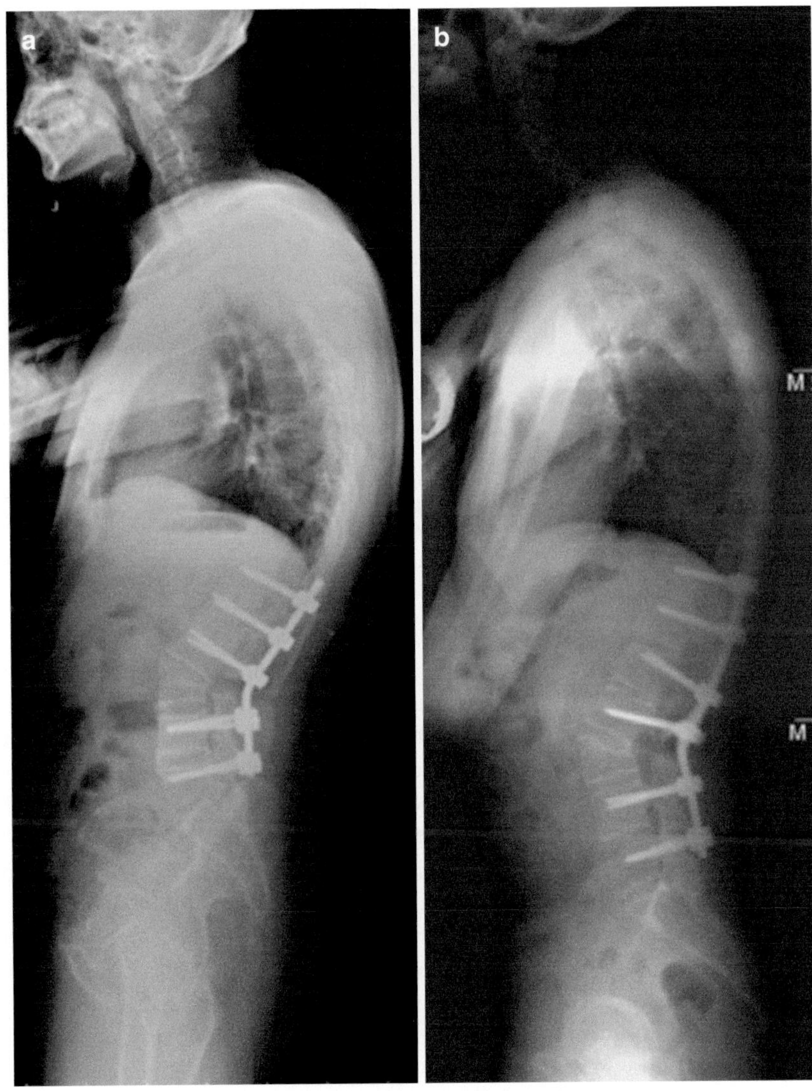

Fig. 9.4 Radiographs of two patients with a single PSO at L3. (**a**) Patient has a UIV at T12; (**b**) Patient has a UIV at T11

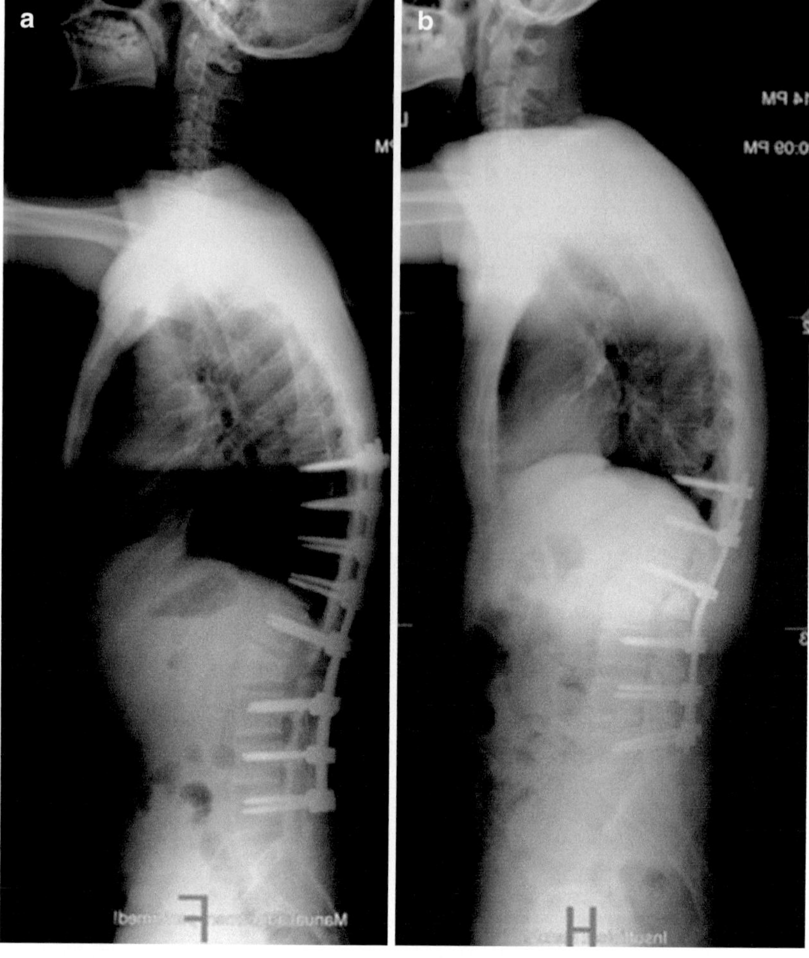

Fig. 9.5 Radiographs of two patients with a single PSO at L2. (**a**) Patient has UIV at T9 that is above apical vertebra T1; (**b**) Patient has a UIV at T11 that is below apical vertebra T10

compared for preoperative and 24-month postoperative radiographic parameters and clinical data. What's more, all the included patients were divided into groups based on the relative position of UIV and apical vertebra (AV), Group AV (the UIV was AV or above) and Group Non-AV, and the abovementioned parameters and data were compared again (Fig. 9.5). We found that during the 29.3 (24–60) months' follow-up, no fixation failure occurred in all patients. Group A and Group B had no significant differences in age and gender composition. The mean instrumented segments of Group A were less than that in Group B. Two groups had similar magnitudes of deformity corrections and functional improvement at the 24-month follow-up. The incidence of complaining about the protrudent sensation in Group A is higher than that in Group B. The incidence of complaining about the protrudent sensation in Group AV was higher than that in Group Non-AV (Fig. 9.6). Thus, we concluded that when PSO or VCD is performed to treat the AS thoracolumbar kyphosis, three vertebrae cranial to the proximal OV are enough for the correction and fixation with low incidence of complaining about the protrudent sensation. However, in patients with a pseudarthrosis, the instrumentation must get across the pseudarthrosis.

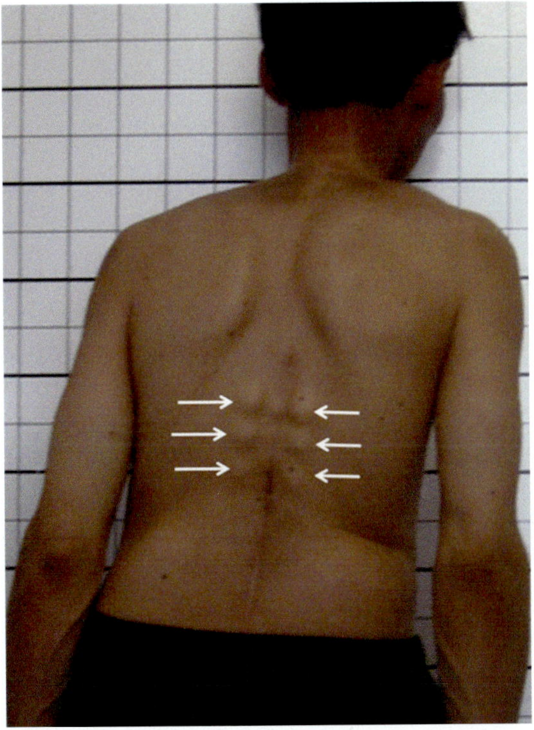

Fig. 9.6 Screw tail remained close to the skin, which resulted in macroscopic protuberances

References

1. Braun J, Sieper J. Ankylosing spondylitis. Lancet. 2007;369(9570):1379–90.
2. Rosenbaum J, Chandran V. Management of comorbidities in ankylosing spondylitis. Am J Med Sci. 2012;343(5):364–6.
3. Chang KW, Chen YY, Lin CC, et al. Closing wedge osteotomy versus opening wedge osteotomy in ankylosing spondylitis with thoracolumbar kyphotic deformity. Spine. 2005;30(14):1584–93.
4. Bridwell KH. Decision making regarding Smith-Petersen vs. pedicle subtraction osteotomy vs. vertebral column resection for spinal deformity. Spine. 2006;31(19 Suppl):S171–8.
5. Xu H, Zhang Y, Zhao Y, et al. Radiologic and clinical outcomes comparison between single- and two-level pedicle subtraction osteotomies in correcting ankylosing spondylitis kyphosis. Spine J. 2015; 15(2):290–7.
6. Chen IH, Chien JT, Yu TC. Transpedicular wedge osteotomy for correction of thoracolumbar kyphosis in ankylosing spondylitis: experience with 78 patients. Spine. 2001;26(16):E354–60.
7. Zheng GQ, Song K, Zhang YG, et al. Two-level spinal osteotomy for severe thoracolumbar kyphosis in ankylosing spondylitis. Experience with 48 patients. Spine. 2014;39(13):1055–8.
8. Wang Y, Bunger CE, Zhang Y, et al. Lowest instrumented vertebra selection in Lenke 3C and 6C scoliosis: what if we choose lumbar apical vertebra as distal fusion end? Eur Spine J. 2012;21(6):1053–61.
9. Wang Y, Bunger CE, Zhang Y, et al. Lowest instrumented vertebra selection for Lenke 5C scoliosis: a minimum 2-year radiographical follow-up. Spine. 2013;38(14):E894–900.
10. Carter S, Lories RJ. Osteoporosis: a paradox in ankylosing spondylitis. Curr Osteoporos Rep. 2011; 9(3):112–5.
11. van Royen BJ, Slot GH. Closing-wedge posterior osteotomy for ankylosing spondylitis. Partial corporectomy and transpedicular fixation in 22 cases. J Bone Joint Surg Br. 1995;77(1):117–21.
12. Zhao Y, Wang Y, Wang Z, et al. Effect and strategy of one-stage interrupted two-level transpedicular wedge osteotomy for correcting severe kyphotic deformities in ankylosing spondylitis. Clin Spine Surg. 2016;30(4):E454–9.
13. Yao Z, Zheng G, Zhang Y, et al. Selection of lowest instrumented vertebra for thoracolumbar kyphosis in ankylosing spondylitis. Spine. 2016;41(7):591–7.

Surgimap Spine for Preoperative Surgical Planning in Patients with Ankylosing Spondylitis

10

Xuesong Zhang, Wenhao Hu, and Yan Wang

1 Introduction

Precise preoperative planning is necessary for any surgical procedure to achieve an optimal therapeutic effect. Retrieving spinal alignment, horizontal vision, and global sagittal balance is recognized as the main surgical purpose for ankylosing spondylitis (AS) patients with kyphosis deformity. Some authors have proved that reasonable restoration of sagittal plane is tightly associated with postoperative quality of life [1, 2]. In an attempt to increase clinical effect, we need to optimize postoperative spinal alignment.

Inadequate preparation is likely to lead to undercorrection or overcorrection. Schwab et al. reported among patients who underwent pedicle subtraction osteotomy (PSO) in the lumbar spine, 23% of realignment procedures failed [3]. In one such study, 22% of patients who underwent PSO in the thoracic spine have poor sagittal alignment postoperatively [4]. Improper realignment often leads to poor functional outcome and major complications, such as pseudarthrosis and fixation failure, which often need revision operations. Smith et al. [5] described the rate of rod breakage is 8.6% in deformity patients and 15.6% in patients who underwent PSO procedure. And the main reason is the remaining sagittal malalignment.

X. Zhang (✉) · W. Hu · Y. Wang
Chinese PLA General Hospital, Beijing, China

2 Surgical Planning

Several authors put forward some mathematical formulas [6–10] and graphical methods [11–14] for surgical planning. Van et al. [13] reported a biomechanical analysis for preoperative planning in AS patients that makes SVA measurements without regard for the position of lower extremities. The effect of the lower limbs on spinal sagittal plane balance was fully considered in this method. There are two main steps involved in the method. First, a standard lateral radiographs of full-length standing spine was made when the patient was relaxed. Then, through rotating the radiograph, the surgeon could speculate the osteotomy angle.

In 2008, Roy et al. [11] proposed a mathematical method with the use of a computational program for surgical planning in AS patients who need osteotomy surgery. During their planning, sacral end plate angle (SEA), sagittal vertical axis (SVA), and chin-brow vertical angle (CBVA) were measured to evaluate the sagittal balance. The patients included in the study have been improved greatly in balance after closing wedge osteotomy. However, it could not be denied that the postoperative sagittal parameters do not completely matched with preoperative planning.

It's noting, the relationship between the sagittal balance of spine and the spino-pelvic

Y. Wang (ed.), *Surgical Treatment of Ankylosing Spondylitis Deformity*,
https://doi.org/10.1007/978-981-13-6427-3_10

parameters is not properly understood, which, the effect of pelvic incidence (PI) and pelvic tilt (PT) were neglected in most methods. Moreover, these are relatively complex for routine clinical use. Surgimap Spine (Nemaris Inc., NY, USA), a free computer program for surgical planning, has become more and more popular among spinal surgeons. It provides a practical graphical method for the planning of osteotomy surgery by combining the spinal-related measurement and surgical planning tools with knowledge from published literature [15]. In this chapter, we would like to introduce the use of Surgimap Spine in surgical planning for patients with AS.

3 Measurement of Preoperative Sagittal Radiographs

Surgimap Spine offers dedicated tools for measurement of coronal and sagittal parameters. The first step is importing the anteroposterior and lateral full-length spine radiographs including the whole spine and pelvis. For patients with AS, the sagittal parameters including SVA, PT, and PI are the key points. SVA is employed to measure the vertical offset between the C7 vertebra and posterosuperior corner of the sacrum. The SVA measure just requires the identification of the center of C7 and the posterosuperior corner of S1 (Fig. 10.1).

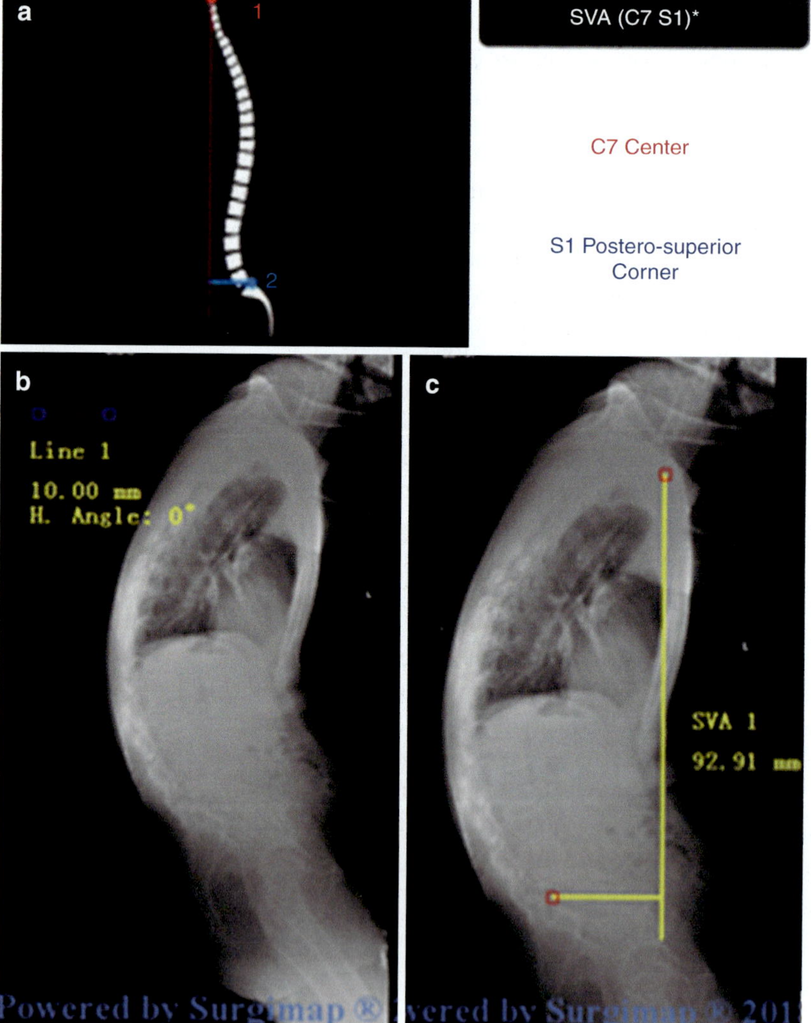

Fig. 10.1 Measurement of sagittal vertical axis (SVA). (**a**) Identification of the center of C7 and the posterosuperior corner of S1. (**b**) Image calibration was performed. (**c**) SVA of this AS case is 92.91 mm

A negative value denotes a plumb line posterior to the posterosuperior corner of S1. Of note, before measuring the length, image calibration must be done. The surveyor should draw a line on the image and then define the actual length of the line. A positive value denotes a plumb line anterior to the posterosuperior corner of S1.

In recognition of the sacrum end plate and two femoral heads, the pelvic parameters PT and PI were calculated automatically (Fig. 10.2). When LL is measured, the S1 superior end plate and the L1 superior end plate need to be outlined, and a small arc appears on the measurement indicating which angle is being measured (Fig. 10.3).

4 Simulation of the Osteotomy

The first step of the simulated procedure is to select the level of osteotomy. We consider some factors when making this decision: the higher the degree of correction, the lower the risk of nerve defect, the sufficient distal fixation, and the preservation of the motor segment. Currently, PSO and vertebral column decancellation (VCD) are most often used for correction of kyphotic deformity with AS. As we know, PSO is a closing wedge osteotomy [16], so we choose the tool "Wedge Osteotomy" in this software. The wedge section is determined by two straight lines consisting of three points. The anterior point was located at the anterior cortex of the vertebral body. The intersection of the upper and lower edge of the pedicle and the vertebral body was selected as the other two points. After choosing the "osteotomy" button, the image changes accordingly: the wedge-shaped part is removed and the posterior column closed (Fig. 10.4). Different from PSO, VCD technique is a "Y" osteotomy instead of a "V" osteotomy. The anterior point of VCD changes from anterior columnar cortex to the intersection of anterior and

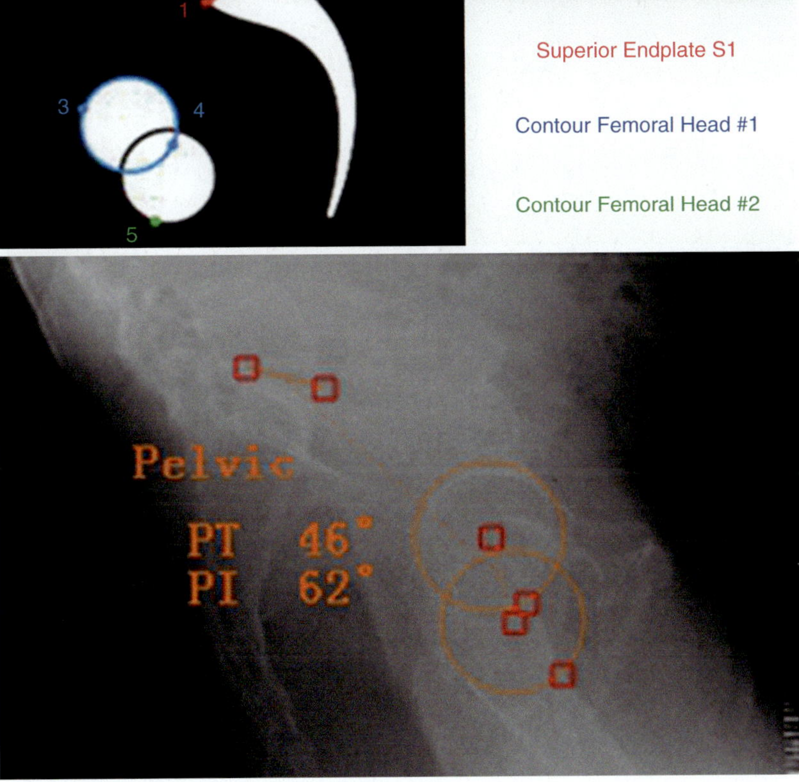

Fig. 10.2 Measurement of pelvic parameters. In recognition of the sacrum end plate and two femoral heads, the pelvic parameters PT and PI were calculated automatically

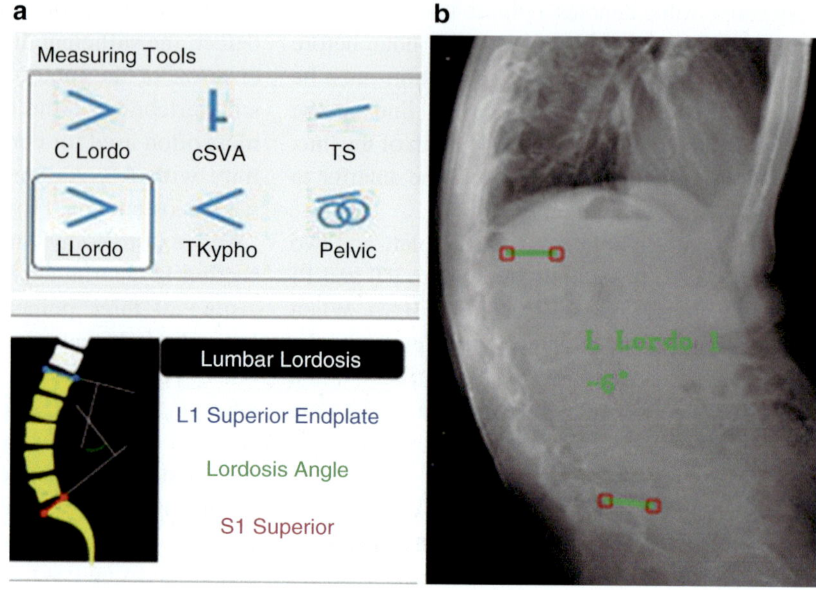

Fig. 10.3 Measurement of lumbar lordosis (LL). (**a**) Select the "LLordo" measurement tool. (**b**) Identification of the S1 superior end plate and the L1 superior end plates

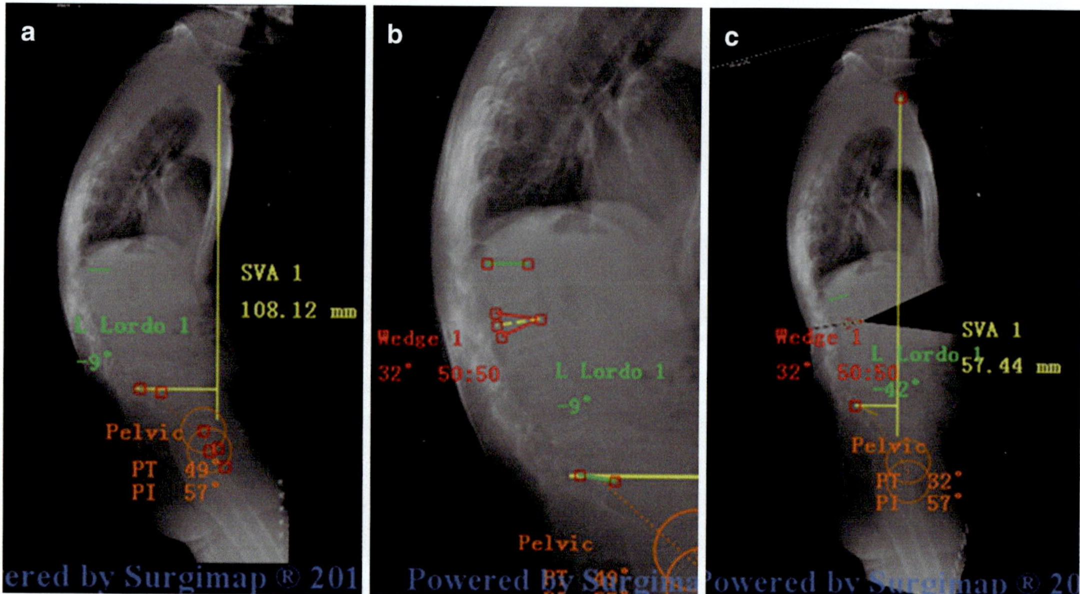

Fig. 10.4 The simulation of PSO in Surgimap for patients with AS. (**a**) Preoperative sagittal parameters were measured and analyzed. (**b**) The osteotomy level was located L2, the 'Wedge Osteotomy' tool was used, and the anterior point was located at the anterior cortex of the vertebral body. (**c**) Radiographic image and parameters were shown after simulated osteotomy

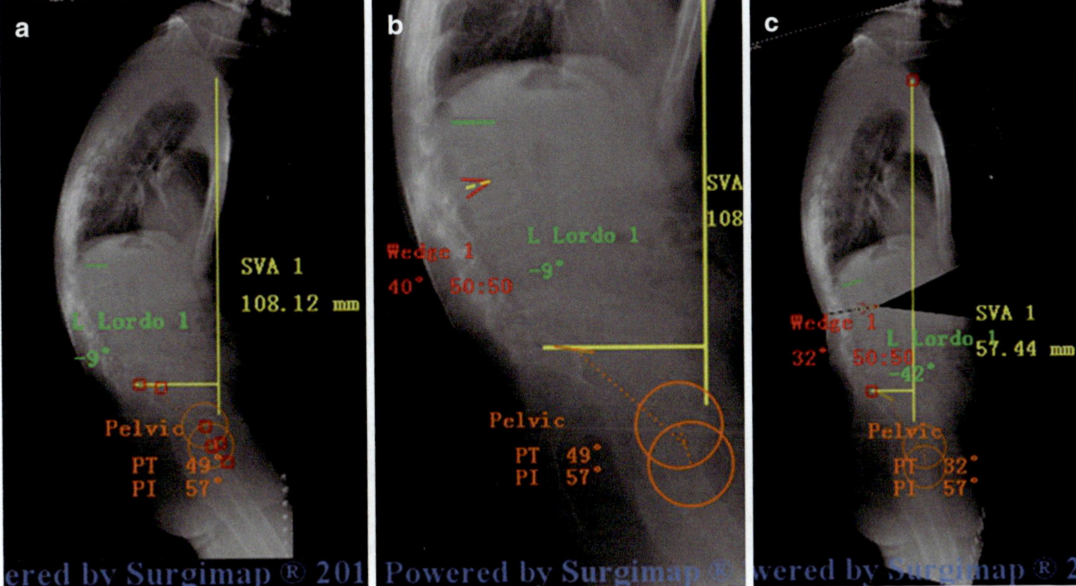

Fig. 10.5 The simulation of VCD in Surgimap for patients with AS. (**a**) Preoperative sagittal parameters were measured and analyzed. (**b**) The osteotomy level was located L2, the 'Wedge Osteotomy' tool was used, and the anterior point was located at the border of the anterior and medial column. (**c**) Radiographic image and parameters were shown after simulated osteotomy

medical column (Fig. 10.5). When the posterior column is closed, the anterior column opens meanwhile.

5 Evaluating Surgimap-Predicted Postoperative Parameters to select the Optimal Technique

After applying the osteotomy in Surgimap, it will depict osteotomy graphically directly on radiographic images. Then, we need to re-measure the key sagittal parameters including SVA, LL, PT, PI, and SS and to check if the osteotomy is suitable for the individual. SVA < 50 mm, PT < 20 mm, and PI-LL < 10° were considered corrective success [17, 18]. If one-level PSO or VCD is insufficient for severe kyphosis, two-level osteotomy is recommended (Fig. 10.6).

A good surgical plan requires an accurate and comprehensive assessment of sagittal alignment, and Surgimap not only measures global and local critical parameters but also considers the compensation mechanisms used to maintain body balance and the impact of spino-pelvic parameters. Surgimap, providing a geometrical method, allows the surgeon to simulate surgical operations on preoperative x-rays to provide estimates of postoperative results. This software offers a virtual preview of surgical outcomes and gives advice to the surgeon about the amount of correction required. Moreover, Surgimap, an effective and practical tool, is easy to operate and easy to learn. Surgimap's ability to predict correct sagittal plane after surgery has proven to be excellent [19]. In 2014, Atici et al. [20] used Surgimap Spine for surgical planning in patients with severe deformity who need two-level PSO osteotomy; however, the result seems less than ideal. They explain the reason may be it is unable to estimate the amount of bleeding and the possible injury of the spinal cord. However, the primary objective of preoperative plan for the spinal deformity surgery program is to analyze changes in the spinal alignment and predict the effect of

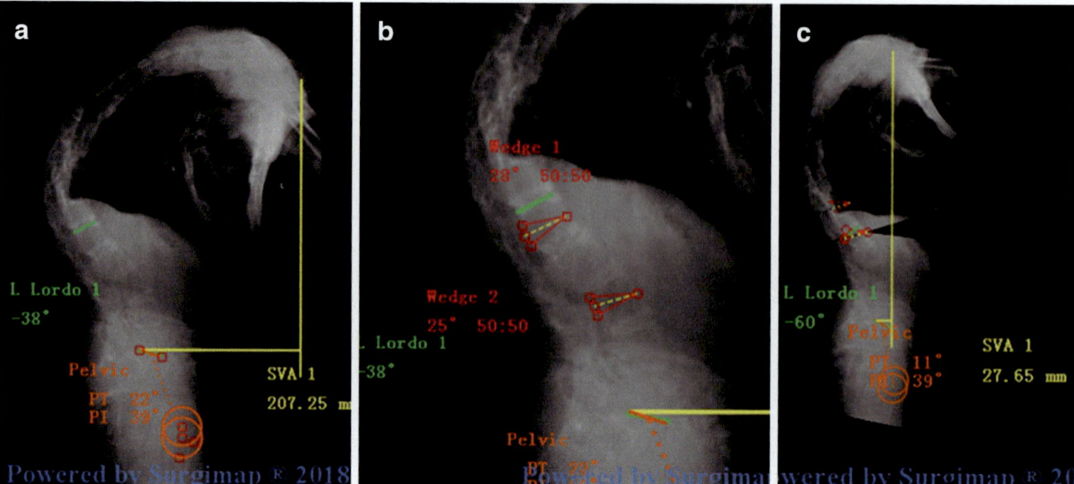

Fig. 10.6 The simulation of two-level osteotomy in Surgimap for patients with AS. (**a**) Preoperative sagittal parameters were measured and analyzed. (**b**) The osteotomy level was located L10 and L1. (**c**) Radiographic image and parameters were shown after simulated osteotomy

surgical techniques in order to select the best operation for a given patient. The amount of bleeding and spinal injury are affected by many factors, including the patient's coagulation function, the duration of surgery, and the surgeon's technique. So, it is inappropriate to require a preoperative planning software to evaluate these indicators. The other weakness of the software is that it is unable to consider the mutual changes that may occur in unused parts [15]. For AS patients, all the spine is fixed, so the influence of adjacent segment is limited. With our experience, all patients obtained satisfactory clinical photographic results as planned before the operation.

6 Conclusion

For correction treatment in AS patients, the Surgimap Spine is a reliable and useful tool. It provides a simple method for measuring and evaluating the spino-pelvic parameters and simulating the osteotomy process. The most suitable surgical method should be selected for individual patients.

This study was conducted with approval from the Ethics Committee of Chinese PLA General Hospital, and all patients provided informed consent for their participation in this study.

References

1. Smith JS, Klineberg EO, Schwab FJ, Shaffrey CI, Moal B, Ames CP, Hostin R, Fu KMG, Kebaish KM, Burton DC. Change in classification grade by the Schwab-SRS adult spinal deformity classification and impact on health-related quality of life measures: prospective analysis of operative and nonoperative treatment. Spine. 2012;12:1663.
2. Blondel B, Schwab F, Ungar B, Smith J, Bridwell K, Glassman S, Shaffrey C, Farcy JP, Lafage V. Impact of magnitude and percentage of global sagittal plane correction on health-related quality of life at 2-years follow-up. Neurosurgery. 2012;71:341.
3. Schwab FJ, Patel A, Shaffrey CI, Smith JS, Farcy JP, Boachie-Adjei O, Hostin RA, Hart RA, Akbarnia BA, Burton DC. Sagittal realignment failures following pedicle subtraction osteotomy surgery: are we doing enough?: Clinical article. J Neurosurg Spine. 2012;16:539–46.
4. Lafage V, Smith JS, Bess S, Schwab FJ, Ames CP, Klineberg E, Arlet V, Hostin R, Burton DC, Shaffrey CI. Sagittal spino-pelvic alignment failures following three column thoracic osteotomy for adult spinal deformity. Eur Spine J. 2012;21:698–704.
5. Smith JS, Shaffrey CI, Ames CP, Demakakos J, Fu KM, Keshavarzi S, Li CM, Deviren V, Schwab FJ, Lafage V. Assessment of symptomatic rod fracture after posterior instrumented fusion for adult spinal deformity. Neurosurgery. 2012;71:862–7.
6. Boulay C, Tardieu C, Hecquet J, Benaim C, Mouilleseaux B, Marty C, Pratpradal D, Legaye J, Duvalbeaupère G, Pélissier J. Sagittal alignment of spine and pelvis regulated by pelvic incidence: standard values and prediction of lordosis. Eur Spine J. 2006;15:415–22.

7. Kim YJ, Bridwell KH, Lenke LG, Rhim S, Cheh G. An analysis of sagittal spinal alignment following long adult lumbar instrumentation and fusion to L5 or S1: can we predict ideal lumbar lordosis? Spine. 2006;31:2343.
8. Schwab F, Lafage V, Patel A, Farcy JP. Sagittal plane considerations and the pelvis in the adult patient. Spine. 2009;34:1828.
9. Lafage V, Schwab F, Vira S, Patel A, Ungar B, Farcy JP. Spino-pelvic parameters after surgery can be predicted: a preliminary formula and validation of standing alignment. Spine. 2011;36:1037.
10. Berjano P, Langella F, Ismael MF, Damilano M, Scopetta S, Lamartina C. Successful correction of sagittal imbalance can be calculated on the basis of pelvic incidence and age. Eur Spine J. 2014;23:587–96.
11. Pigge RR, Scheerder FJ, Smit TH, Mullender MG, van Royen BJ. Effectiveness of preoperative planning in the restoration of balance and view in ankylosing spondylitis. Neurosurg Focus. 2008;24:E7.
12. Ondra SL, Marzouk S, Koski T, Silva F, Salehi S. Mathematical calculation of pedicle subtraction osteotomy size to allow precision correction of fixed sagittal deformity. Spine. 2006;31:E973.
13. Van Royen BJ, De GA, Smit TH. Deformity planning for sagittal plane corrective osteotomies of the spine in ankylosing spondylitis. Eur Spine J. 2000;9:492.
14. Le HJ, Leijssen P, Duarte M, Aunoble S. Thoracolumbar imbalance analysis for osteotomy planification using a new method: FBI technique. Eur Spine J. 2011;20(Suppl 5):669.
15. Akbar M, Terran J, Ames CP, Lafage V, Schwab F. Use of Surgimap spine in sagittal plane analysis, osteotomy planning, and correction calculation. Neurosurg Clin N Am. 2013;24:163.
16. Hu WH, Wang Y. Osteotomy techniques for spinal deformity. Chin Med J (Engl). 2016;129:2639.
17. Legaye J, Duval-Beaupère G, Hecquet J, Marty C. Pelvic incidence: a fundamental pelvic parameter for three-dimensional regulation of spinal sagittal curves. Eur Spine J. 1998;7:99–103.
18. Schwab F, Patel A, Ungar B, Farcy JP, Lafage V. Adult spinal deformity-postoperative standing imbalance: how much can you tolerate? An overview of key parameters in assessing alignment and planning corrective surgery. Spine. 2010;35:2224.
19. Langella F, Villafañe JH, Damilano M, Cecchinato R, Pejrona M, Ismael M, Berjano P. Predictive accuracy of Surgimap™ surgical planning for sagittal imbalance: a cohort study. Spine. 2017;42:E1297.
20. Atici Y, Akman YE, Balioglu MB, Kargin D, Kaygusuz MA. Two level pedicle substraction osteotomies for the treatment of severe fixed sagittal plane deformity: computer software-assisted preoperative planning and assessing. Eur Spine J. 2015;25(8):2461–70.

Cervical Osteotomy in Ankylosing Spondylitis

11

Geng Cui, Ningtao Ren, Yuan Li, Chao Chen, and Xuesong Zhang

Ankylosing spondylitis (AS) is an inflammatory disease in which joints become arthritic and eroded, followed by autofusion (ankylosis). AS typically affects the axial spine with the initial onset of sacroiliitis, followed by involvement of the lumbar spine with progression cranially to involve the rest of the spinal column. A thoracolumbar kyphosis is the most common deformity which causes hard standing, walking, looking horizontally, and so on. Although thoracolumbar kyphotic deformities are most common, the cervical and/or upper thoracic spine can also be involved. If the primary deformity has been determined to be in the cervical spine, the patient is unable to see straight ahead. Patients with these deformities, in addition to the problems with horizontal gaze, also can experience other debilitating symptoms, including limitation of chewing, speaking, or swallowing. The only available treatment is an osteotomy at the cervicothoracic junction. The chin-brow angle is of paramount importance when planning a corrective osteotomy in the cervicothoracic region [1]. The aim of surgery is to restore horizontal gaze and sagittal balance, improve function, diminish social disability, and provide durable correction. A key point is not to overcorrect the horizontal gaze because this can lead to inability of patients to see the floor ahead of them [2–4].

G. Cui (✉) · N. Ren · Y. Li · C. Chen · X. Zhang
China PLA General Hospital (301 Hospital), Beijing, China

1 Characteristics of AS Cervicothoracic Kyphosis and Surgical Indications

Severe cervicothoracic kyphosis (CTK) of ankylosing spondylitis (AS) is rare. CTK can cause significant disability due to loss of horizontal gaze, functional limitation, and chin-on-chest deformity. Patients with this deformity can experience dysphagia and problems related to poor oral intake, neck pain, weakness due to the spinal cord stretched over the apex or neuroforamina stenosis, and increases in the risk of fall-related injuries. Cervicothoracic kyphosis (CTK) ankylosing spondylitis can cause hyperreflexia, bipedal sensorimotor dysfunction, and gait abnormalities. Severe CTK can lead to gait disorders and quadriparesis. The patients are prone to pathological cervical vertebra bone fracture due to spinal stiffness, sagittal imbalance, and osteoporosis [1].

Surgical indications include: (1) severe limita tion of horizontal gaze; (2) significant neck pain; (3) severe limitation of daily living ability (such as difficulty in swallowing and jaw opening); (4) occurrence of neurological impairment, positive pathological signs; and (5) patients having a

Y. Wang (ed.), *Surgical Treatment of Ankylosing Spondylitis Deformity*, https://doi.org/10.1007/978-981-13-6427-3_11

strong psychological need for correction surgery and a psychological preparation for accepting the risk of surgery.

Surgical contraindications include (1) concurrence with other serious systemic diseases, (2) cervical spinal canal stenosis, and (3) older patients [2–11].

2 Selection of Osteotomy and Internal Fixation Methods

2.1 C7–T1 SPO Extension Osteotomy (Fig. 11.1)

In 1958, Urist [12] first described an extension osteotomy, which is the most common surgical approach for correction of the symptomatic deformity, at the cervicothoracic junction. Since the initial description of an extension osteotomy, surgical techniques have evolved affecting both radiographic and clinical outcomes. In recent years, although there has been a continuous report on the improvement of surgical methods, C7–T1 extension osteotomy is still one of the standard surgical procedures for the osteotomy of cervicothoracic kyphosis [13, 14]. There are three reasons for the selection of osteotomy in C7–T1: (1) The canal at this level is quite large and reduces the risk of spinal cord compression due to the closure of osteotomy surface. (2) At this segment, the C8 nerve root is quite mobile compared with the upper cervical roots. Even if the C8 nerve root is damaged during the operation, the impact on the function of the hand is relatively small. (3) The resulting correction occurred below the entrance of the vertebral arteries into the transverse foramens, making damage of vertebral arteries less risky.

After a wide and lengthy exposure from C6 to T1, a wide cervical decompression at C7 and T1 is performed. A complete C7 laminectomy and partial laminectomies involving the inferior portion of C6 and the superior portion of T1 were then performed to ensure that the C8 nerve roots are not compressed after the correction. Spinal cord monitoring was performed throughout the

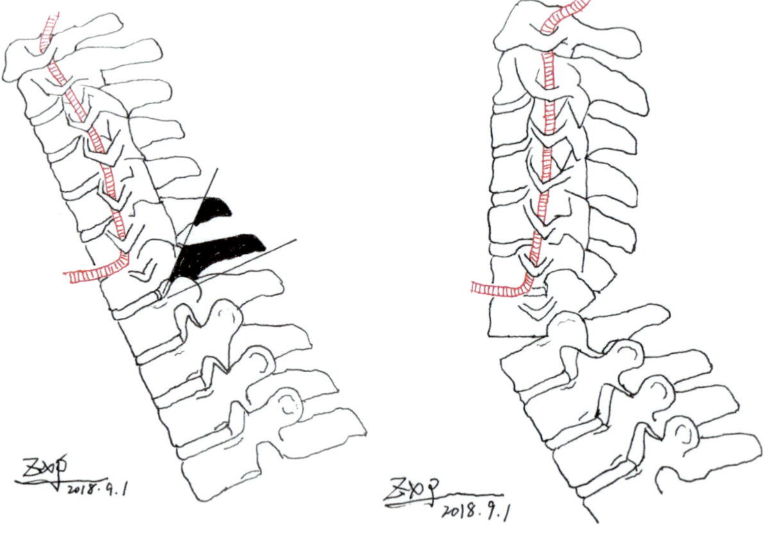

Fig. 11.1 C7–T1 SPO extension osteotomy (Reprint with permission from reference Tokala DP, Lam KS, Freeman BJ, et al. C7 decancellisation closing wedge osteotomy for the correction of fixed cervicothoracic kyphosis. European Spine Journal, 2007, 16(9):1471–1478)

procedure. A wake-up test is performed after correction. Osteotomy surface was closed slowly by the adjustment of position, and the kyphotic deformity was corrected. After operation, patients would interfere with the halo-vest in the corrected position until the osteotomy becomes stable and gets bone fusion. Recently, many surgeons preferred to use internal fixation instead of halo-vest.

The advantages of C7–T1 SPO extension osteotomy are as follows: (1) The operation is relatively simple and safe. (2) The angle of osteotomy in single segment SP osteotomy can be well controlled on the sagittal plane. (3) The hinge axis is located in the middle column, short spinal cord contraction, and large osteotomy angle. (4) It is suitable for severe sagittal deformity.

The disadvantage of C7–T1 SPO extension osteotomy are as follows: (1) Due to the small area of the osteotomy contact surface, it is easy to be instability after the operation; (2) There are more symptoms of C8 nerve root; (3) Opening of the anterior intervertebral space can lead to the pseudoarthrosis in the osteotomy site; (4) Opening of the anterior column after osteotomy can also lead to the injury of trachea, esophagus and large vessel [13].

2.2 C7 Pedicle Subtraction Osteotomy (Fig. 11.2)

The angle of C7 pedicle subtraction osteotomy (PSO) was based on the preoperative design. After a wide and lengthy exposure (at least including upper and lower three vertebrae around C7), cervical lateral mass or pedicle fixation and thoracic vertebral pedicle fixation were performed. A complete C7 laminectomy and partial laminectomies involving the inferior portion of C6 and the superior portion of T1 were then performed to ensure that the pedicle was exposed. Firstly, one side of the pedicle screw connection rod was installed for temporary fixation. Secondly, on the other side, pedicle subtraction osteotomy was performed, and then, a small amount of cancellous bone was pushed to the anterior 1/4 of the vertebral body to maintain the continuity of the anterior wall when the osteotomy surface was closed. Finally, complete the

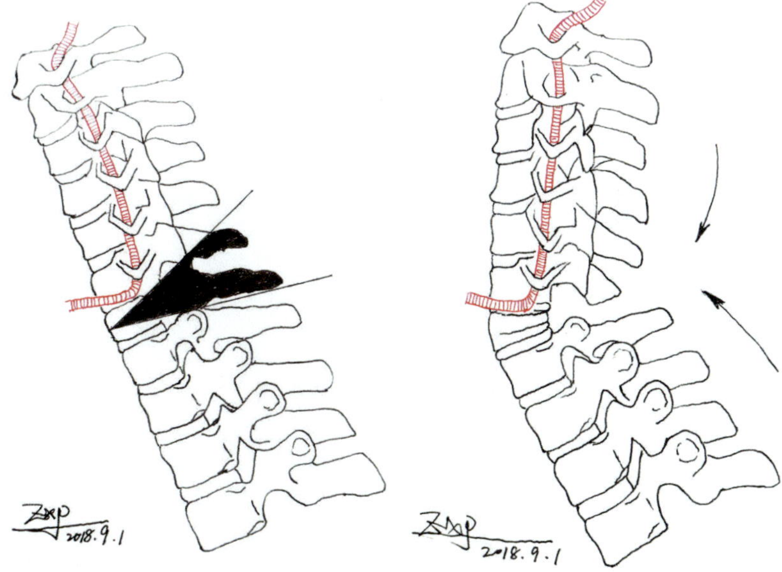

Fig. 11.2 C7 pedicle subtraction osteotomy (Reprint with permission from reference Tokala DP, Lam KS, Freeman BJ, et al. C7 decancellisation closing wedge osteotomy for the correction of fixed cervico-thoracic kyphosis. European Spine Journal, 2007, 16(9):1471–1478)

opposite side with the same method. The vertebral body forms the "eggshell" shape after the pedicle subtraction osteotomy. The compression fracture of C7 was caused by the adjustment of position and implants pressure. Osteotomy surface was closed slowly, and the kyphotic deformity was corrected [15, 16].

The advantages of C7 pedicle subtraction osteotomy are as follows: (1) The large area of the osteotomy contact surface can prevent the spondylolisthesis and instability of the spine. (2) It can reduce the risk of the anterior longitudinal ligament and vascular tear. (3) The hinge axis is located in the front column. (4) It is suitable for mild sagittal imbalance.

The disadvantages of C7 pedicle subtraction osteotomy are as follows: (1) The operation is complicated. (2) Spinal cord contraction is relatively large and high possibility of nerve injury. (3) Due to the anatomical limitations, the angle of the osteotomy is limited [16–19].

The following figures and cases are obtained with patients' consent.

2.3 Case 1

Patient characteristics: Male, 34 years old. Thoracolumbar pain, limited mobility for 13 years, increased with spinal deformity for 3 years. Diagnosed of AS in 2001. Double hip replacement surgery in 2011. So far, kyphosis worsens as the disease progresses. Diagnosis: Ankylosing spondylitis; chin-on-chest deformity. Preoperative pictures (Figs. 11.3 and 11.4).

Intraoperative position and surgical procedure (Figs. 11.5, 11.6, 11.7, 11.8, 11.9, and 11.10).

Comparison of preoperative and postoperative data and follow-up (Figs. 11.11, 11.12, and 11.13).

Unfortunately, the patient didn't accept the scheduled lumbar osteotomy because of his

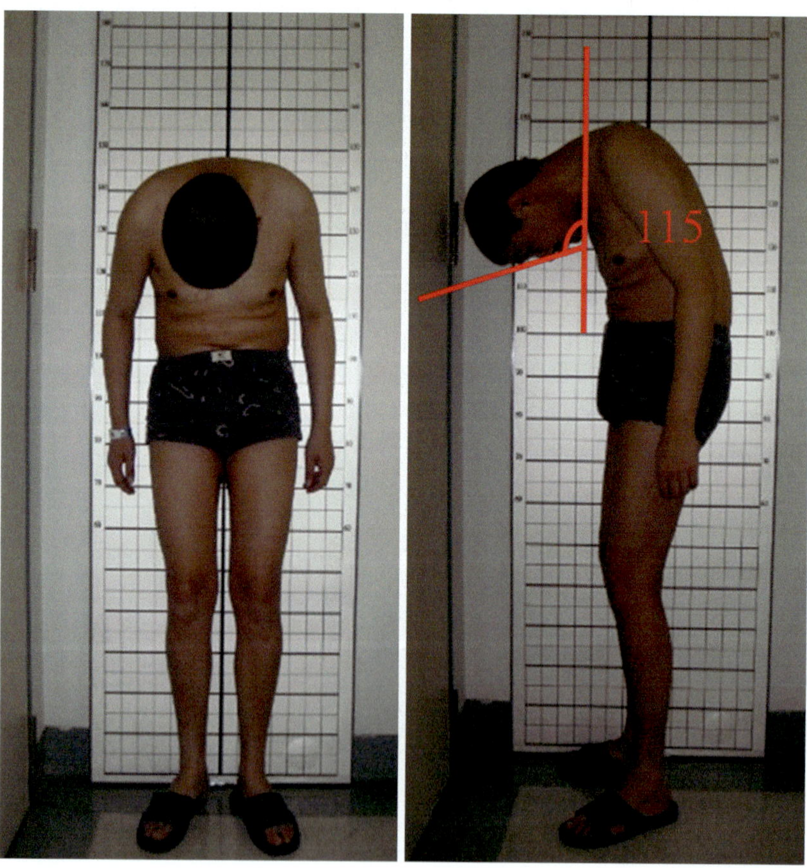

Fig. 11.3 Preoperative clinical appearance (original height, 183 cm; present height, 141 cm; sitting height, 64 cm; CBVA = 115°)

personal reason in 3 months after the first operation. The rod breakage was found at 6-month follow-up (Fig. 11.14). Then second operation was performed (Fig. 11.15).

The first and second postoperative X-ray comparison (Figs. 11.16 and 11.17).

Anterior cervicothoracic fusion was performed in the third operation (Fig. 11.18). Postoperative X-ray, clinical appearance, and follow-up (Figs. 11.19, 11.20, 11.21, 11.22, and 11.23).

Appearance changes from the first operation to the third operation (Figs. 11.24 and 11.25).

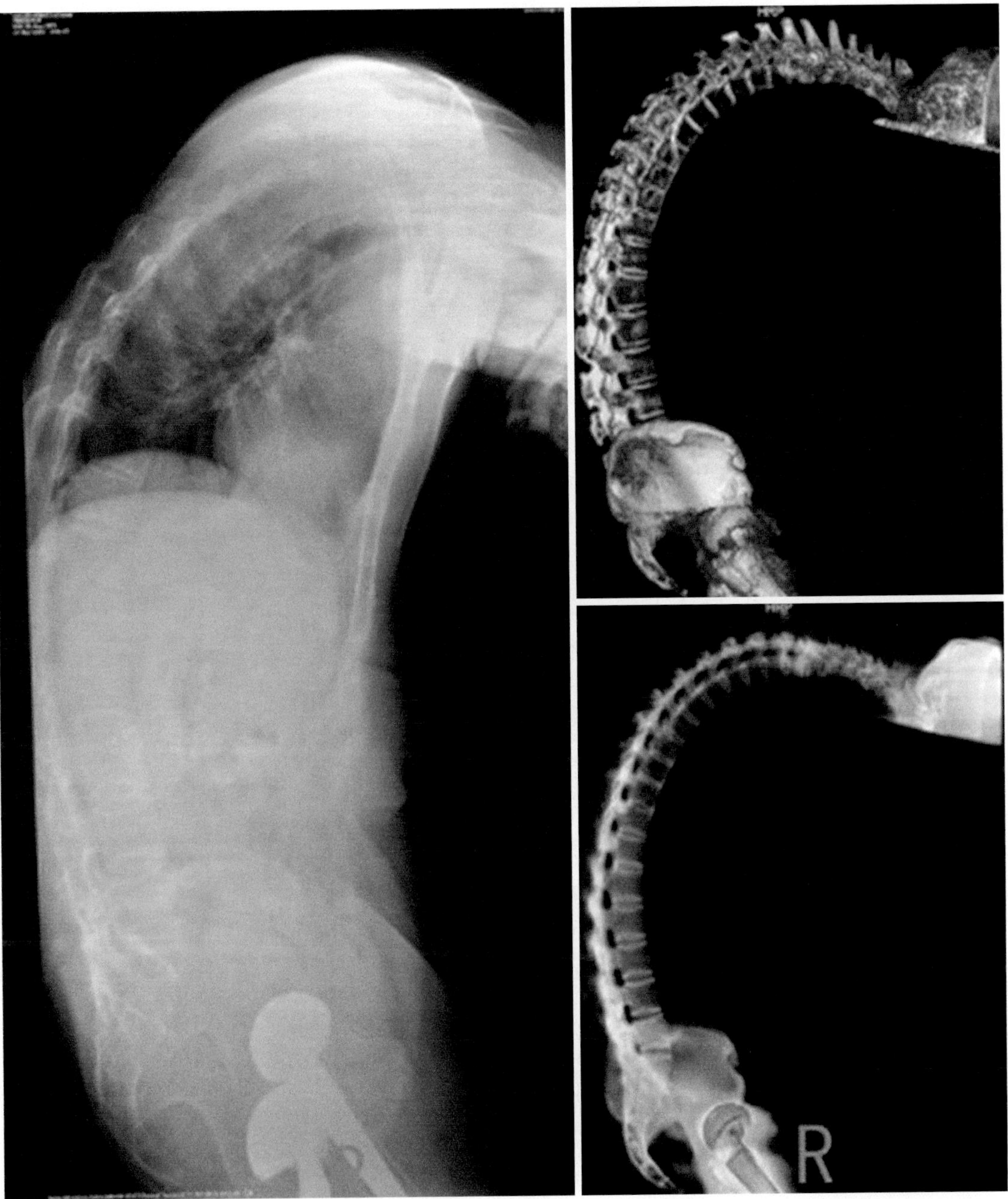

Fig. 11.4 Preoperative X-ray and CT. Cobb(C2–C7) = 40°, Cobb(T2–T5) = 28°, Cobb(C2–T5) = 85°, Cobb(T5–T12) = 49.3°, Cobb(T10–L2) = 28.1°, Cobb(L1–S1) = 10.7°, SS = 5°, PI = 45°, PT = 40°, t PT = 9.7°

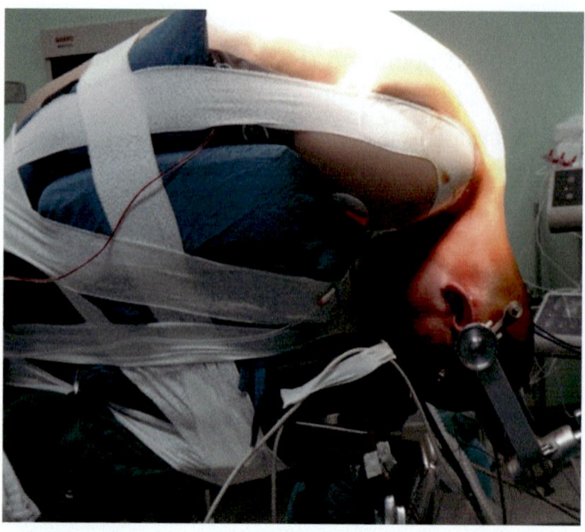

Fig. 11.5 C7–T1 SPO extension osteotomy intraoperative position

2.4 Case 2

Patient characteristics: Male, 33 years old. Ankylosing spondylitis for 20 years, kyphotic deformity for 20 years. Double hip replacement surgery in 2007 and 2014. So far, kyphosis worsens as the disease progresses. Normal life and work were obviously affected. Diagnosis: ankylosing spondylitis; preoperative pictures (Figs. 11.26, 11.27, and 11.28).

Intraoperative position and surgical procedure (Figs. 11.29 and 11.30).

Comparison of preoperative and postoperative data (Figs. 11.31, 11.32, and 11.33).

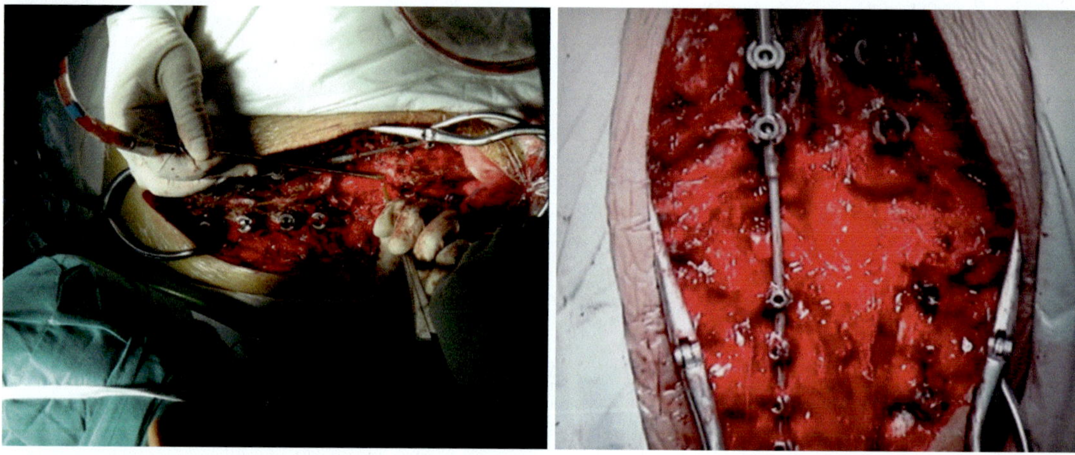

Fig. 11.6 Remove the laminae and spinous processes from C6 to T1 and C7 pedicle; osteotomy width is about 5.5 cm; place rods

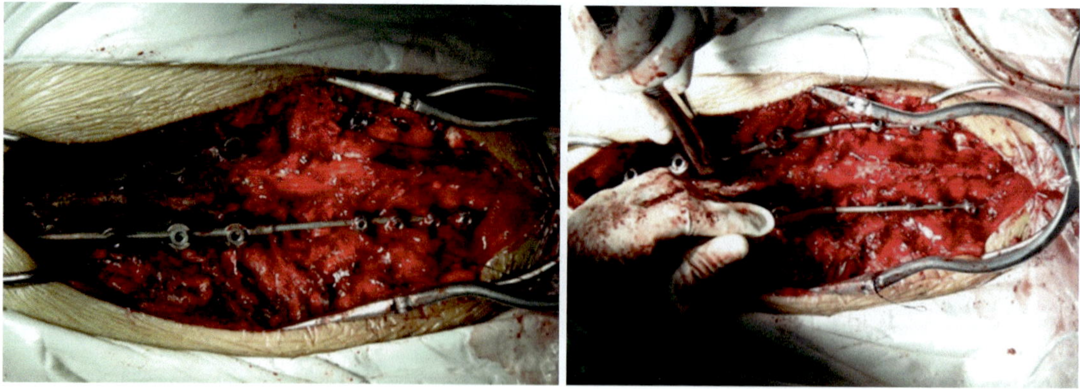

Fig. 11.7 The patient's head is extended to create an avulsion fracture of the anterior and middle columns of the ankylosed cervical spine with the instantaneous axis of rotation at the C7 pedicle base

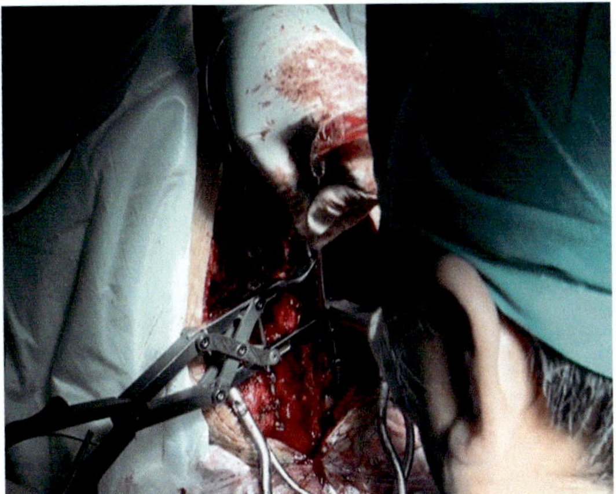

Fig. 11.8 Raise head gradually

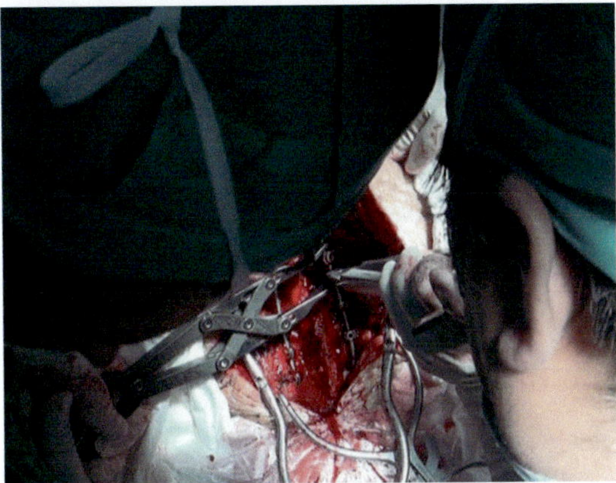

Fig. 11.9 Osteotomy surface was closed

3 Cervical Osteotomy Effect Analysis

Cervical thoracic osteotomy can greatly improve the vision of patients with kyphosis of AS. And it could also improve personal hygiene and survival ability in daily life especially in the appearance significantly. Measuring the angle between the patient's jaw and vertical line (the chin-brow vertical (CBV) angle) can assess the degree of correction [8, 11]. The average total correction angle of CBV reported by McMaster [9] was 54° (30°–71°). The follow-up of 18 months showed that the average degree of correction loss was 6° (0–20°). Simmons et al. [11] reported that CBV of the early 114 patients from 1967 to 1997 (conventional technique group) was corrected from preoperative 56° (30°–146°) to postoperative 4°(0–60°), and CBV of 17 patients from 1997 to 2003 (current technique group) was corrected from preoperative 49° (30°–90°) to postoperative 12° (3°–15°). They recommended that overcorrection should also be avoided, and retaining about 10° flexion allows patients to stand up right when they are looking at the front horizontally and the ground. They can sit in front of the table reading and also driving in daily lives.

Most patients' neck pain was relieved after operation, and the ability of daily life was also obviously improved. Belanger et al. [15] reported

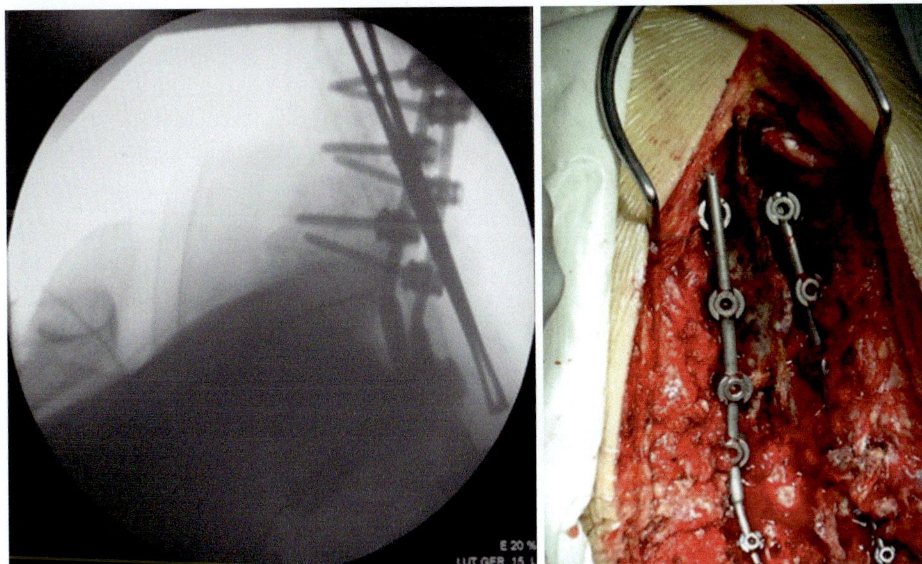

Fig. 11.10 Intraoperative X-ray and image. Corrective about 60° (operation time 5 h, Blood loss 800 ml)

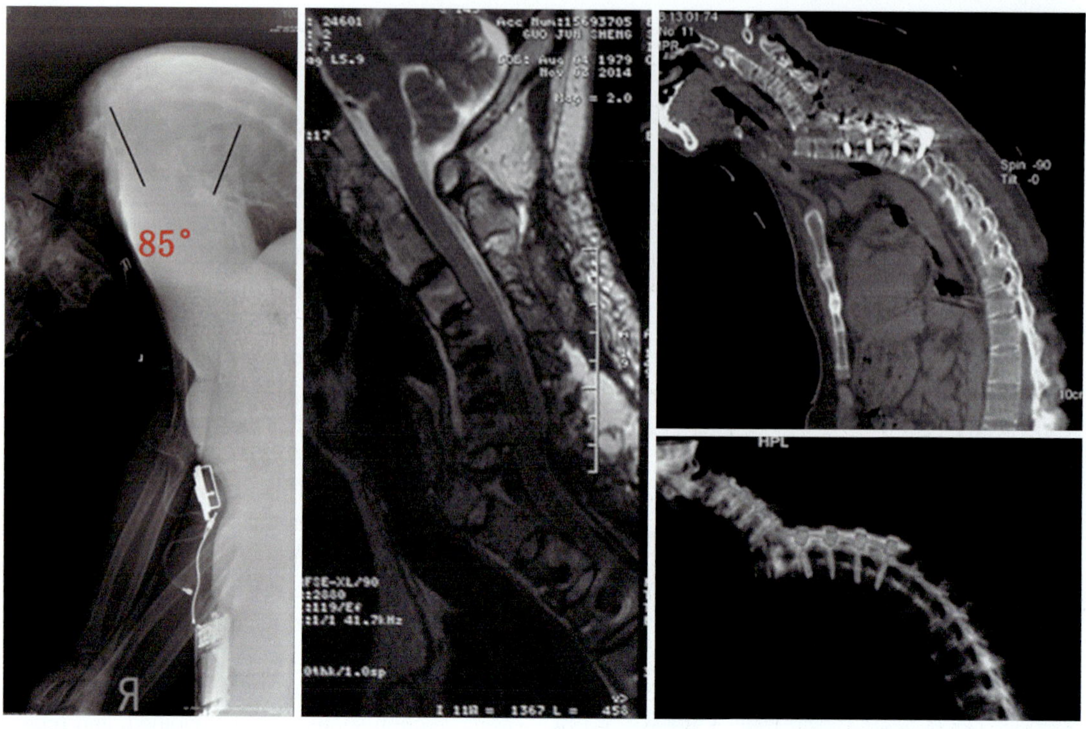

Fig. 11.11 Preoperative and 1-week postoperative image data. Severe sagittal translation occurred at osteotomy site (C67)

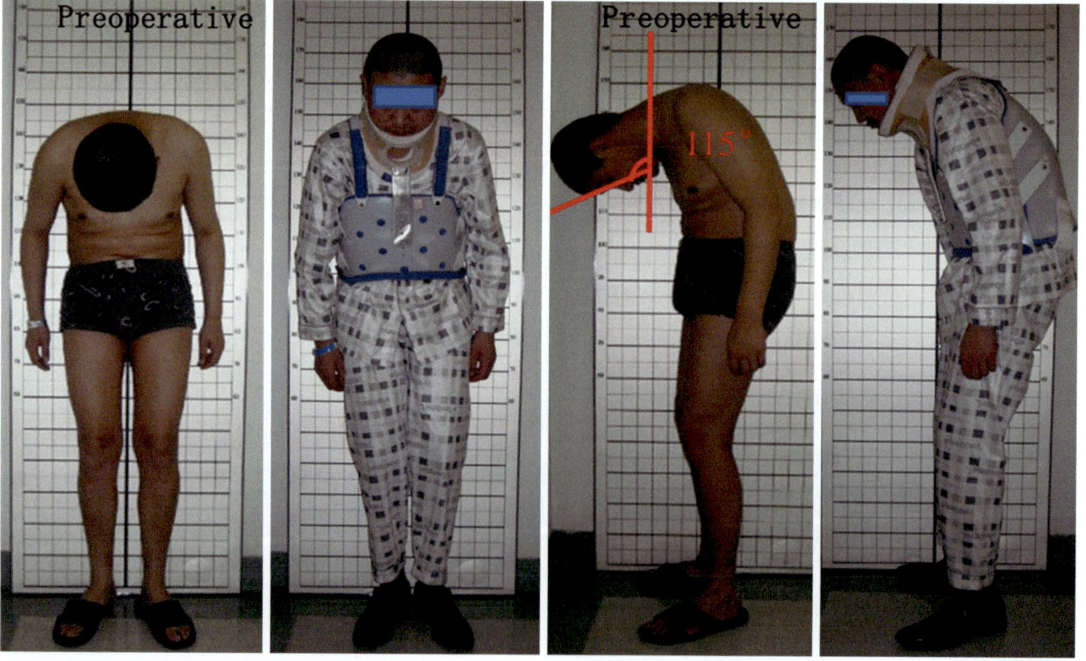

Fig. 11.12 Preoperative and 1-week postoperative appearance. Postoperative 24-h weakness of hand intramuscular occurred, transient neurological dysfunction of C8 nerve root symptomatic treatment gradually relieved, the basic recovery of hand intramuscular after 3 months

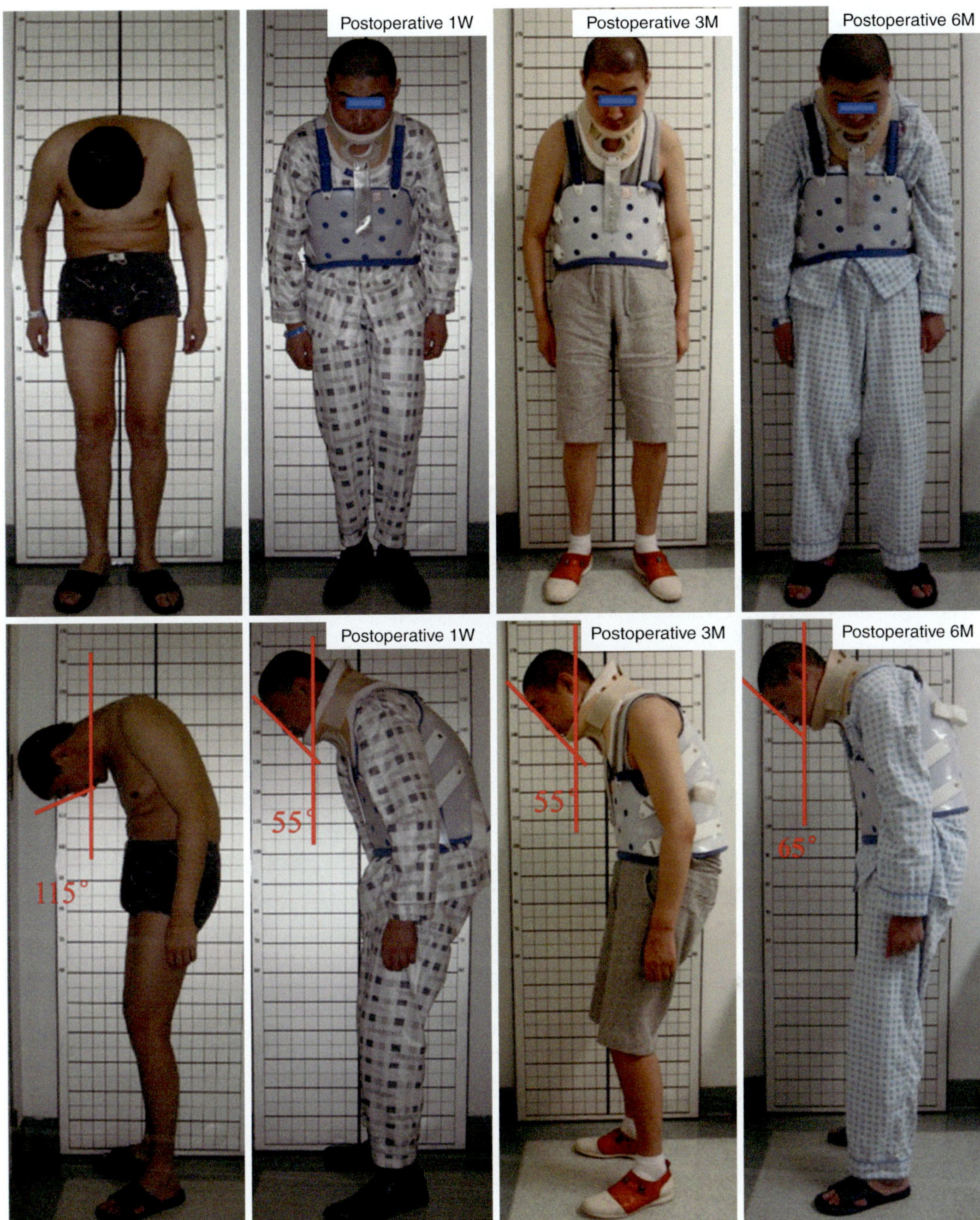

Fig. 11.13 Preoperative and postoperative 1 W, 3 M, and 6 M appearances

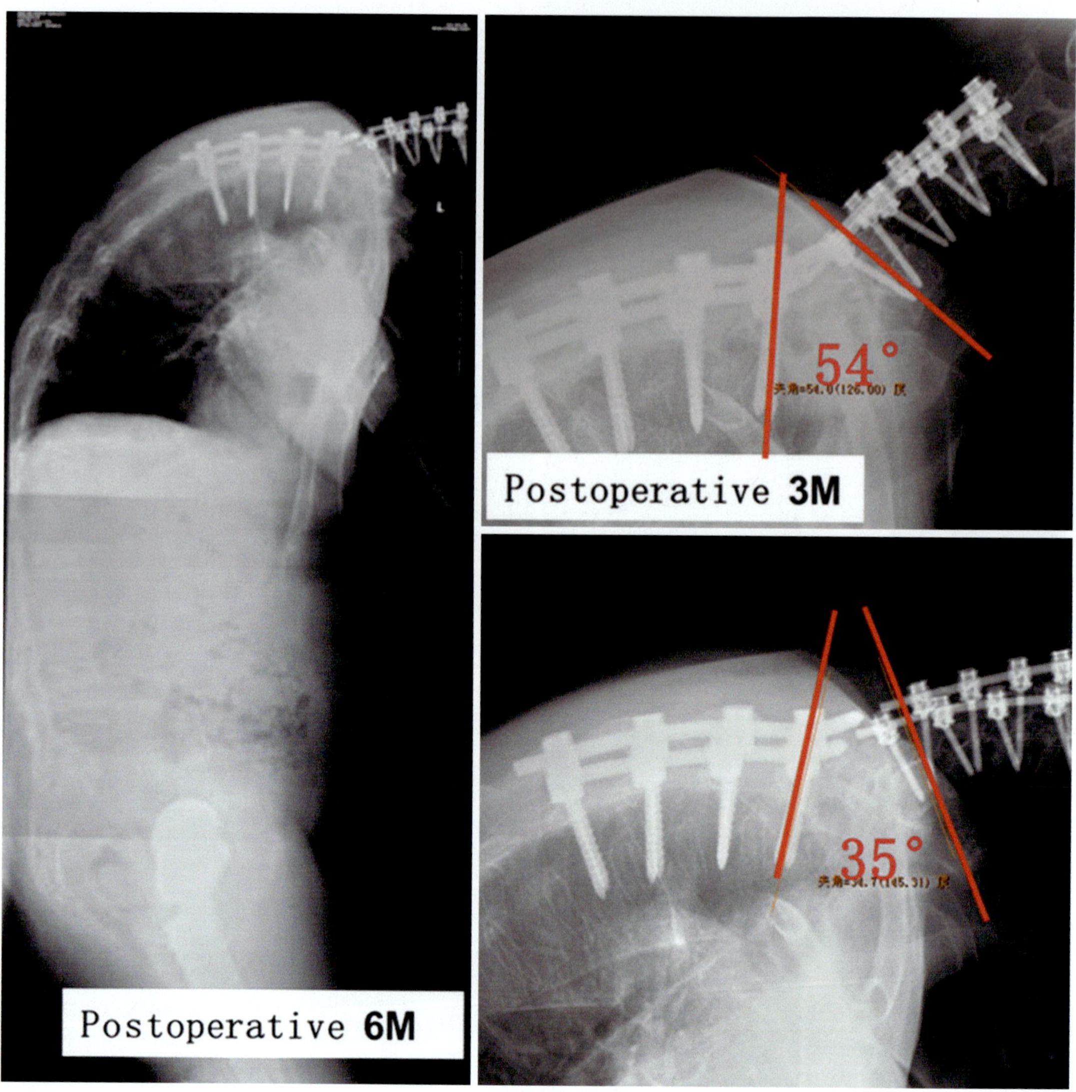

Fig. 11.14 Rod breakage in postoperative 6-month follow-up. Because of the small area of the osteotomy contact surface and global saggital imbalance, it is easy to be instability after the operation

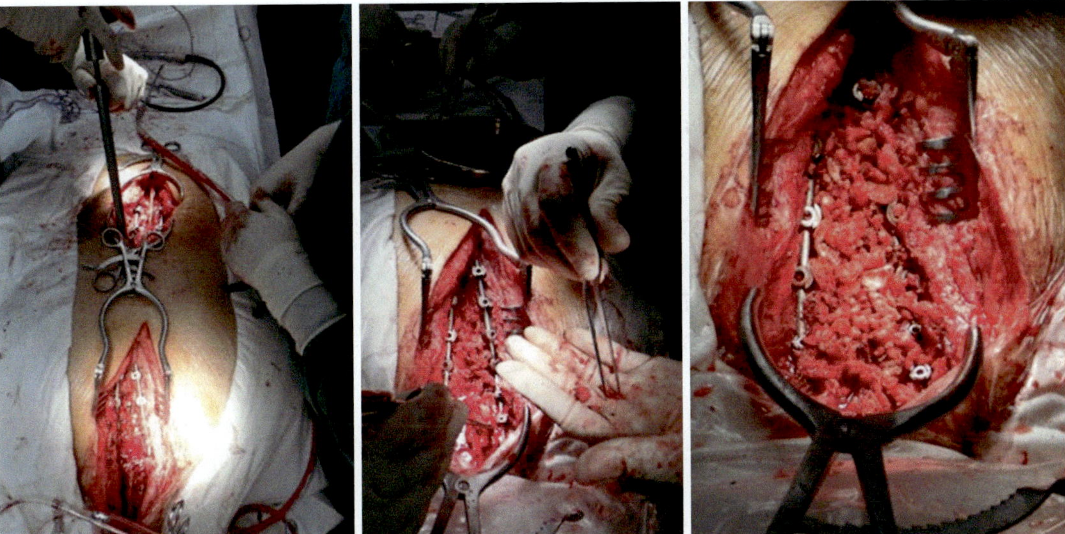

Fig. 11.15 Second operation. One-stage cervicothoracic revision and thoracolumbar osteotomy. VCD osteotomy in the lumbar 2. Change the rod in cervicothoracic and posterior bone graft in lumbar and cervical osteotomy site

26 cases of AS neck kyphotic deformity. They divided the preoperative neck pain into three grades: mild, moderate, and severe. 21 patients' pain were improved at least 1 grade after operation, and 8 of them neck pain disappeared. In 19 patients with preoperative dysphagia, 18 significantly improved. McMasterd [9] reported 15 cases AS of neck kyphotic kyphosis couldn't participate in the work before surgery, and 4 patients returned to work after surgery. Tokala et al. [7] asked eight patients to write satisfaction questionnaire with excellent, good, satisfactory, unchanged, unsatisfactory, and poor as options. Three patients responded excellent, and five patients responded good. One hundred thirty-one patients reported by Simmons et al. [11] also expressed satisfaction after osteotomy.

4 Operative Complications

AS cervicothoracic junction osteotomy has great risk and many complications. Postoperative complications include death, nerve injury, sagittal displacement, and pseudoarthrosis.

There are 5 clinical papers included 227 patients shows that 6 (2.6%) patients died after the operation and all of them were died of cardiac and respiratory complications [7–9, 11, 15]. 16 cases were reported by Langeloo and one of them was a young patient about 30 old years had cardiac arrest after operation 4 days later [8]. He died of hypoxic schemic encephalopathy after 6 weeks. Although the patient had no obvious symptoms of cardiovascular system, AS is a chronic systemic inflammatory disease. It often affects the cardiac conduction system and causes conduction block, atrial fibrillation, and other arrhythmias. Surgery may stimulate potential heart damage triggering cardiac arrest [20].

Simmons' report is the largest sample of cervical and thoracic osteotomy orthopedic study so far [11]. And 4 of 131 patients died within 3 months after operation. Two of them died of heart disease, respectively, on the second day and 21st day after operation. One patient died of pulmonary embolism on 13th day after operation, and one patient died of severe pulmonary infection on 77th day after operation. They thought the main cause of postoperative death was heart and lung disease.

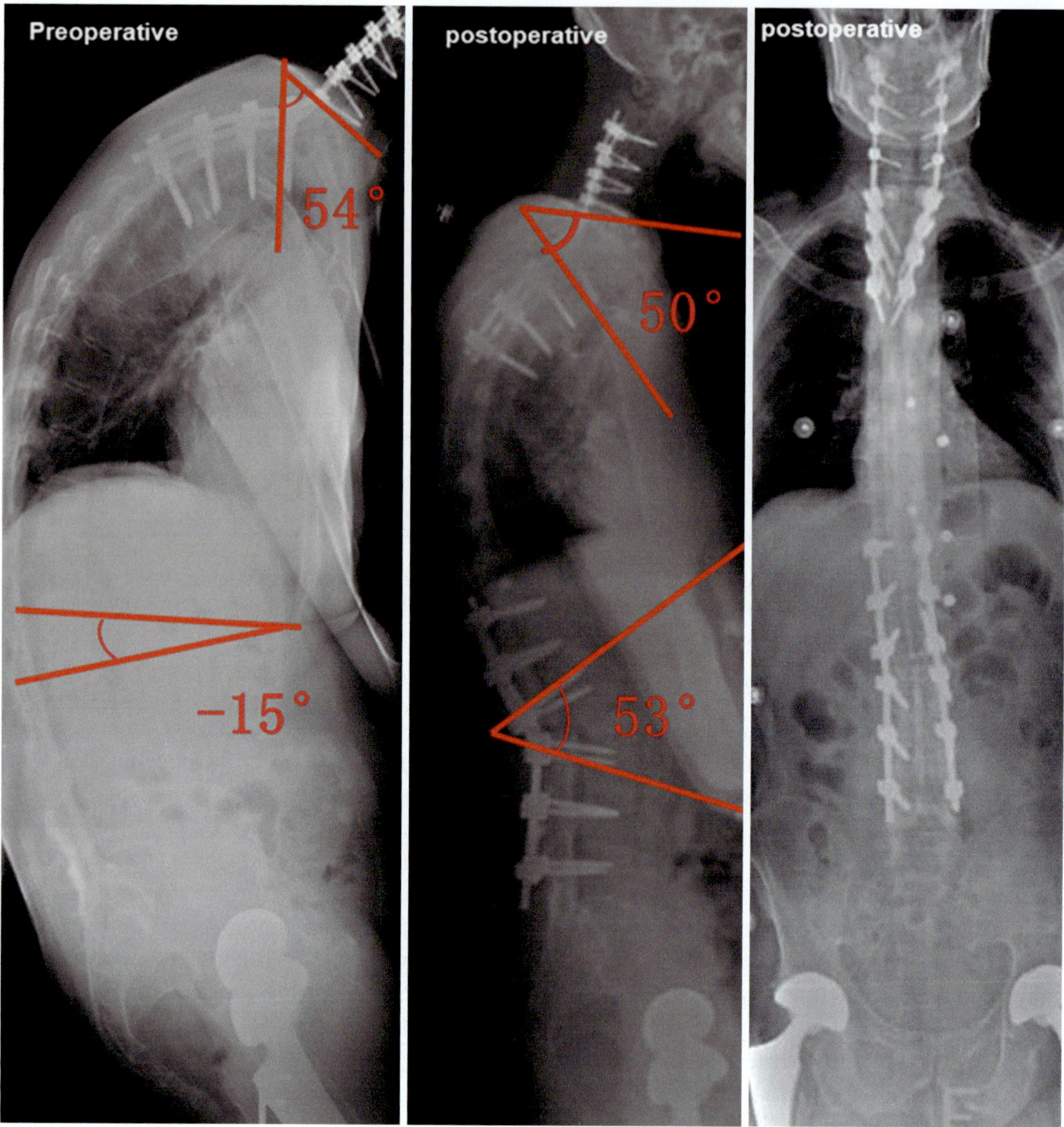

Fig. 11.16 Second postoperative. Before rod breakage, Cobb(C6–T2) = 54°; after rod breakage, Cobb(C6–T2) = 35°; after revision, Cobb(C6–T2) = 50°; lumbar 2 VCD osteotomy correction angle, (−15°) + 53° = 68°

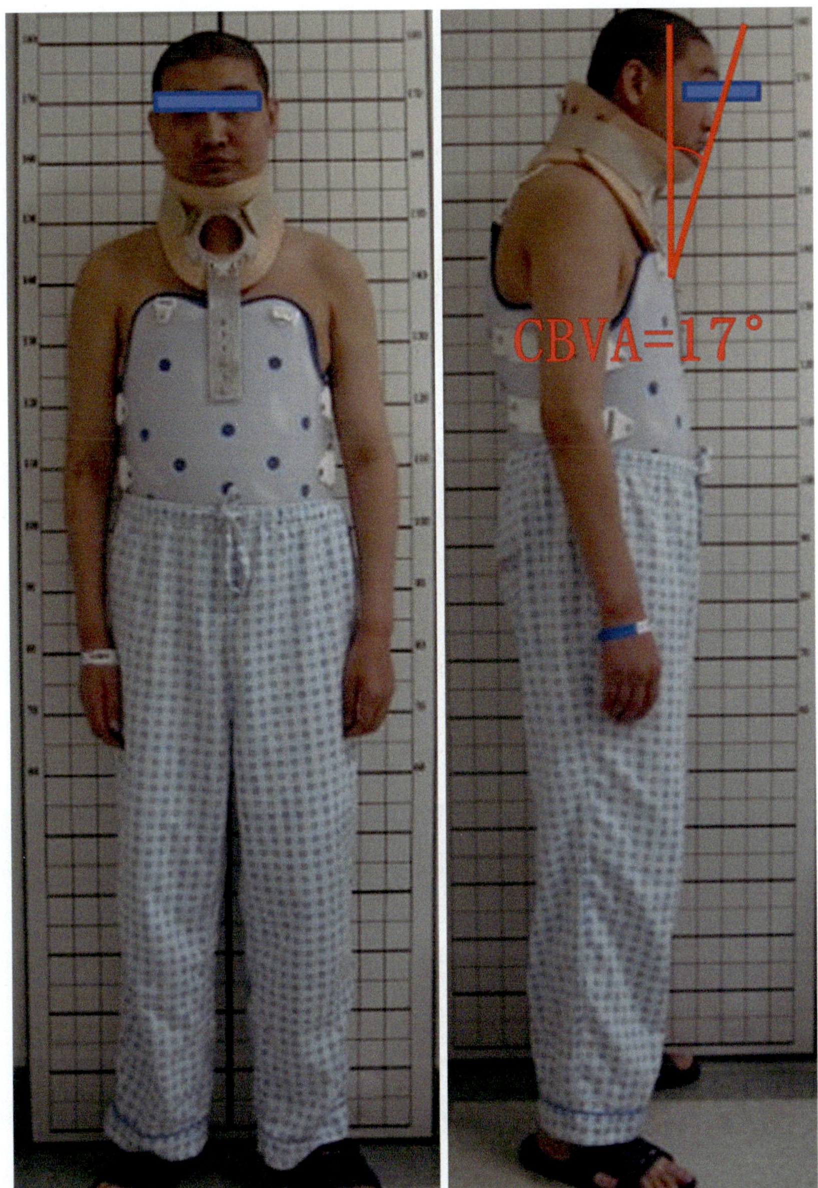

Fig. 11.17 Second postoperative CBVA = 17°

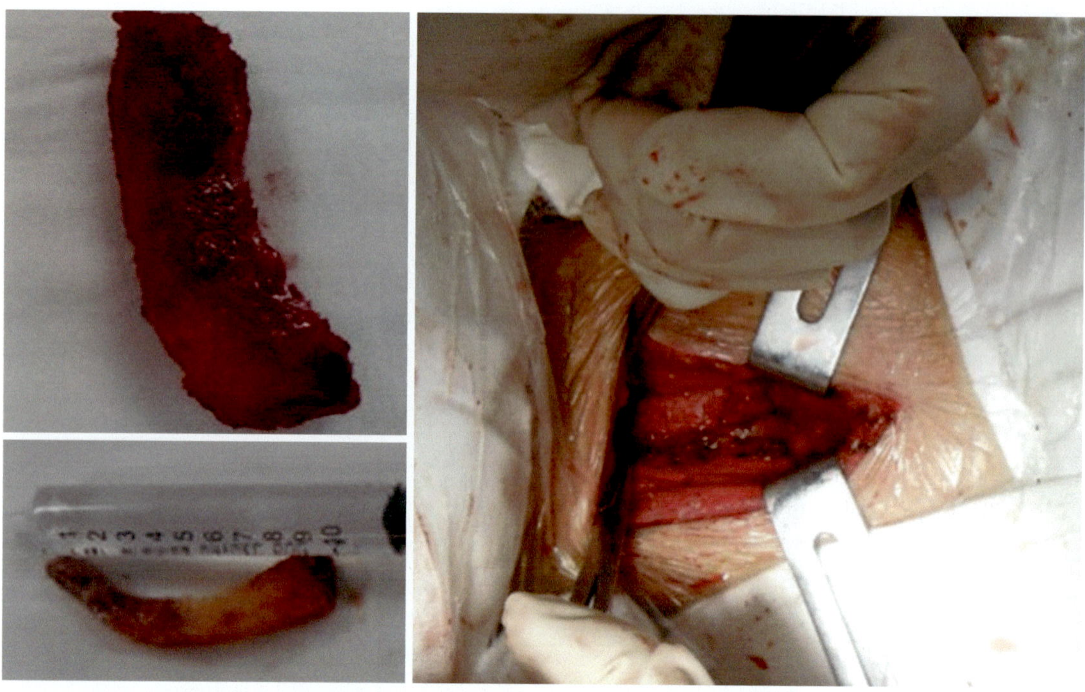

Fig. 11.18 Third operation: anterior cervicothoracic fusion. Anterior C6–T1 vertebral body slotting autogenous iliac bone graft fusion

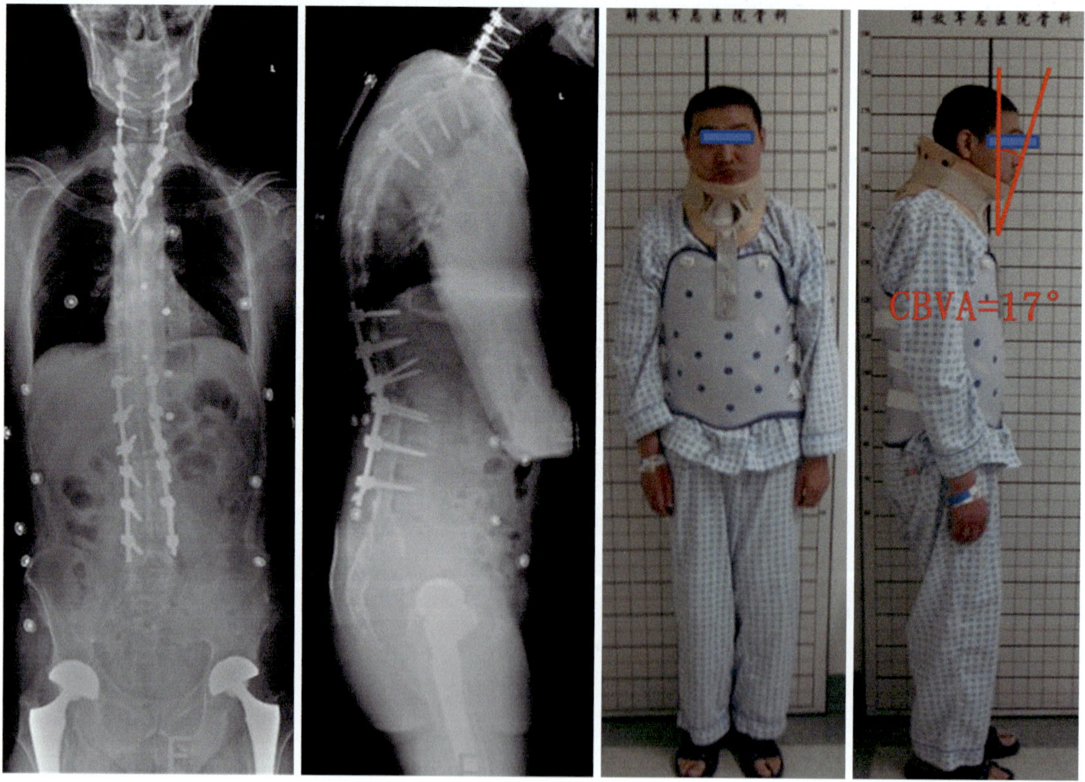

Fig. 11.19 After anterior cervicothoracic fusion

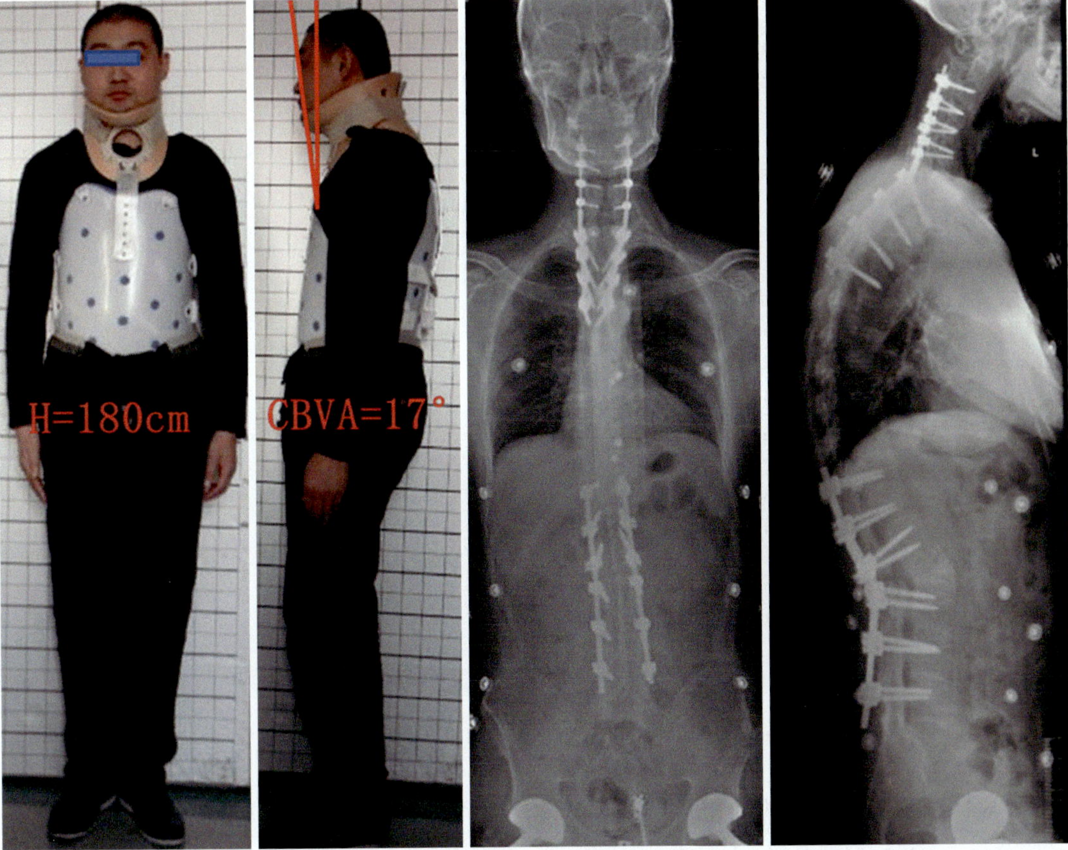

Fig. 11.20 The postoperative follow-up of 3 months

However, these cases occurred before 1997. With the development of mature technique, anesthesia, and postoperative monitoring and the improvement of nursing level, no cases of postoperative death occurred in recent years.

Osteotomy always around the nerve tissue, and it is likely to damage nerve. The temporary instability during osteotomy increased the risk of neurological complications. The possible causes of neurological complications are as follows [21]: (1) osteotomy method is incorrect or sagittal translation during osteotomy. Spinal nerve tissue damaged in the process of drawing; (2) the amount of osteotomy in the intervertebral foramen is not enough. The osteotomy surface compress the C8 nerve root; (3) rupture of the anterior longitudinal ligament osteotomy caused instability or even subluxation. The incidence of neck-thoracic kyphosis postoperative neurological complications in patients was 23.4%. Most of them were mild and temporary C8 nerve root injury symptom [4].

Simmons et al. [11] said halo could be used to relieve the compression of C8 nerve roots' intervertebral foramen. Most patients would be completely relieved after a few months. Belanger [15] reported that three cases of upper limb pain and feeling diminished occurred immediately after operation, and the symptoms were completely relieved within 6 months after the operation.

In about 227 patients enrolled in the five series of clinical trials, only 8 cases (3.5%) had permanent neurological complications including quadriplegia, hemiparesis, and C6 spinal cord permanent damage [7–9, 11, 15]. Simmons et al. [11] reported three patients with severe

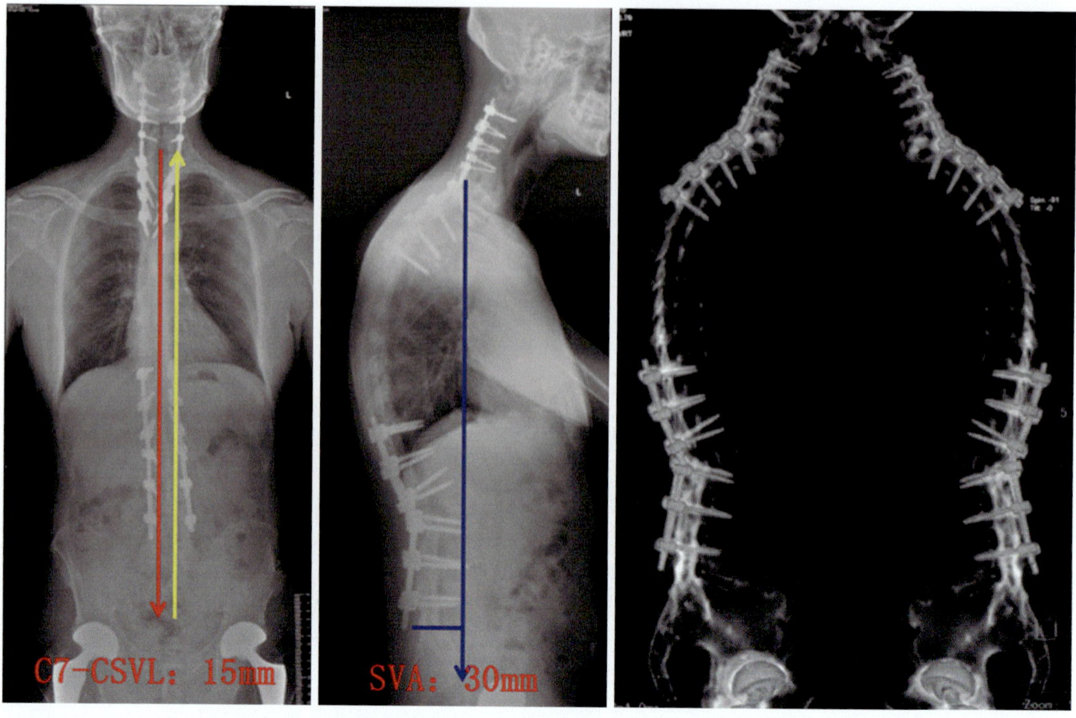

Fig. 11.21 The postoperative 6-month follow-up of X-ray and CT

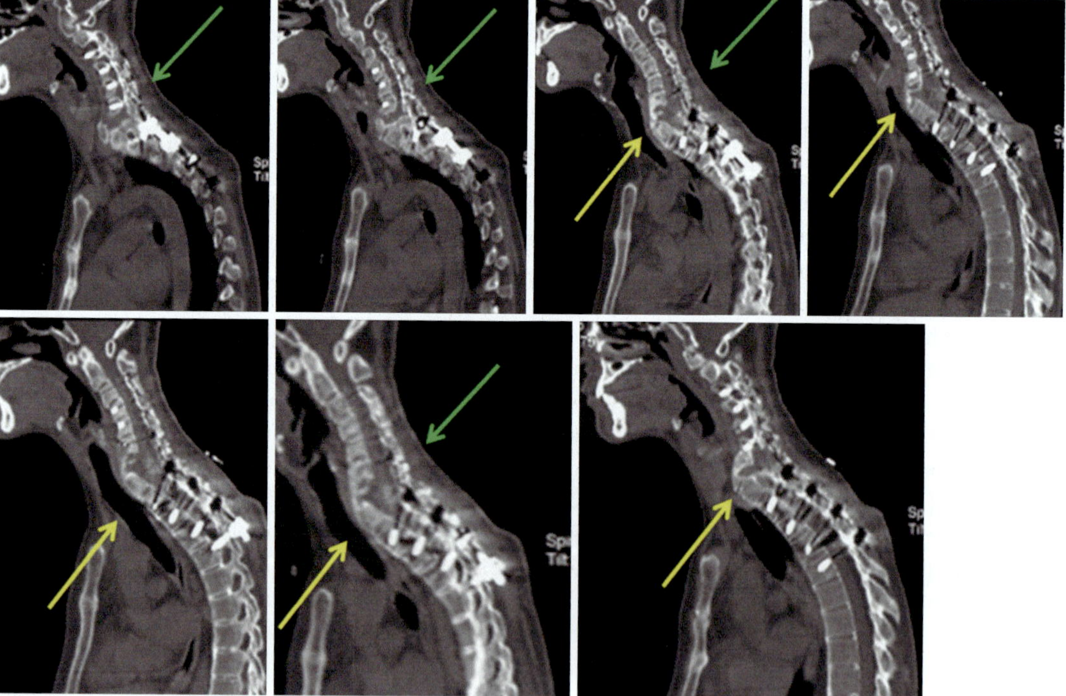

Fig. 11.22 The postoperative 6-month follow-up, good autograft bone fusion

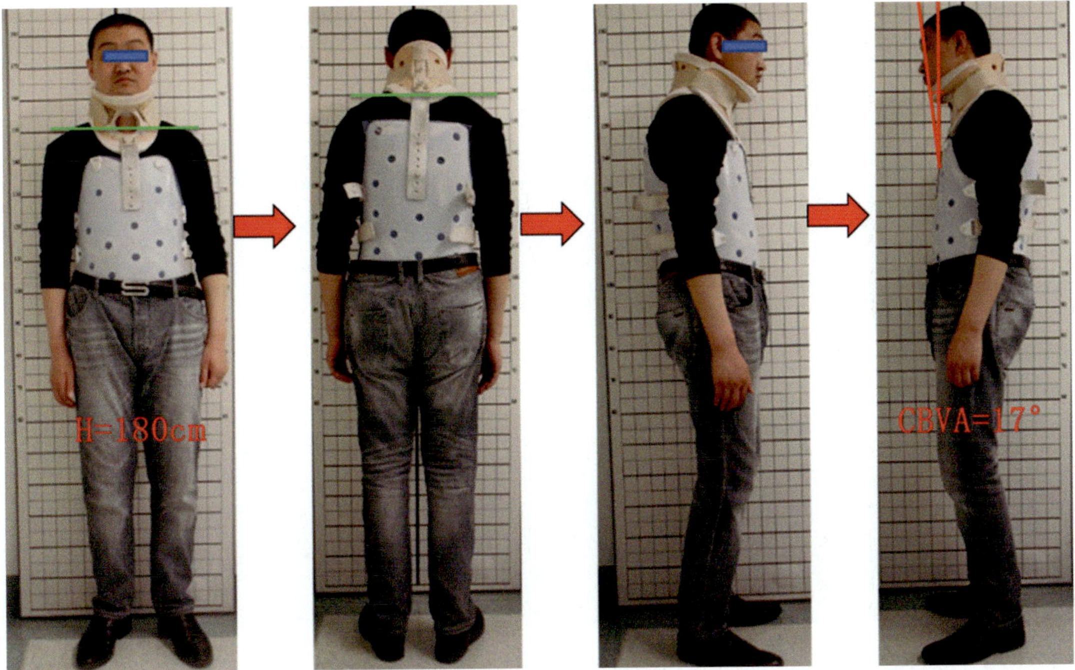

Fig. 11.23 The postoperative 6-month follow-up of clinical appearance

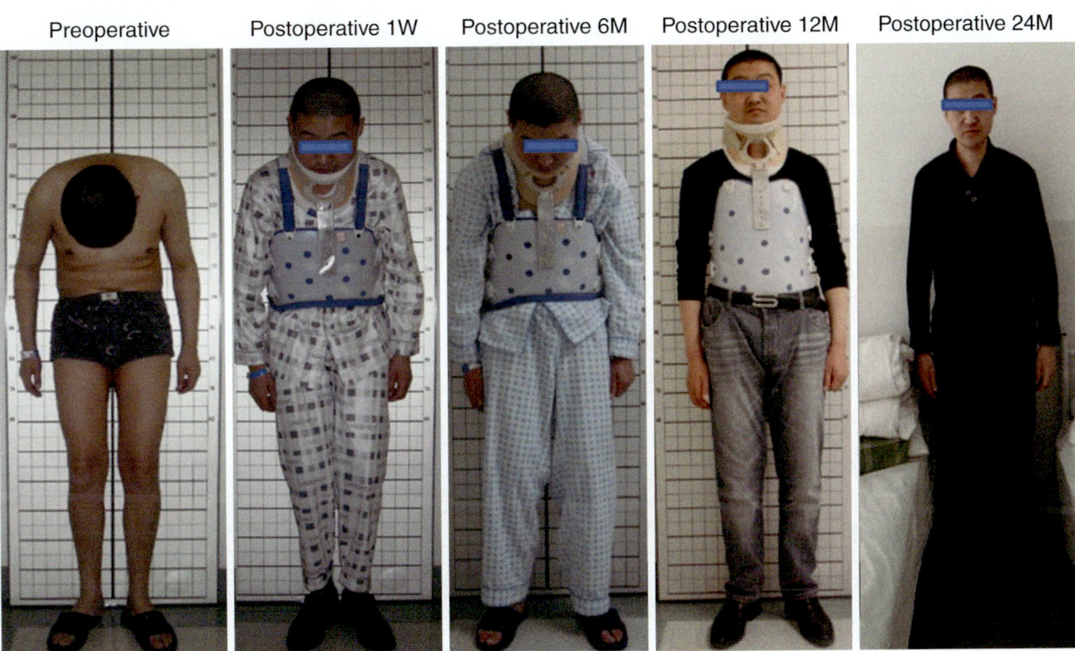

Fig. 11.24 Preoperative and postoperative clinical appearance

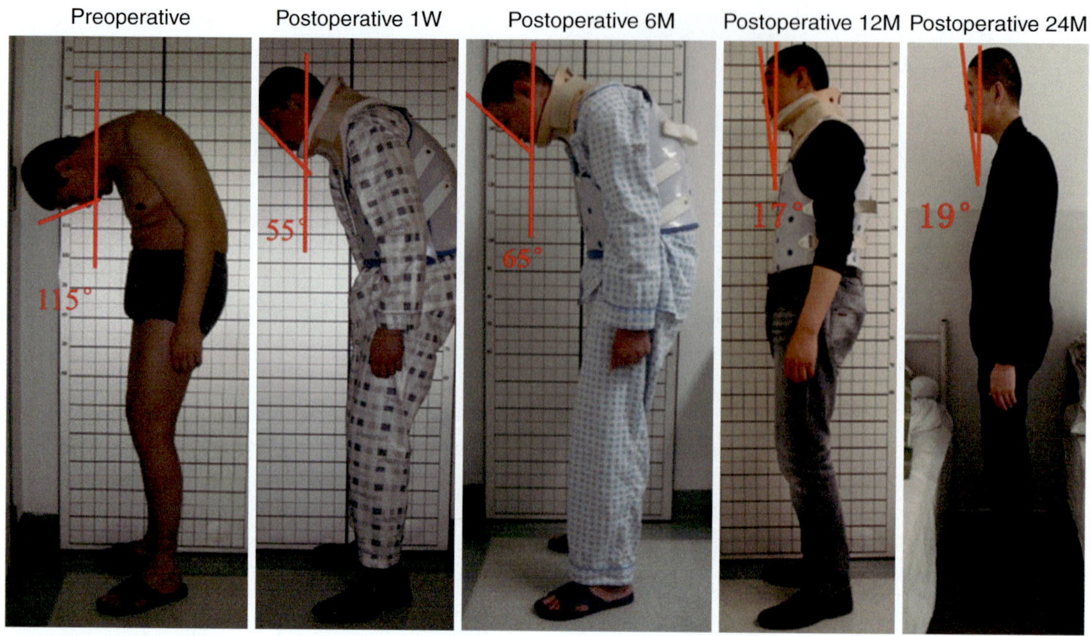

Fig. 11.25 Preoperative and postoperative CBVA data

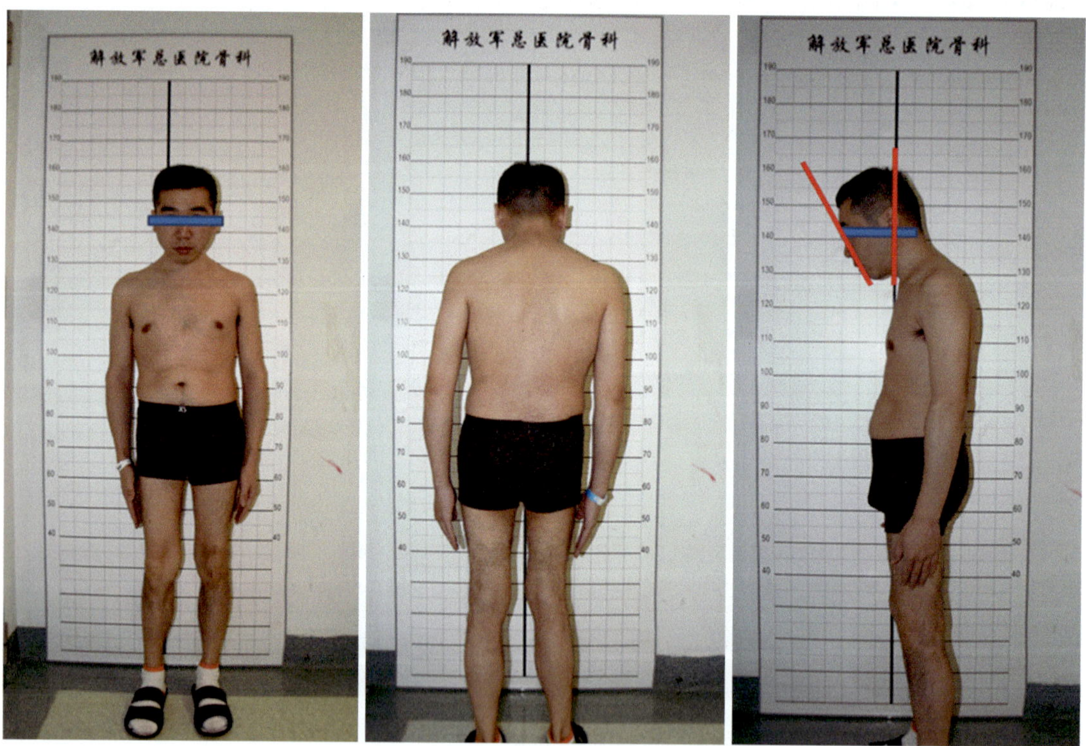

Fig. 11.26 Preoperative clinical appearance (present height, 161 cm; CBVA = 30°)

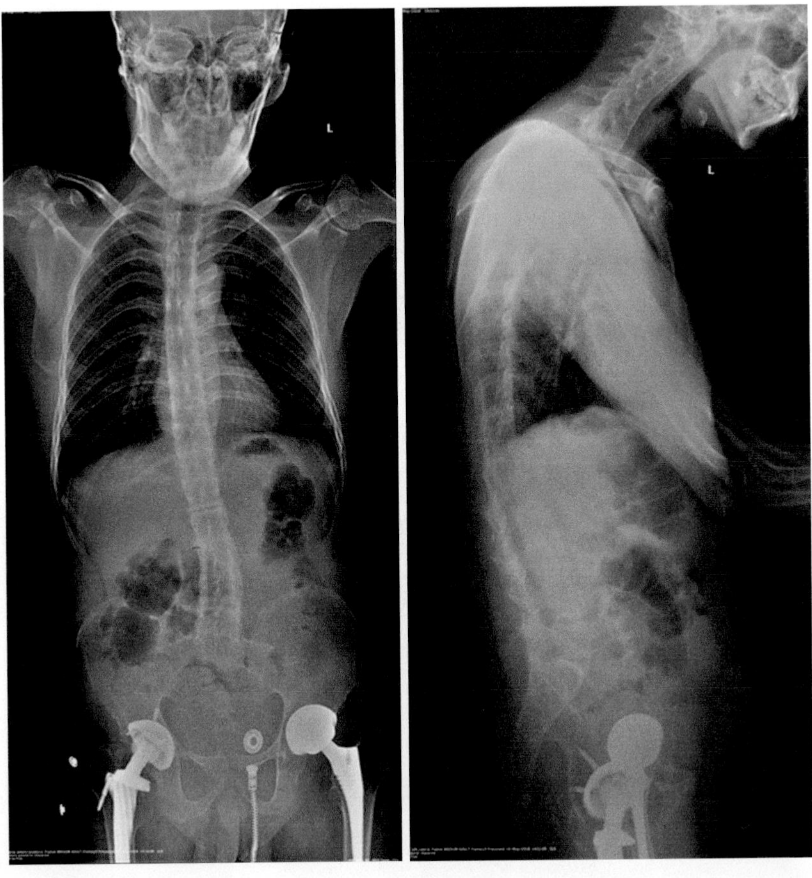

Fig. 11.27 Preoperative X-ray

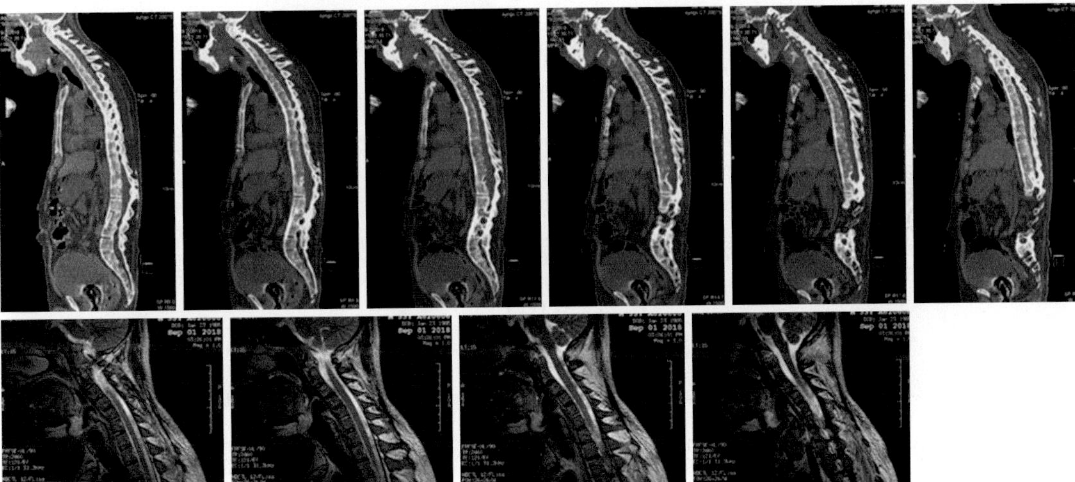

Fig. 11.28 Preoperative CT and MRI

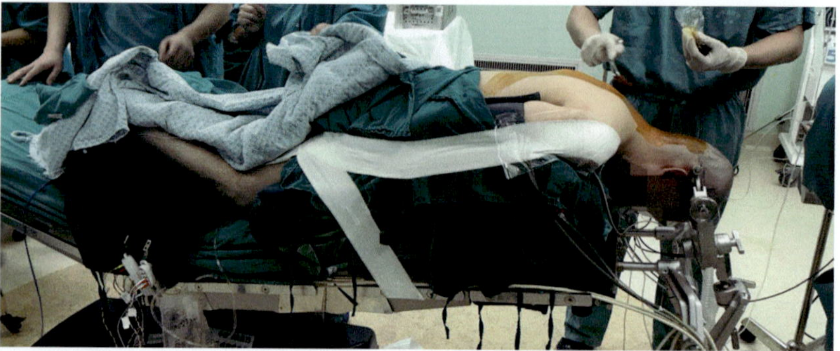

Fig. 11.29 C7 pedicle subtraction osteotomy intraoperative position

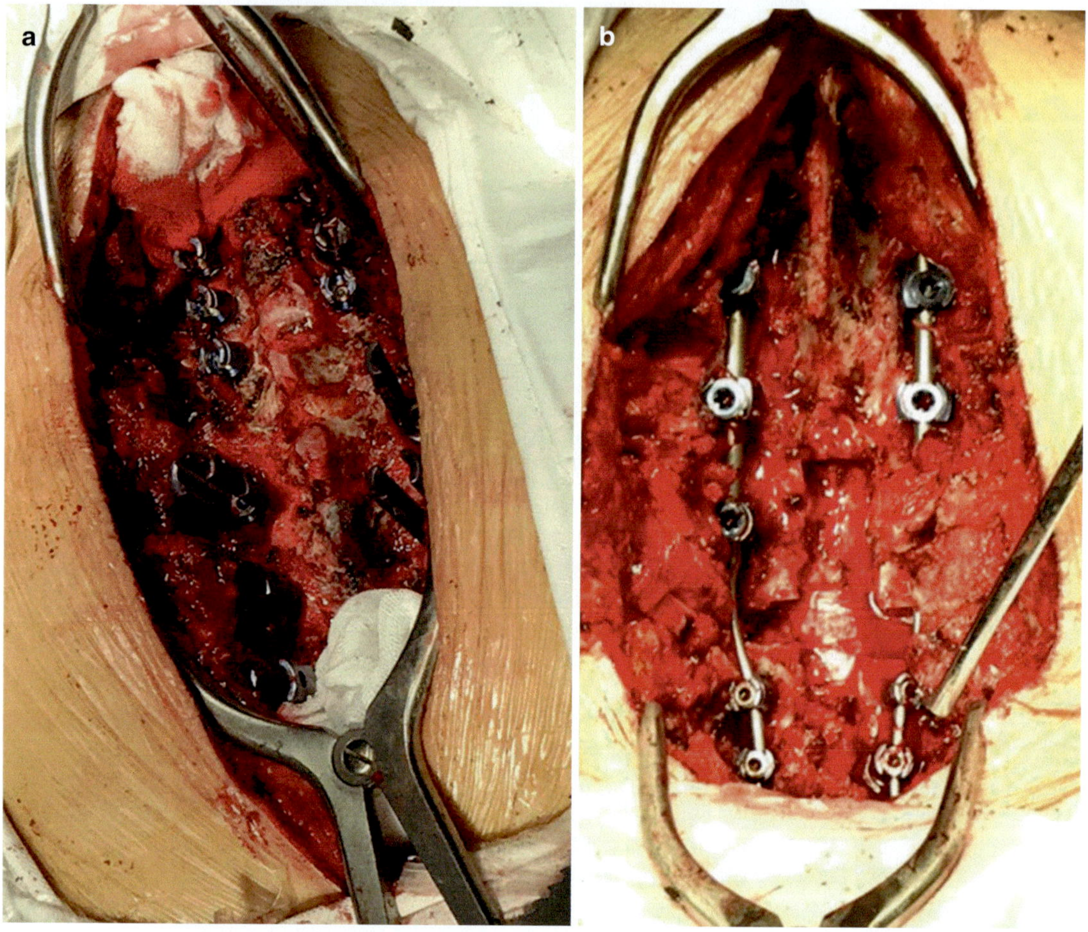

Fig. 11.30 Because the patient needs small orthopedic angle, C7 pedicle subtraction osteotomy was chosen. (**a**) A wide and lengthy exposure (from C3 to T4). C3–C5 lateral mass fixation and T2–T4 pedicle fixation were performed. (**b**) A complete C7 laminectomy and partial laminectomies involving the inferior portion of C6 and the superior portion of T1. Osteotomy surface was closed

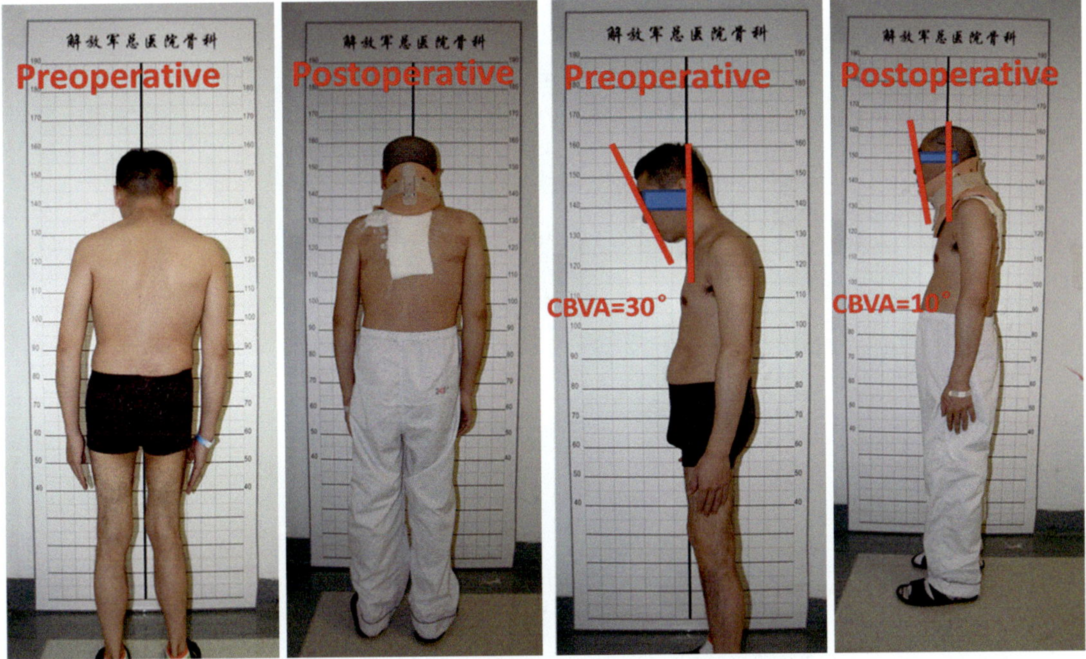

Fig. 11.31 Preoperative and postoperative appearance. No obvious complications occurred after operation

neurological complications. One patient developed paraplegia after operation, and he could stand but not walk. Surgical exploration found ruptured dura ruled. One patient had general paralysis during operation. Surgical exploration in local anesthesia found that the folds of the dura oppressed the spinal cord. After incision decompression, nerve function recovery during operation. McMaster [9] reported one case of a patient having four limbs paralyzed without obvious cause on the seventh day after operation. Not using internal fixation and halo-vest external fixation loose may lead to osteotomy site displacement causing high spinal cord injury. Langeloo [8] reported that an 82 years old patient with preoperative myelopathy was found C6 spinal cord during operation by MEP monitoring. They did anterior cervical decompression immediately, but the neurological function wasn't improved. The movement and sensory function of right C6 and left C7 nerve root-dominated area were lost permanently after surgery.

The incidence of pseudoarthrosis is 0–13.3%. Cases of pseudoarthrosis were treated without internal fixation. The possible reason may be the unstable external fixations caused by subluxation of osteotomy site and the formation of pseudarthrosis [10, 21]. Simmons et al. [11] had documented six patients with the formation of pseudarthrosis, and all of them had re-fusion. McMaster [9] reported two cases of dislocation of the osteotomy site when detected by X-ray 1 week after surgery. After several months of halo head ring traction, there was no improvement in imaging examination. And they did anterior cervical spine graft at the fourth and sixth month, respectively. One of them achieved stable fusion with bone fusion and another fusion failed due to deep infection. They believe that 50% of patients with subluxation of osteotomy site will develop into pseudoarthrosis and they need anterior fusion surgery.

Simmons et al. [11] recorded 131 patients with Cervicothoracic kyphosis deformity, five of them had postoperative pneumonia, 4 cases had deep vein thrombosis resulting in pulmonary embolism, and 15 patients had halo nail infection. McMaster [9] reported three cases of

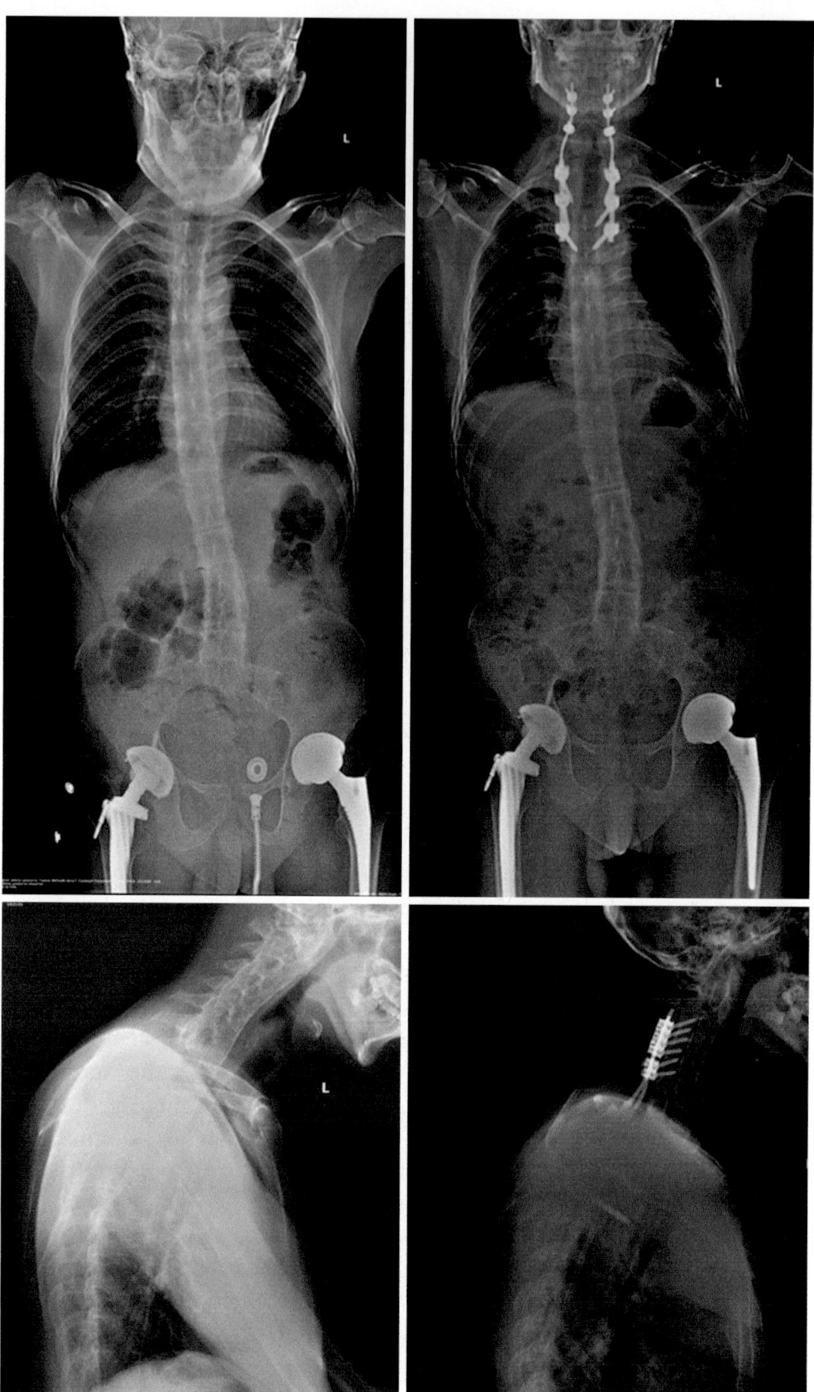

Fig. 11.32 Preoperative and postoperative X-ray

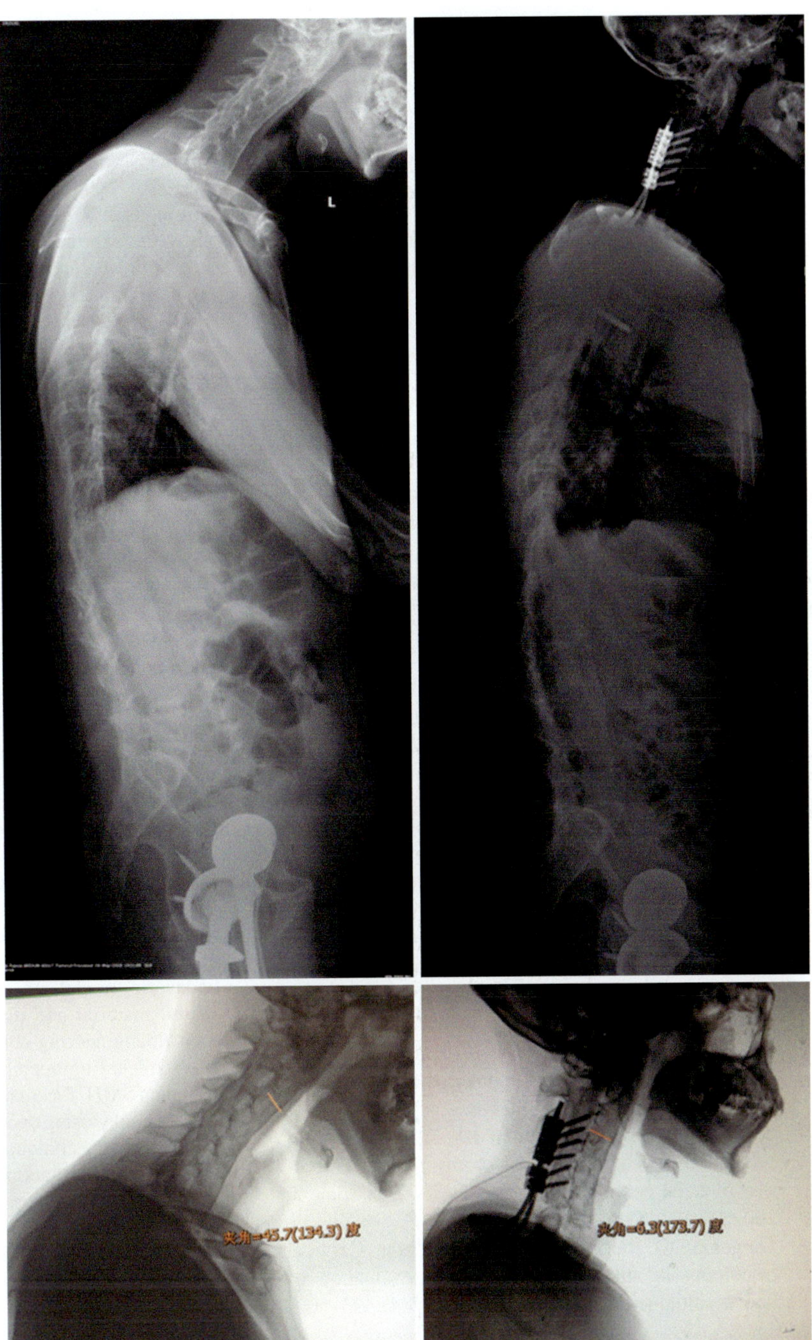

Fig. 11.33 Preoperative Cobb(C3–T4) = 45.7° and postoperative Cobb(C3–T4) = 6.3°

temporary postoperative swallowing difficulty, and they recovered after 10 days. One case had hematemesis and took conservative treatment.

Langeloo et al. [8] reported two deep incision infection cases and one case of viral meningitis. The main reason of deep tissue infection may be the use of hormones and immunosuppression by anti-inflammatory drugs in AS patients and a variety of systemic complications.

References

1. Mehdian SM, Boreham B, Hammett T. Cervical osteotomy in ankylosing spondylitis. Eur Spine J. 2012;21(12):2713–7.
2. Koller H, Meier O, Zenner J, et al. Non-instrumented correction of cervicothoracic kyphosis in ankylosing spondylitis: a critical analysis on the results of open-wedge osteotomy C7-T1 with gradual halo-thoracic-cast based correction. Eur Spine J. 2013;22:819–32.
3. Mehdian S, Arun R. A safe controlled instrumented reduction technique for cervical osteotomy in ankylosing spondylitis. Spine (Phila Pa 1976). 2011;36(9):715–20.
4. Mummaneni PV, Mummaneni VP, Haid RW Jr, et al. Cervical osteotomy for the correction of chin-on-chest deformity in ankylosing spondylitis. Technical note. Neurosurg Focus. 2003;14(1):e9.
5. Chin KR, Ahn J. Controlled cervical extension osteotomy for ankylosing spondylitis utilizing the Jackson operating table: technical note. Spine (Phila Pa 1976). 2007;32(17):1926–9.
6. El Maghraoui A, Bensabbah R, Bahiri R, et al. Cervical spine involvement in ankylosing spondylitis. Clin Rheumatol. 2003;22(2):94–8.
7. Tokala DP, Lam KS, Freeman BJ, et al. C7 decancellisation closing wedge osteotomy for the correction of fixed cervico-thoracic kyphosis. Eur Spine J. 2007;16(9):1471–8.
8. Langeloo DD, Journee HL, Pavlov PW, et al. Cervical osteotomy in ankylosing spondylitis: evaluation of new developments. Eur Spine J. 2006;15(4):493–500.
9. McMaster MJ. Osteotomy of the cervical spine in ankylosing spondylitis. J Bone Joint Surg Br. 1997;79(2):197–203.
10. Etame AB, Than KD, Wang AC, et al. Surgical management of symptomatic cervical or cervicothoracic kyphosis due to ankylosing spondylitis. Spine (Phila Pa 1976). 2008;33(16):E559–64.
11. Simmons ED, DiStefano RJ, Zheng Y, et al. Thirty-six years experience of cervical extension osteotomy in ankylosing spondylitis: techniques and outcomes. Spine (Phila Pa 1976). 2006;31(26):3006–12.
12. Urist MR. Osteotomy of the cervical spine; report of a case of ankylosing rheumatoid spondylitis. J Bone Joint Surg Am. 1958;40-A(4):833–43.
13. Sengupta DK, Khazim R, Grevitt MP, et al. Flexion osteotomy of the cervical spine: a new technique for correction of iatrogenic extension deformity in ankylosing spondylitis. Spine. 2001;26(9): 1068–72.
14. Schneider PS, Bouchard J, Moghadam K, et al. Acute cervical fractures in ankylosing spondylitis: an opportunity to correct preexisting deformity. Spine. 2010;35(7):248–52.
15. Belanger TA, Milam RA, Roh JS, et al. Cervicothoracic extension osteotomy for chin-on-chest deformity in ankylosing spondylitis. J Bone Joint Surg Am. 2005;87(8):1732–8.
16. Gill JB, Levin A, Burd T, et al. Corrective osteotomies in spine surgery. J Bone Joint Surg Am. 2008;90(11):2509–20.
17. Scheer JK, Tang JA, Buckley JM, et al. Biomechanical analysis of osteotomy type and rod diameter for treatment of cervicothoracic kyphosis. Spine. 2011;36(8):519–23.
18. Scheer JK, Tang JA, Deviren V, et al. Biomechanical analysis of cervicothoracic junction osteotomy in cadaveric model of ankylosing spondylitis: effect of rod material and diameter. In: ASME 2010 summer bioengineering conference. American Society of Mechanical Engineers; 2010.
19. Mehdian SMH, Freeman BJC, Licina P. Cervical osteotomy for ankylosing spondylitis: an innovative variation on an existing technique. Eur Spine J. 1999;8(6):505–9.
20. Rosenbaum J, Chandran V. Management of comorbidities in ankylosing spondylitis. Am J Med Sci. 2012;343(5):364.
21. Hoh DJ, Khoueir P, Wang MY. Management of cervical deformity in ankylosing spondylitis. Neurosurg Focus. 2008;24(1):E9.

Part IV

Complication and Nursing in AS Patients

12 Intraoperative Nursing and Position in Spinal Osteotomy

Chunguo Wang and Youhao Zhang

Spinal kyphosis deformity is the secondary posture change caused by the late stage of ankylosing spondylitis. The deformity of the spine in the sagittal plane seriously affects the life quality of AS patients. Satisfactory surgical position is significant for the degree of kyphosis correction related with ankylosing spondylitis. Intraoperative position nursing care is the key to ensure the safety of patients, reduce surgical complications, and improve the effect of surgical correction.

1 Introduction

Ankylosing spondylitis (AS) is an unidentified systemic disease characterized by chronic inflammatory reaction of the axial skeleton and affects mostly among young adults in their second through fourth decades of life. The ratio of the prevalence of AS in male and female is 3:1. The main clinical manifestations are stiffness or pain in the lower back. Spinal lesions are progressively aggravated so that the rigidity, deformity, and dysfunction of spinal column seriously affect life quality of the late-stage patients [1]. The secondary posture change caused by ankylosing spondylitis is kyphotic deformity or flexion contracture of hips which significantly worsen with duration of the disease. Torso appearance of the patients with severe AS may be C-shaped or even L-shaped, resulting in impairment of the ability to stand upright and reduction of the visual field, respiratory function, balance, sitting position, swallowing function, and ambulation [2]. Osteotomy is the main treatment of late-stage AS to remove the physical or mental anguish of patients caused by deformity and dysfunction of spine and joints. Prone position is commonly used in spinal operation, with advantages of full field of vision and facilitating relevant surgical operations. But this position may lead to such physiological changes as circulatory and respiratory disorders and nerve and skin compression injury. Satisfactory surgical position could maintain smooth breathing and good circulation as well as avoid peripheral nerve injury and excessive traction of skeleton and muscles.

2 Preoperative Care

2.1 Preoperative Visit

Routine visits were usually made to relieve the anxiety of the patients, and the patients were given a certain understanding of the surgical operation through explanations so that the patient could actively cooperate with medical personnels. Grasp the patient's general

C. Wang · Y. Zhang (✉)
Department of Orthopedics, Chinese PLA General Hospital, Beijing, China
e-mail: zhangyouhao@allinmd.cn

Y. Wang (ed.), *Surgical Treatment of Ankylosing Spondylitis Deformity*,
https://doi.org/10.1007/978-981-13-6427-3_12

information by communicating with the surgeon, and make a preliminary assessment of the patient's physical condition, nutritional status, skin condition, surgical indication, and estimated operating time. Make a knowledge about the extent of the patient's disease, the patient's posture, the segment of the lesions (thoracolumbar spine or combined with hip joints), the degree of kyphosis, the activity of the cervical spine and limbs, or whether there is any chronic disease (such as diabetes, cardiovascular disease, etc.). Make a good preoperative evaluation by understanding the patients' body mass, height, daily activity, and functional position of the lesion segment in the patient's prone position to establish a safety criterion for postanesthetic position placement (Fig. 12.1).

2.2 Preoperative Preparation

On the day of surgery, cushioning the patient's ankle and knee joints, ilium, and armpits, the operating room nurse could send the patient to the operating room on the mobile sickbed with active position (usually in lateral decubitus position). The operating room temperature should be set between 22 and 26 °C. A vein channel is established in the left forearm to ensure that the infusion tubes are unbended and the fluid is unobstructed in the prone position. Circuit nurses cooperate with the anesthesiologist to perform internal jugular vein catheterization and radial artery invasive blood pressure monitoring. Patients cannot lie flat because of kyphotic deformity and stiff joints. Therefore, when the patient lies supine, the front part of the

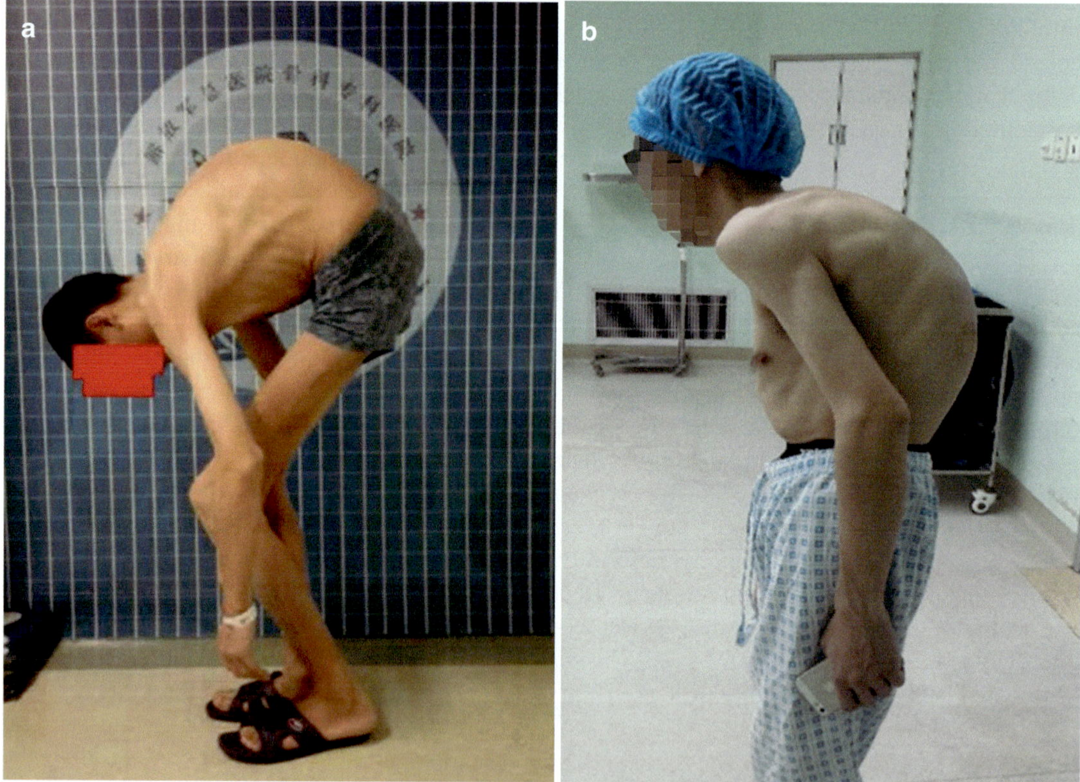

Fig. 12.1 (**a**, **b**) Visiting nurses should know about the different degrees of kyphosis, the activity of spine and large joints, and the segment of lesions during preoperative visit

sickbed should be lifted up and the patient's head and lower limbs cushioned with sponge pads. With his head and lower limbs padded, the patient could maintain the functional position of the vertebral alignment (Fig. 12.2). Tracheal intubation may be performed with patients of good cervical motion and large mouth opening in this position. If necessary, they can be intubated or transnasally intubated with fiber-optic bronchoscopes. After intubation, remove the pillow under the patient's buttocks, and place another one behind his back in a semi-sitting position.

3 Operative Position Nursing Care

When placed in prone position, the patient's own body mass has a great impact on the respiratory system, and severe cases such as refractory hypoxia and carbon dioxide accumulation may occur. At the same time, a prone position may increase abdominal pressure. Changes in abdominal pressure may influence airway pressure and cause intraoperative blood loss as a result of epidural venous congestion [3]. The main stress points are ribs, the anterior superior iliac spine, the bilateral knees, and the anterior border of tibia in this bow-shaped prone position. The smaller area is less tolerated since the entire weight of the body is concentrated on these sites where bone bulges or thin muscles and fat adhere to. These parts should be scrupulously protected to avoid pressure sores caused by longtime compression. All surgeries were performed with somatosensory-evoked potentials and transcranial motor-evoked potentials for neurophysiologic monitoring to detect whether there exists spinal cord injury or not [4].

In case of spinal cord injury, each part of the patient's body should be carefully supported to enable the head, neck, and vertebral column to remain in the functional position and rotate synchronously when the body position is changed, for the patient's whole muscles being relaxed under general anesthesia. Small gaskets should be properly placed on these sites to prevent skin pressure injury, where often bone bulges or thin muscles and fat adhere to, such as the front side of the acromion, bilateral ribs, anterior superior iliac spine, knees, etc. Pay attention to protecting the head, neck, shoulders, and elbows. Padded with a sponge under the armpit, the upper limbs are flexed and placed on braces fixed on both sides of the operating table [5].

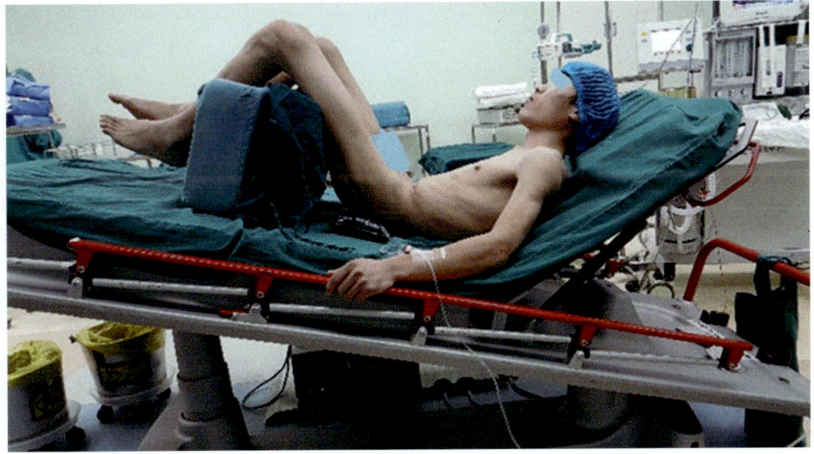

Fig. 12.2 Patient positioning supine on the sickbed with lower limbs, buttocks, and head padded to maintain the functional position of the vertebral alignment

Do not abduct the shoulders more than 90° to prevent pressure or stretch on the brachial plexus to avoid nerve injuries. Bilateral breasts of female patients should be protected from being compressed whereas external genitalia of male patients being crushed to avoid injury (Fig. 12.3).

Put adequate soft pillows under the chest and abdomen according to the degree of kyphosis, ensuring the stability of this position and the safety of the follow-up operation. If necessary, the cushions could be added or reduced depending on demands of the surgery (Fig. 12.4).

The patient lies prone with his head put on the headrest. The head tilts slightly forward, and the neck is straightened to avoid overextension or overflexion which could cause obstruction of the respiratory tract. If the head is twisted 90° to the side, the contralateral vertebral artery will be completely occluded to be prone to cerebral ischemia and cerebral thrombosis. Adjust the height of the headrest and the

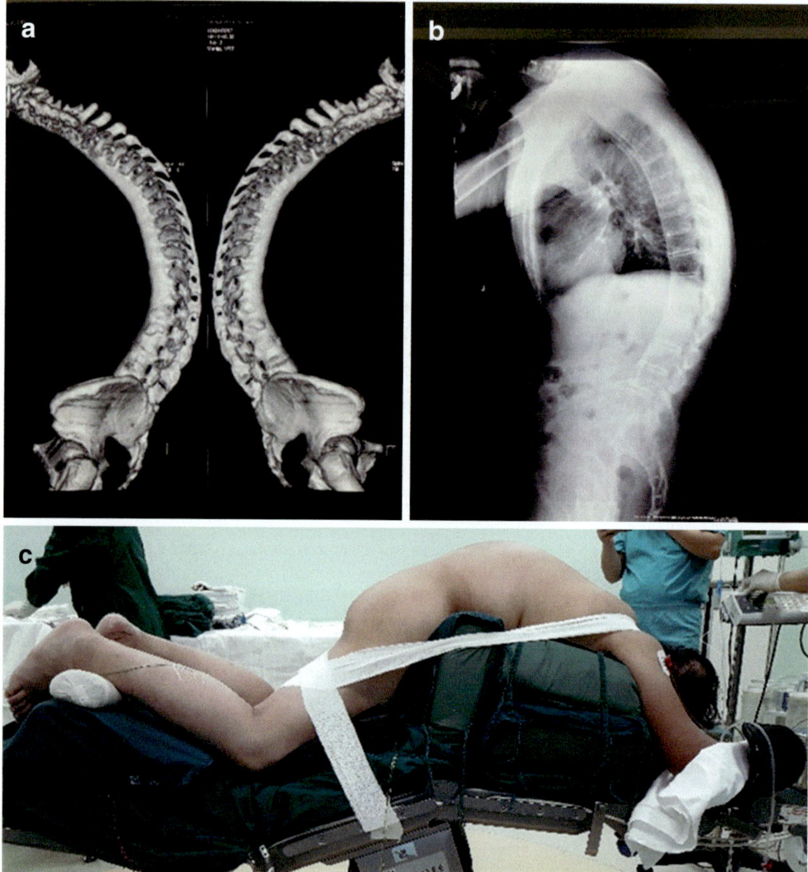

Fig. 12.3 A 35-year-old man was admitted with mild AS kyphosis deformity. (**a**) A preoperative CT three-dimensional reconstruction view that clearly shows bony anatomy of kyphosis. (**b**) A preoperative lateral radiograph of patient with single thoracolumbar stiffness treated with VCD osteotomy. (**c**) Under general anesthesia, the patient was placed prone on a radiolucent operating table depending on the degree of fixed kyphosis

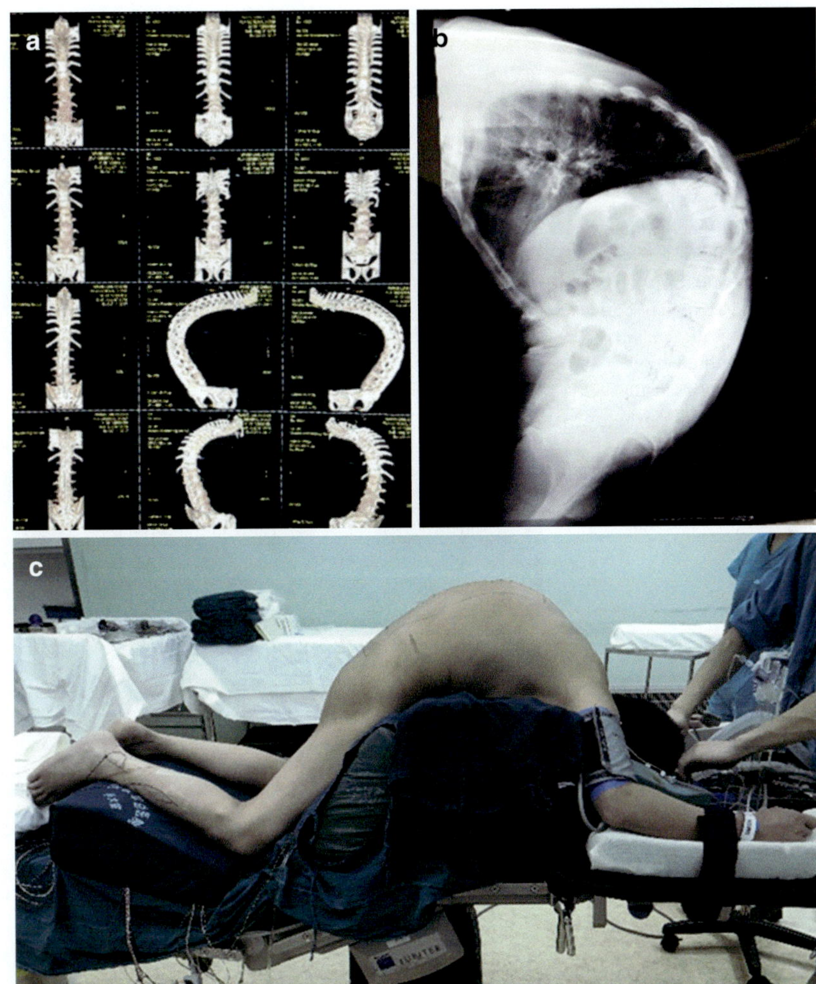

Fig. 12.4 Severe AS kyphosis deformity of a 39-year-old man. (**a**) Preoperative CT three-dimensional reconstructions best delineate the anatomical pathology. (**b**) A preoperative standing lateral radiograph in patient with AS. (**c**) According to the significant thoracolumbar curve, position the patient prone on an operating table with the arms carefully supported and the elbows padded

prone position bracket to an appropriate one depending on the cervical curve. Select the forehead, cheeks, and mandible to be the supporting points of the head and the face to avoid direct compression of the malar bone. At the same time, the patient's lips should be protected when his jaw is supported. Carefully pad the pressure points. The upper pads of the frame should rest on the chest and not in the axilla to avoid pressure on any nerves from the brachial plexus [6] (Fig. 12.5).

Adjust the stress points according to pressure conditions. Apply chlortetracycline ointment and protection film for eye protection. Put the cotton balls into the external auditory meatus to prevent the active iodine from dripping into the ear when the patient's skin is disinfected. In the prone position, venous congestion in the head leads to insufficient blood supply of the visual organs. If the eyelids are in contact with the headrest with the eyeballs pressed for a long time, it will cause congestion and edema of the conjunctiva and

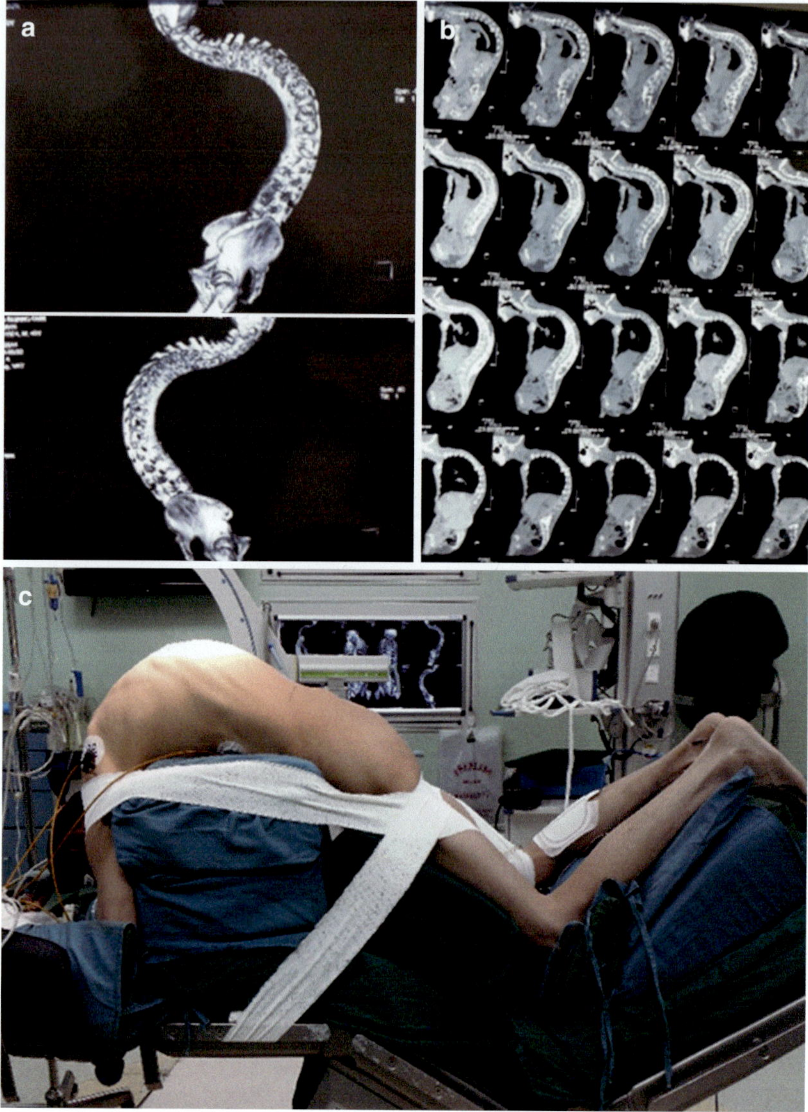

Fig. 12.5 A 40-year-old man with mild cervical and thoracolumbar stiffness. (**a**) Preoperative CT three-dimensional reconstruction evaluation of what was presumed to be routine AS scheduled for surgical osteotomy. (**b**) A preoperative CT scan in patient with AS. (**c**) Padded with cushions and fixed with elastic bands, the patient was positioned on an operating table to fit the curve of superior segment of vertebral column

even blindness in spite of the fact that to be blind is a rare complication after surgery. What we need is a half-hour inspection of the patient's eyes to see whether they are under pressure or not to avoid injury of eyes and distortion of the endotracheal tube. Tongs would be used to make the patient's head fixed to the operating table when it comes to the fact of severe cervical and thoracolumbar kyphosis deformity (Fig. 12.6).

Lateral decubitus position would be used in patient with severe thoracolumbar stiffness and hip rigidity before hip replacement is performed (Fig. 12.7). It will easily lead to upper airway obstruction if the patient's neck is flexed excessively when placed in the kneeling prone position [7]. When placing the body position, the neck and chest should be avoided from compression. The patient's upper limb should be placed on

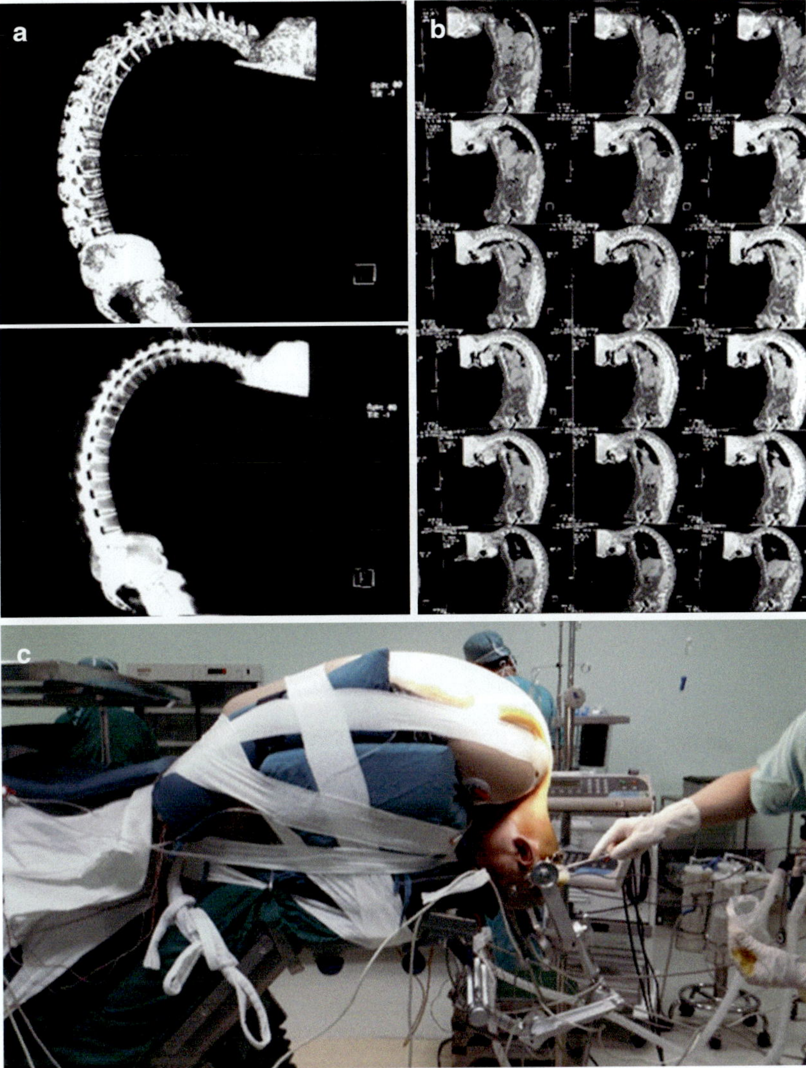

Fig. 12.6 A 34-year-old man with severe cervical stiffness. (**a**) Preoperative CT three-dimensional reconstruction evaluation has been described to offer guidance with bony osteotomy in deformity. (**b**) A preoperative CT scan in patient delineating the anatomical pathology. (**c**) The patient was placed prone with tongs applied to fix the head to the operating table because of severe cervical and thoracolumbar kyphosis deformity

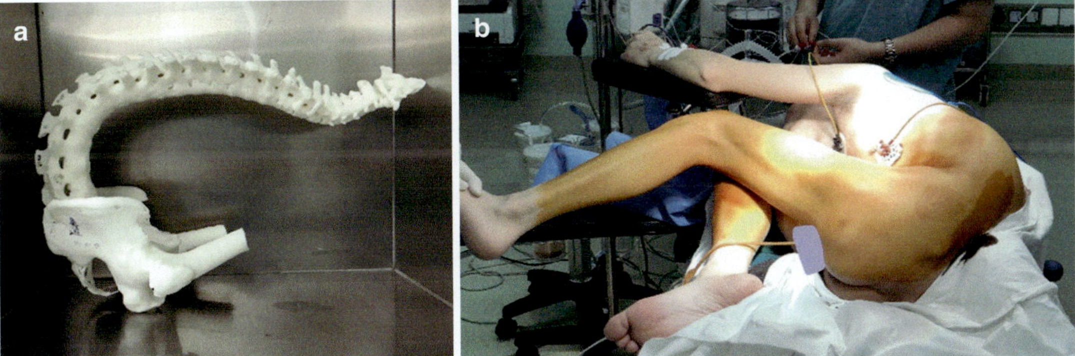

Fig. 12.7 A 36-year-old man with severe thoracolumbar stiffness and hip rigidity. (**a**) A model of the patient's spinal column and hip joints with the use of 3D printing technology. (**b**) The patient positioning on the operating table

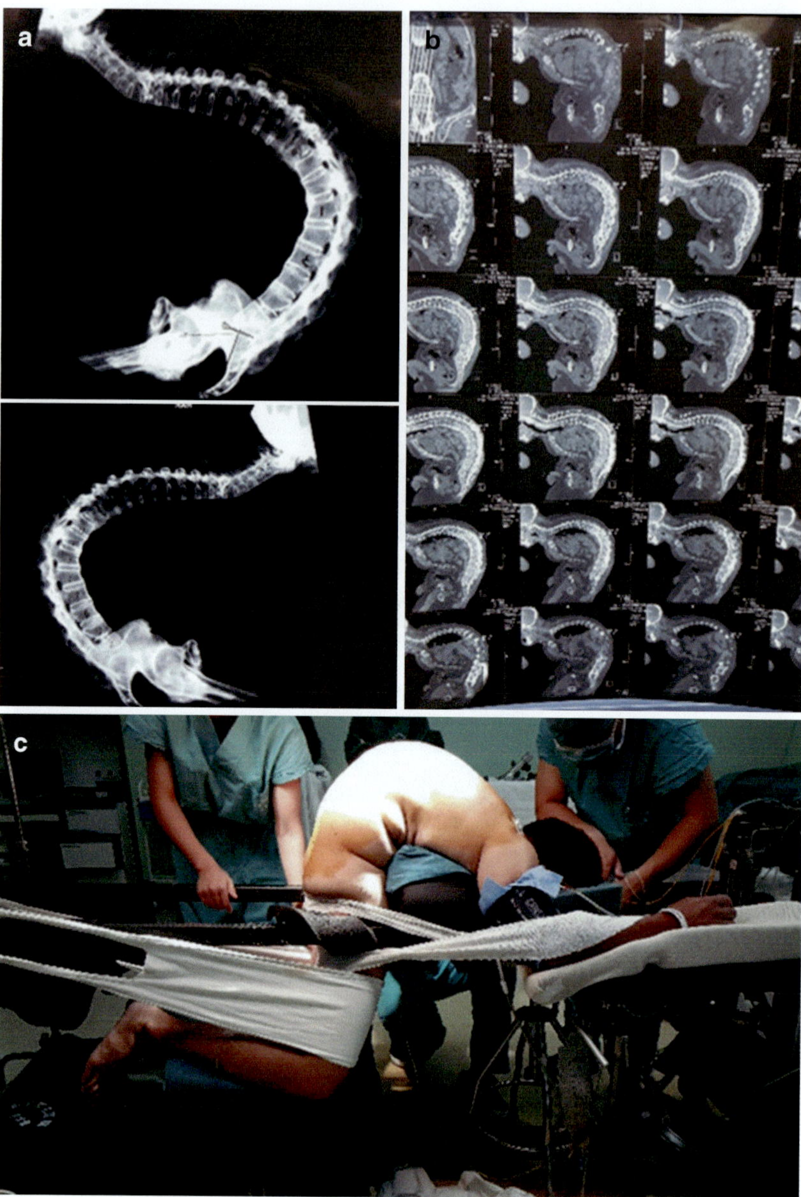

Fig. 12.8 Severe AS kyphosis deformity of a 32-year-old man. (**a**) Preoperative CT three-dimensional reconstructions delineating the anatomical pathology. (**b**) A CT scan in patient with thoracolumbar kyphosis deformity. (**c**) According to the significant thoracolumbar curve, position the patient kneeling prone on an operating table with the arms carefully supported and the elbows padded

both sides or placed on the palm rest. So a soft pad would be used to support the patient's chest and abdomen and a hip support frame to prop up the patient's buttocks, exposing the lumbosacral region [8] (Fig. 12.8).

4 Conclusion

Surgical position is directly related to the extent of operation visual field when the patient is undergoing surgery. It is advantageous to perform operation, reduce the difficulty, and shorten the time of operation, which is vital to the patient's safety. Prolonged operation time can cause skin indentation, redness, blisters, and even skin necrosis. Circulation and respiration will be affected due to ventral compression, lower limb sagging, and hyperextension and hyperflexion of the neck. The correct surgical position could not only reveal the operative field well but also has a close relationship with the success of surgery and the recovery of patients after surgery.

This study was approved by the Institutional Review Board of the hospital, and all participating subjects provided written informed consent for the study.

References

1. Kubiak EN, Moskovich R, Errico TJ, Di Cesare PE. Orthopaedic management of ankylosing spondylitis. J Am Acad Orthop Surg. 2005;13(4):267–78.
2. Hu W, Yu J, Liu H, Zhang X, Wang Y. Y shape osteotomy in ankylosing spondylitis, a prospective case series with minimum 2 year follow-up. PLoS One. 2016;11(12):e0167792.
3. Koh JC, Lee JS, Han DW, Choi S, Chang CH. Increase in airway pressure resulting from prone position patient placing may predict intraoperative surgical blood loss. Spine (Phila Pa 1976). 2013;38(11):E678–82.
4. Kamel I, Zhao H, Koch SA, Brister N, Barnette RE. The use of somatosensory evoked potentials to determine the relationship between intraoperative arterial blood pressure and intraoperative upper extremity position-related neurapraxia in the prone surrender position during spine surgery: a retrospective analysis. Anesth Analg. 2016;122(5):1423–33.
5. Khandelwal A, Mahajan C, Sameera V, Prabhakar H, Kapoor I. Intraoperative blood pressure discrepancy between arms during prone position! J Neurosurg Anesthesiol. 2018;30(1):80–1.
6. Jahangiri FR, Holmberg A, Vega-Bermudez F, Arlet V. Preventing position-related brachial plexus injury with intraoperative somatosensory evoked potentials and transcranial electrical motor evoked potentials during anterior cervical spine surgery. Am J Electroneurodiagnostic Technol. 2011;51(3):198–205.
7. Benfanti PL, Geissele AE. The effect of intraoperative hip position on maintenance of lumbar lordosis: a radiographic study of anesthetized patients and unanesthetized volunteers on the Wilson frame. Spine (Phila Pa 1976). 1997;22(19):2299–303.
8. Lang SS, Eskioglu E, Mericle RA. Intraoperative angiography for neurovascular disease in the prone or three-quarter prone position. Surg Neurol. 2006;65(3):283–9; discussion 289.

13 Sagittal Translation During Osteotomy

Xuesong Zhang, Fanqi Hu, Yongyu Hao, and Yan Wang

1 Definition

Sagittal translation (ST) is an accidental event that surgeons commonly encounter during spinal osteotomy in ankylosing spondylitis kyphosis. As a displacement developed at the level of osteotomy intraoperatively and postoperatively, sagittal translation (ST) had been recorded in all of the osteotomy methods [1–4] since Chang et al. [5] first reported it in spinal osteotomy surgery (Fig. 13.1).

For example, in the procedures of PSO, the correction is obtained through closing the osteotomy wedge which hinges at the anterior column of the vertebral body. However, this procedure releases three column of the spine and leads to unrestricted movement of the anterior column hinge. If the hinge moved during surgery, a displacement of vertebral column called sagittal translation (ST) might occur at the osteotomy site (Fig. 13.2).

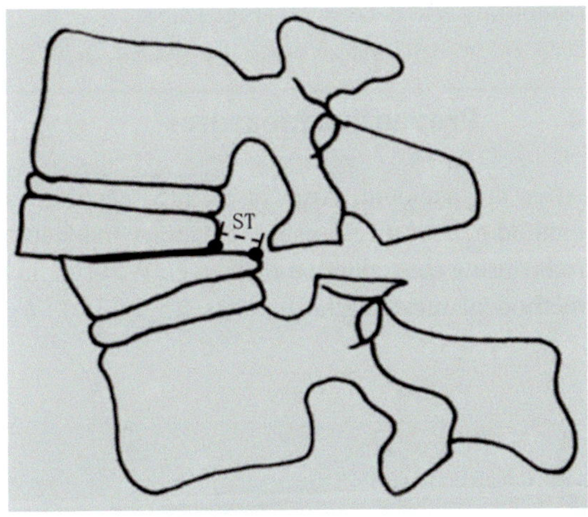

Fig. 13.1 Radiographs in a patient with kyphosis due to ankylosing spondylitis after pedicle subtraction osteotomy to correct the deformity. Significant sagittal translation (ST) was observed after closure of the osteotomized vertebra

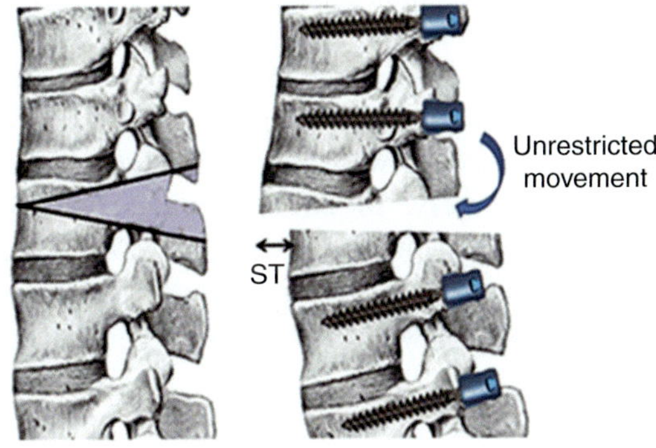

Fig. 13.2 Mechanism of ST in PSO and illustration of the cage method. *Left* A V-shaped wedge resection in PSO. *Right* The osteotomy gap and anterior column hinge are unrestricted, and ST happens after sagittal movement of the osteotomy site during closure

X. Zhang (✉) · F. Hu · Y. Hao · Y. Wang
Chinese PLA General Hospital, Beijing, China

Y. Wang (ed.), *Surgical Treatment of Ankylosing Spondylitis Deformity*,
https://doi.org/10.1007/978-981-13-6427-3_13

2 Risk of Sagittal Translation

The intraoperative neurophysiological monitoring of patients with persistent neurologic complications often occurred after osteotomy procedure [6, 7]. Therefore, the closure procedure of the osteotomy wedge is probably the main cause of the nerve injury. It has been recognized that once ST occurs as the osteotomy site is closed, the nerve roots are vulnerable to being pinched because of the displacement [8, 9]. Thus, neurovascular complications are more likely to appear in management with ST than that without ST [10]. Even catastrophic consequences can be brought by neurovascular complications [11–13]. In 2009, O'Shaughnessy et al. reported that one patient who experienced segmental translation during PSO had a decline in intraoperative somatosensory-evoked potentials. Kao-Wha Chang et al. believed that the risk of nerve root injury in AS patients with ST was substantial. Qian et al. [14] suggested that if the sagittal translation (ST) between posterior inferior edge of the cranial vertebral body and the posterior superior edge of the caudal body at the osteotomized level was more than 5 mm, the patient was considered to have vertebral subluxation (VS) at the osteotomy site. Once intraoperative VS was visually confirmed through intraoperative fluoroscopy, remedial measures were reported to ensure the safety of surgery. In 2011, Arun et al. [15] described a patient who underwent OWO died intraoperatively due to aortic injury and catastrophic bleeding secondary to ST.

3 Cause of Sagittal Translation

After osteotomy procedure, the original kyphosis spine is transformed into a lordosis spine at the apex of the osteotomy wedge, so the spinal cord, cauda equina, and dural sac crinkle and move forward to the posterior wall of the vertebral body in the relatively narrow osseous spinal canal. Although the posterior vertebral lamina has been removed, the posterior wall of the vertebral body is very close to the posterior wall of the vertebral body. Inadequate latent decompression of the spinal canal and lamina can also lead to compression of the spinal cord, cauda equina, and nerve root, which leads to neurological symptoms. In order to prevent the happening of sagittal translation, we systematically reviewed the postoperative imaging; we found a few causes which may contribute to the happening of ST. First, the depth of pedicle screws in the cranial centrum is different from the screws in the cranial centrum (Fig. 13.3). Second, the hinge point of the orthopedic rod is not at the same level as the osteotomy wedge (Fig. 13.4). Third, the sagittal diameter of the upper and lower osteotomy surface in the osteotomy site is (A $\neq$ B) (Fig. 13.5).

4 Preventive Measures

After the accident, Arun et al. [15] reported a method to prevent ST using temporary malleable rods during the reduction maneuver. We used this method in most of the patients (Fig. 13.6). We

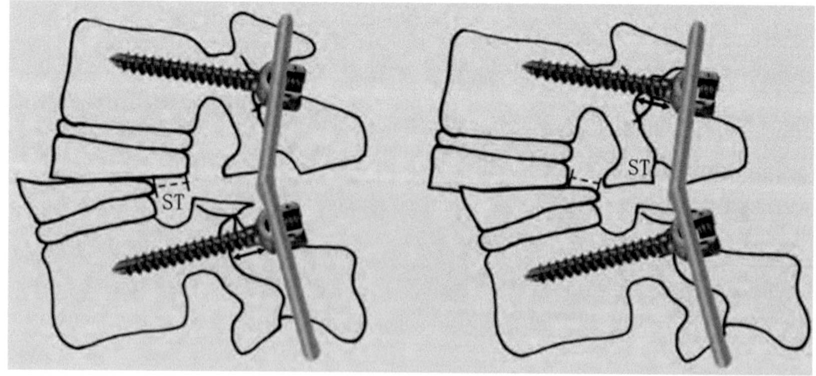

Fig. 13.3 The depth of pedicle screws in the cranial centrum is different from the screws in the cranial centrum

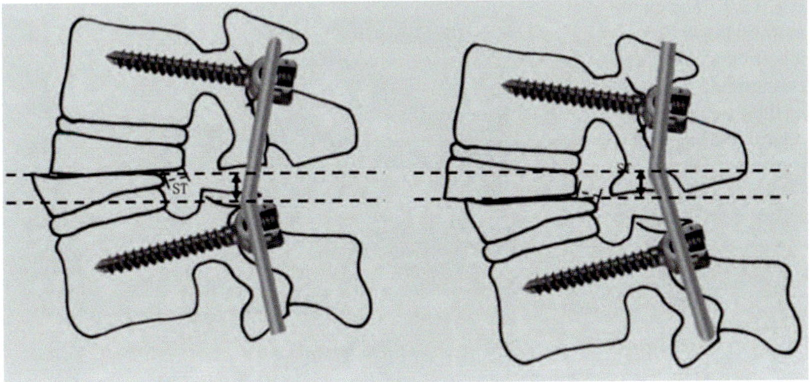

Fig. 13.4 The hinge point of the orthopedic rod is not at the same level as the osteotomy wedge

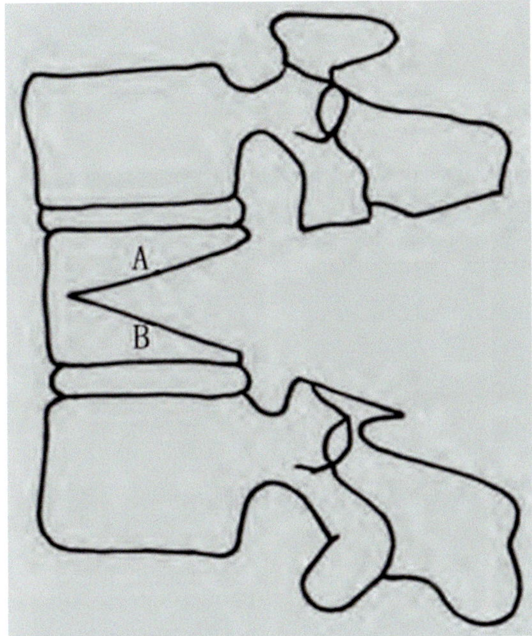

Fig. 13.5 The sagittal diameter of the upper and lower osteotomy surface in the osteotomy site (A ≠ B)

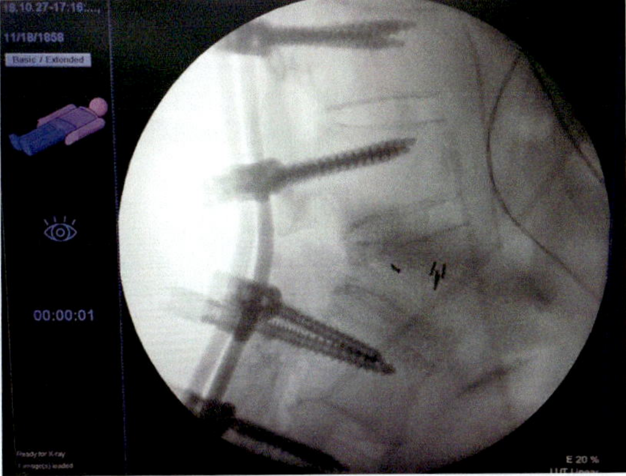

Fig. 13.6 Intraoperative imaging showing that correction of the deformity at the osteotomy segment was obtained, with a temporary rod in place

found that this method plays an important role in preventing ST before the reduction maneuver finished. But also according to our experience, most of the STs happen because of the unrestricted movement of the osteotomy site after the fracture of the anterior cortex during closing procedure. However, the temporary rods should be removed before the osteotomy gap being closed. It could not completely avert ST using temporary rods for correction of AS kyphosis and the neurovascular complications caused by ST. That could be critical for a few patients. Recently, we have proposed a method of PSO with a cage. We insert cage with the bone autograft into the osteotomy space at the anterior column of osteotomized vertebra (Fig. 13.7). The cage sinks into the cancellous bone of the cranial and caudal sides of the osteotomized site immediately. It provides a stable hinge to close the osteotomy gap, restricts the movement of the cranial or caudal of the osteotomy site, and reduces the possibility of ST after the anterior cortex fracture. Only in this way the cage can make the closure process more stable because the force of the osteotomy during closure is mainly focused on the cage located in the anterior column. It helps to avoid sagittal displacement and ensures the safety of the procedure (Fig. 13.8).

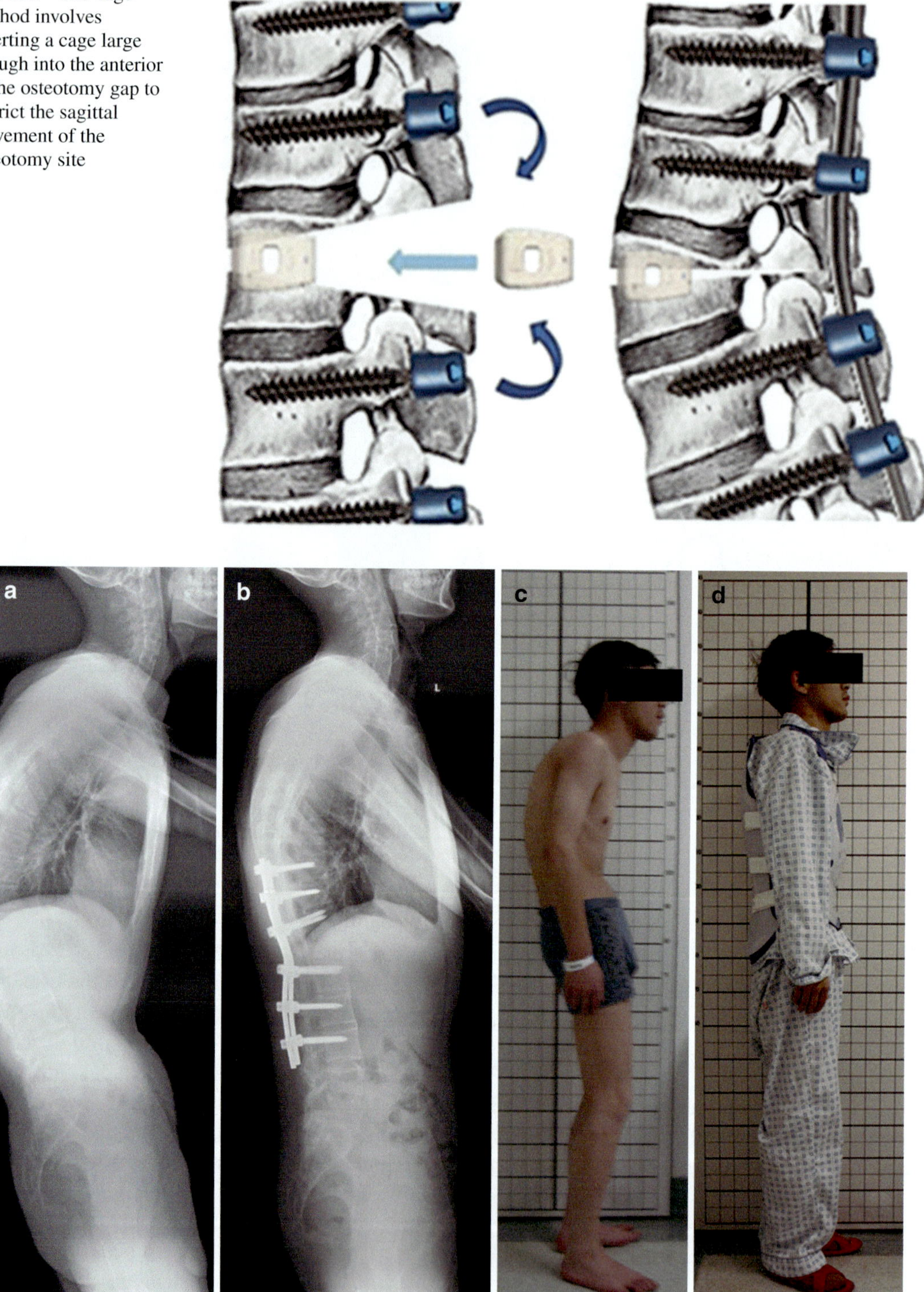

Fig. 13.7 The cage method involves inserting a cage large enough into the anterior of the osteotomy gap to restrict the sagittal movement of the osteotomy site

Fig. 13.8 A 27-year-old male patient suffering from ankylosing spondylitis kyphosis complained of severe back pain for over 4 years that hardly alleviated with analgesics. Preoperative radiograph showed a remarkable kyphosis in thoracolumbar spine with a global kyphosis of 64° (**a**). PSO with a cage was performed at L1. The sagittal profile was significantly improved without sagittal translation, as shown in the 2-year follow-up images (**b**). Pre- and postoperative lateral view shows that the cosmetic disfigurement was improved obviously (**c**, **d**)

This study was conducted with approval from the Ethics Committee of Chinese PLA General Hospital, and all patients provided informed consent for their participation in this study.

5 Emergency Actions Following Sagittal Translation

Intraoperative ST can be visually confirmed through intraoperative fluoroscopy. Once it happened, several emergency actions should be initiated, involving manual adjustment favoring translation reduction as well as checking of intraoperative neuro-monitoring signals instantly. If the somatosensory-evoked potential (SEP) and motor-evoked potential (MEP) monitoring were found to be abnormal during operation, we recommend that a wake-up test should be performed to confirm whether the motor function of the lower limbs was intact or not. Simultaneously, performing extensive laminectomy was the most important remedy according to our experience. And it should be performed when ST was irreversible, especially in patients with intraoperative neurological deficits. In addition, with regard to patients with both irreversible significant ST and intraoperative neurological deficits, surgeons were recommended to remove the instrumentations, even though the removal could lead to loss of kyphosis correction.

References

1. Chang KW, Cheng CW, Chen HC, Chang KI, Chen TC. Closing-opening wedge osteotomy for the treatment of sagittal imbalance. Spine (Phila Pa 1976). 2008;33(13):1470–7.
2. O'shaughnessy BA, Kuklo TR, Hsieh PC, Yang BP, Koski TR, Ondra SL. Thoracic pedicle subtraction osteotomy for fixed sagittal spinal deformity. Spine (Phila Pa 1976). 2009;34(26):2893–9.
3. Wang Y, Zhang Y, Mao K, et al. Transpedicular bivertebrae wedge osteotomy and discectomy in lumbar spine for severe ankylosing spondylitis. J Spinal Disord Tech. 2010;23(3):186–91.
4. Zhang X, Zhang Z, Wang J, et al. Vertebral column decancellation: a new spinal osteotomy technique for correcting rigid thoracolumbar kyphosis in patients with ankylosing spondylitis. Bone Joint J. 2016;98-B(5):672–8.
5. Chang KW, Chen HC, Chen YY, Lin CC, Hsu HL, Cai YH. Sagittal translation in opening wedge osteotomy for the correction of thoracolumbar kyphotic deformity in ankylosing spondylitis. Spine (Phila Pa 1976). 2006;31(10):1137–42.
6. Zhang N, Li H, Xu ZK, Chen WS, Chen QX, Li FC. Computer simulation of two-level pedicle subtraction osteotomy for severe thoracolumbar kyphosis in ankylosing spondylitis. Indian J Orthop. 2017;51(6):666–71.
7. Hu W, Yu J, Liu H, Zhang X, Wang Y. Y shape osteotomy in ankylosing spondylitis, a prospective case series with minimum 2 year follow-up. PLoS One. 2016;11(12):e0167792.
8. Yang J, Huang Z, Grevitt M, Li J, Li F, Yang J. The precise bending rod technique: a novel method for precise correction of ankylosing spondylitis kyphosis. Clin Spine Surg. 2016;29(9):E452–6.
9. Zhao Y, Xu H, Zhang Y, Wang Z, Zhang X, Wang Y. Comparison of two surgeries in treatment of severe kyphotic deformity caused by ankylosing spondylitis: Transpedicular bivertebrae wedge osteotomy versus one-stage interrupted two-level transpedicular wedge osteotomy. Clin Neurol Neurosurg. 2015;139:252–7.
10. Yıldız F, Akgül T, Ekinci M, Dikici F, Şar C, Domaniç Ü. Results of closing wedge osteotomy in the treatment of sagittal imbalance due to ankylosing spondylitis. Acta Orthop Traumatol Turc. 2016;50(1):63–8.
11. Qian BP, Wang XH, Qiu Y, et al. The influence of closing-opening wedge osteotomy on sagittal balance in thoracolumbar kyphosis secondary to ankylosing spondylitis: a comparison with closing wedge osteotomy. Spine (Phila Pa 1976). 2012;37(16):1415–23.
12. Gavaskar AS, Naveen CT. Pedicle subtraction osteotomy for rigid kyphosis of the dorsolumbar spine. Arch Orthop Trauma Surg. 2011;131(6):803–8.
13. Hyun SJ, Kim YJ, Rhim SC. Spinal pedicle subtraction osteotomy for fixed sagittal imbalance patients. World J Clin Cases. 2013;1(8):242–8.
14. Qian BP, Mao SH, Jiang J, Wang B, Qiu Y. Mechanisms, predisposing factors, and prognosis of intraoperative vertebral subluxation during pedicle subtraction osteotomy in surgical correction of thoracolumbar kyphosis secondary to ankylosing spondylitis. Spine (Phila Pa 1976). 2017;42(16):E983–90.
15. Arun R, Dabke HV, Mehdian H. Comparison of three types of lumbar osteotomy for ankylosing spondylitis: a case series and evolution of a safe technique for instrumented reduction. Eur Spine J. 2011;20(12):2252–60.

14 Andersson Lesion-Complicating Ankylosing Spondylitis

Xuesong Zhang, Yao Wang, and Yan Wang

Ankylosing spondylitis (AS) is a chronic inflammatory disease which, for the most part, negatively impacts the spine and sacroiliac joints and causes pain and stiffness and kyphotic deformity [1–4]. When the disease develops into the late phase, osteoporotic changes can make the spine fragile and vulnerable to trauma [5, 6]. A minor trauma could induce Andersson lesion (AL), which is a transvertebral, discovertebral or transdiscal fracture of an ankylosed spine. As a result of Andersson lesion, the localized progressive painful kyphotic deformity can lead to severe disturbances of posture and neurologic abnormalities [7]. Andersson lesion was first proposed by Andersson in 1937 [8]. The exact incidence of this disorder was reported in the literature to be between 1.5% and 28% [5].

Surgical treatment by instrumentation and fusion should be taken into consideration as the principal method to manage symptomatic AL when the conservative treatment fails. Such surgical procedure is to achieve restoration of spinal stability, decompression of the spinal canal, facilitation of fracture healing and restoration of sagittal balance [5]. Several surgical treatment methodologies for Andersson lesion have been raised, including posterior or anterior fusion and combined procedures [6, 9].

This article reviews the etiology, imaging features and treatment strategies of Andersson lesion-complicating ankylosing spondylitis. All patients provided informed consent for their participation in this study.

1 The Etiology of Andersson Lesion

Since Andersson's [8] first description of the lesion in patient with ankylosing spondylitis in 1937, multiple possibilities for etiology of Andersson lesion have been described, including infection, inflammation, trauma and mechanical stress. Meanwhile, many different terms have been used to refer to these localized lesions of the spine, including the 'Andersson lesion' (AL), 'discovertebral lesion', 'vertebral lesion', 'destructive vertebral lesion', 'spondylodiscitis', 'discitis', 'diskitis', 'sterile diskitis', 'pseudarthrosis' or '(stress) fracture', which indirectly reflect that the exact etiology is still controversial [10–14].

Cawley [12] in 1972 firstly divide the Andersson lesions into localized lesions and extensive lesions. Localized lesions were further subdivided according to the exact location: the discal surface of the vertebral rim or the cartilaginous part of the vertebral endplate. Extensive lesions involved both locations and were exclusively seen in patients with an

X. Zhang (✉) · Y. Wang · Y. Wang
PLA General Hospital, Beijing, China

Y. Wang (ed.), *Surgical Treatment of Ankylosing Spondylitis Deformity*,
https://doi.org/10.1007/978-981-13-6427-3_14

ankylosed spine. The localized lesions were assumed to support an inflammatory mechanism because of their occurrence in the early course of ankylosing spondylitis. Park et al. [15] subdivided the Andersson lesions into inflammatory and traumatic types. The inflammatory types were always multiple and part of the natural history of ankylosing spondylitis itself. The traumatic types were usually single lesions, associated with prolonged disease duration and a history of trauma and nonunion of fractures of the posterior column. Bron et al. [5] divided Andersson lesions into three groups according to radiological characteristics: localized lesions, extensive lesions with fractured posterior elements and extensive lesions without fractured posterior elements. Regardless of the exact etiology, mechanical factors in the ankylosed spine will prevent healing of extensive lesions and promote the formation of pseudarthrosis.

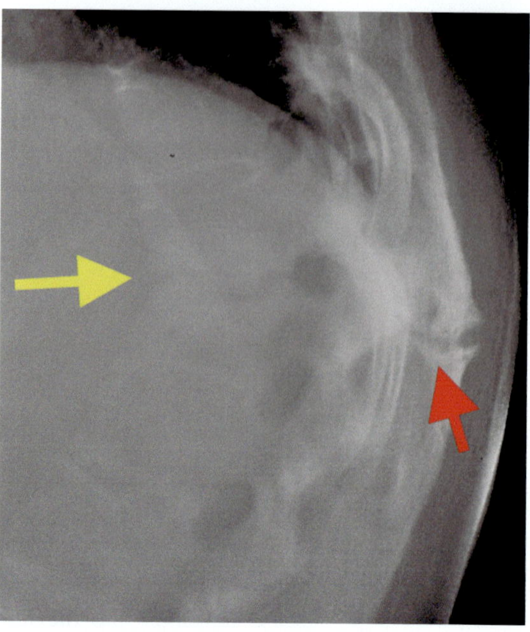

Fig. 14.1 Radiographs showing a traumatic Andersson lesion at T12-L1 with intervertebral disc destruction, osteolysis of the vertebral body (yellow arrow) and fractures of the posterior elements (red arrow)

2 Imaging Performance

2.1 Radiography

Conventional radiographs are usually the initial choice. The exact level of the lesion can be reliably determined when the lowest rib is included in the image [5]. The typical manifestations of Andersson lesion on X-ray are osteolytic destruction with a surrounding zone of reactive sclerosis and vertebral osteophytes and may be accompanied by fractures of the posterior elements [16] (Fig. 14.1). Fang [6] analysed the imaging data of 40 cases of Andersson lesion. Ununited fractures through either ankylosed discs in 37 cases and through vertebral bodies in three cases were found in the research. Corresponding fractures were seen in the posterior column in 34 cases. On the plain radiograph, the circumscribed defect in one or two neighbouring vertebral bodies with varying degrees of narrowing of the intervening disc space, angular kyphosis of the affected spinal segment and an area of reactive sclerosis in the vertebral cancellous bone surrounding the defect were thought to be the major characteristics that differentiated Andersson lesion from an inflammatory spondylodiscitis in Dihlmann's observation [17].

2.2 Computed Tomography Imaging

In observing the extent of lesions, computed tomography (CT) is superior to conventional radiographs, especially on CT sagittal reconstruction, which clearly shows the fractures of the posterior elements and the unfused facet joints [18] (Fig. 14.2). Chan et al. [18] compared CT scans in 18 patients with 22 pseudarthroses with the results of conventional radiographs. CT scans provided data that were missed on conventional radiography in 77% of the lesions. The characteristics of lesions may

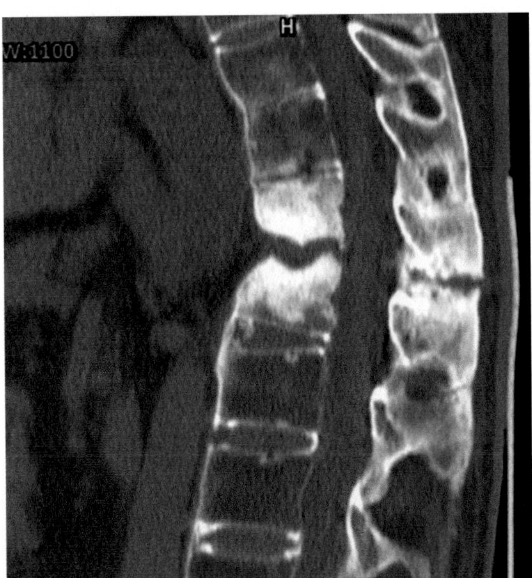

Fig. 14.2 CT sagittal reconstruction image demonstrated disc-space widening and adjacent bony sclerosis, with the fracture of the posterior elements

be more easily found on CT scans than on X-ray radiographs. Irregular discovertebral osteolysis with reactive sclerosis and more frequently detected the vacuum phenomenon and paraspinal swellings can be shown on the CT images. Zhang et al. [2] found spinal stenosis secondary to the formation of osteophyte around the facet joint.

2.3 Magnetic Resonance Imaging

Magnetic resonance imaging (MRI) is considered the most sensitive imaging method for detecting Andersson lesion without radioactive side effects. The MRI signal intensity of inflammatory Andersson lesion in the adjacent vertebra may vary according to the duration of the inflammation [15]. The traumatic Andersson lesion usually shows hypointensity on both T1- and T2-weighted images at either endplate of the lesion site (suggesting sclerosis) or mixed intensity in adjacent vertebral bodies (reduced on T1-weighted images and increased on T2) (Fig. 14.3). The MRI may be used to differentiate pseudoarthrosis from infectious or neoplastic disease. Identification of any abnormalities of the dura, ligaments and soft tissue is most helpful when correlated with clinical presentations [9]. Spinal stenosis is mostly due to the hypertrophy of the ligamentum flavum and facet joint. In addition, MRI can be used for the early detection of the destruction of the posterior column.

3 Treatment

3.1 Conservative Treatment

The principal treatment for patients with Andersson lesion is local stabilization. Conservative treatment including medication, plaster and external fixation is often the first step of treatment. There is no evidence that treatment with drugs, including non-steroidal anti-inflammatory drugs, and anti-tumour necrosis factor-α therapy with infliximab, etanercept and adalimumab is beneficial in the treatment of symptomatic AL [19]. Shen et al. [18] proposed that for the pseudarthrosis occurred in the upper thoracic spine, reliable stability to prevent kyphosis could be provided by the sternal rib complex, as the 'fourth column'. However, conservative management is not always effective on the cervical and thoracolumbar lesions due to greater mobility [5, 6]. Without solid fixation gained from surgery, minimal persistent motion at the Andersson lesion might hinder fracture healing and union. Neither brace immobilization nor halo jacket immobilization could eradicate this minimal persistent motion [20].

3.2 Surgical Strategy

When conservative treatment fails to effectively resolve progressive thoracolumbar kyphotic deformity, sagittal imbalance, intractable pain

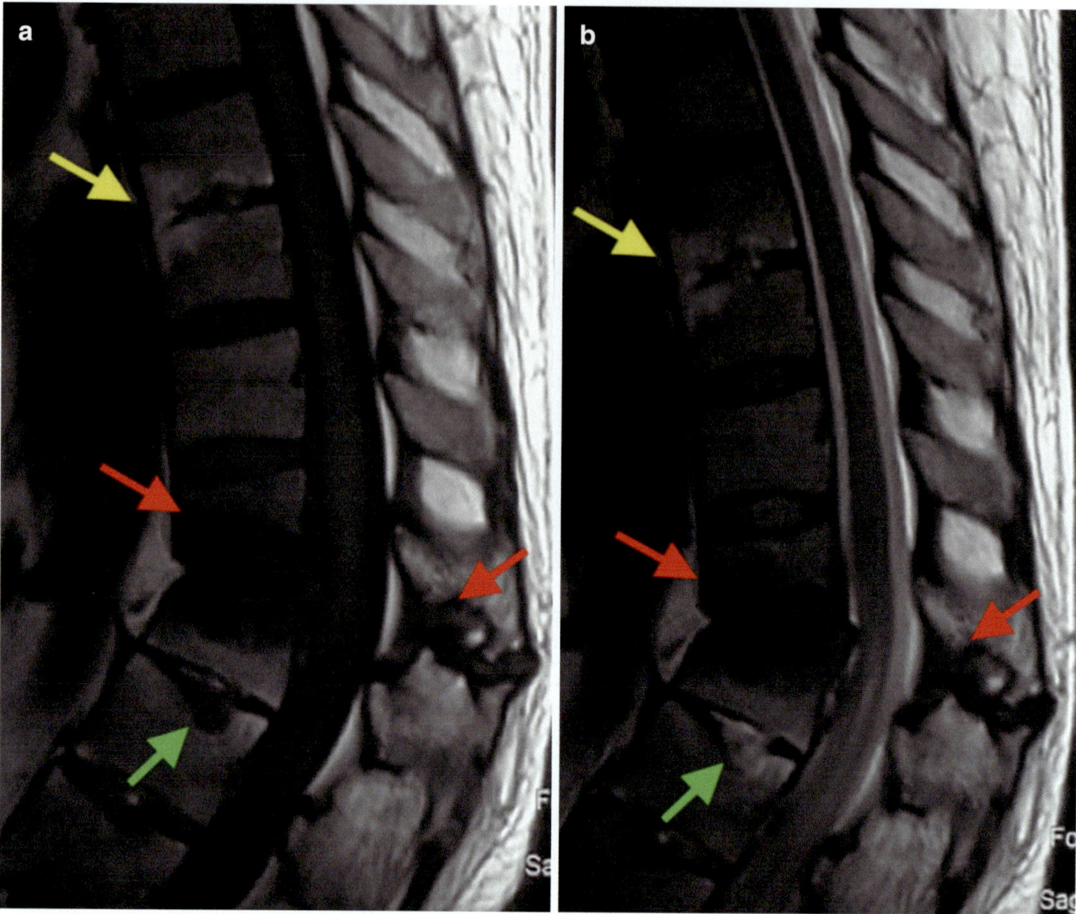

Fig. 14.3 T1 (**a**)- and T2 (**b**)-weighted sagittal MR images. *Red arrow:* a traumatic Andersson lesion with posterior column fracture and spinal canal stenosis at T12-L1. Both images revealed hypointense signal intensity of the pseudarthrosis. *Yellow arrow*: an old inflammatory Andersson lesion at T9-T1O with reactive fatty degeneration of the bone marrow. *Green arrow*: florid inflammatory Andersson lesions at L1-L2 with acute inflammation

and neurological deficit caused by symptomatic Andersson lesion, one should consider surgical instrumentation and fusion as the principal path.

Adoption of the surgical procedures aims to decompress the spinal canal, to remediate spinal stability, restore sagittal balance and promote healing and fusion.

Both instrumented and non-instrumented stabilization utilizing anterior, posterior or combined approach [5] are among the many surgical procedures that have been proposed. Nevertheless, till now, there is no ideal surgical option till now that is one-size-fits-all.

In the previous studies, Fang et al. had suggested anterior fusion, considering that its direct access to the anterior lesion, complete curettage and ideal biomechanical characteristics for repairing the lesion provide advantages [6, 11]. However, the inability in correcting the global kyphosis is the drawback of this procedure [4, 21]. Chang et al. conducted a research using posterior opening wedge osteotomy, in which an average correction of 38° was created

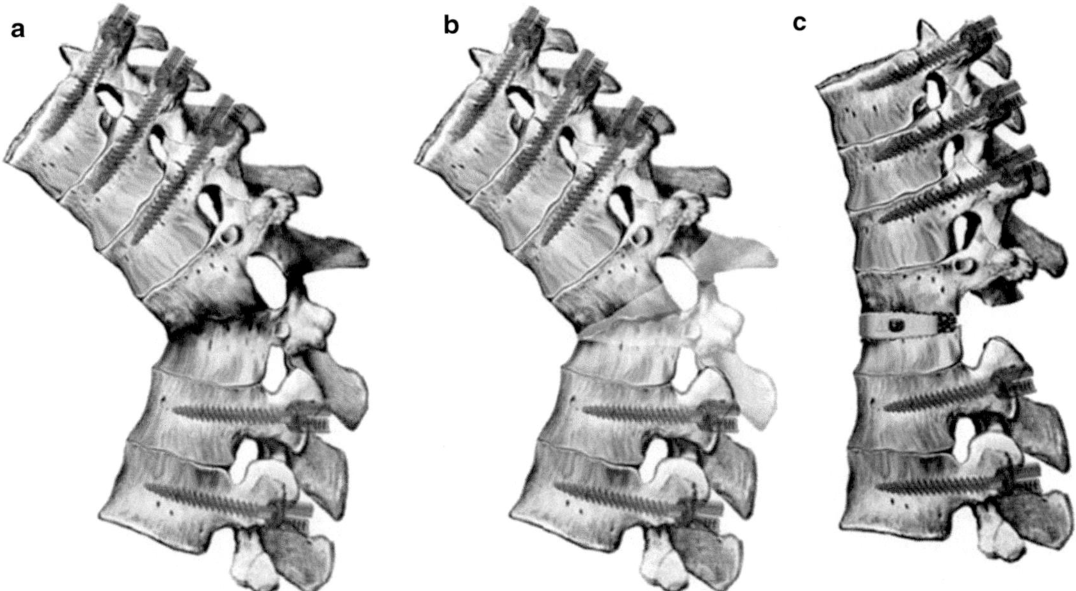

Fig. 14.4 Transpedicular subtraction and disc resection osteotomy. (**a**) The Andersson lesion area of an ankylosed spine. (**b**) The resection of a large part of the pedicles, the lesion disc with both endplates. (**c**) After the insertion of a cage with autograft bone, bone-on-bone solid fusion was finally obtained. (Reprinted, with permission, from: Zhang, X., Wang, Y., Wu, B. et al. Eur Spine J (2016) 25: 2587. https://doi.org/10.1007/s00586-015-4213-6)

and maintained at the final follow-up in 30 patients [21]. Chen et al. and several authors recommended the usage of combined approach with both anterior and posterior surgical procedures to treat Andersson lesion with kyphotic deformity secondary to advanced AS. Encouragingly, the combined approach has achieved successful fusion and positive clinical result [4, 11, 22]. On the flip side, whether in one- or two-stage surgical procedure, the approach has increased surgical risk, driven by potential larger amount of blood loss and longer duration of surgery.

Speaking from our experience, we performed one-stage transpedicular subtraction and disc resection osteotomy, and satisfactory rehabilitation was reported from all patients (Figs. 14.4, 14.5 and 14.6).

Different from the osteotomies in other disease or an inflexible spine without pseudarthrosis [23], the Andersson lesion plane sets a limit on the chosen level of the osteotomy procedure. In transpedicular subtraction and disc resection osteotomy technique, a cage is put at the anterior column acting as a hinge. Precontoured rods were utilized to stabilize the osteotomy area. By gently applying pressure on the pedicle screws at both sides of the osteotomy site, appropriate correction could be finally obtained, and this can be adjusted more conveniently during the process than traditional closed-wedge osteotomy like pedicle subtraction osteotomy (PSO) technique.

Among the steps of the osteotomy, surfaces of normal cancellous bone need to be exposed by resection of osteolysis with surrounding reactive sclerosis on both eroded endplates. By insertion of a cage with autograft bone, the osteotomy area could be solidly fused at the final follow-up.

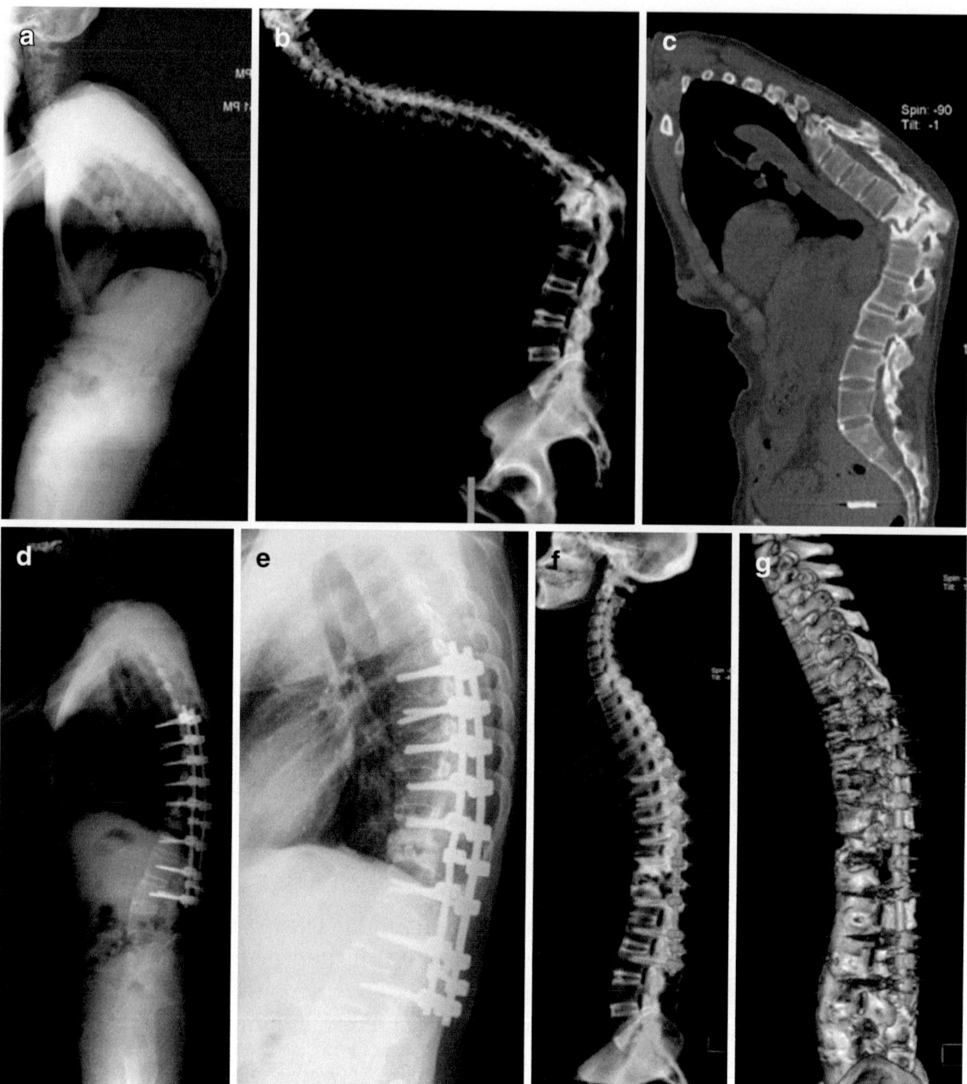

Fig 14.5 A female patient (47 years old) suffering from Andersson lesion. (**a**–**c**) Preoperative X-ray demonstrated global kyphosis (101°) and regional kyphosis (65°) at T11/12 level. Sagittal 3D-CT image showed three-column fractures with irregular discovertebral osteolysis surrounded by reactive sclerosis. (**d**) Immediately after surgery, postoperative X-ray showed the regional kyphosis was corrected to 11° by transpedicular subtraction and disc resection osteotomy performed at T11/12. (**e**–**g**) 3.5 years after surgery, postoperative radiograph and 3D-CT demonstrated that the correction was maintained and solid fusion obtained. (**h**–**k**) The cosmetic deformity was corrected obviously. (Reprinted, with permission, from: Zhang, X., Wang, Y., Wu, B. et al. Eur Spine J (2016) 25: 2587. https://doi.org/10.1007/s00586-015-4213-6

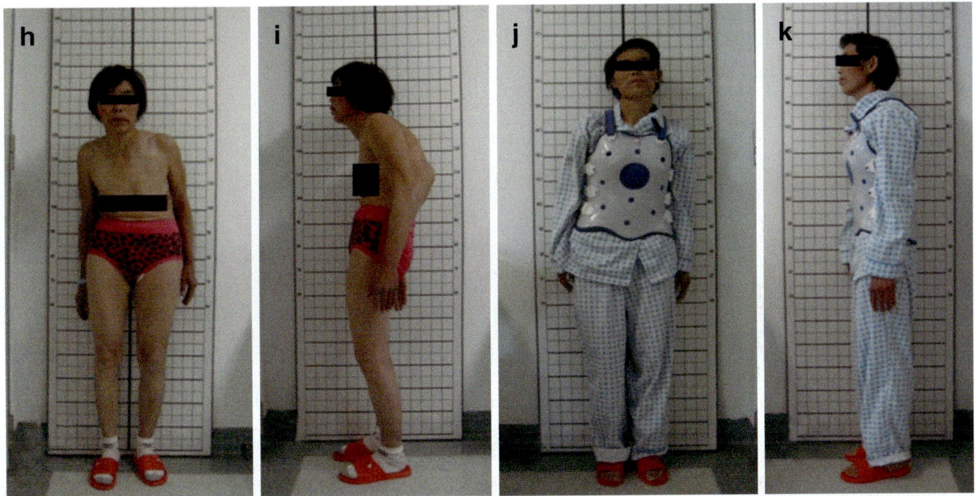

Fig. 14.5 (continued)

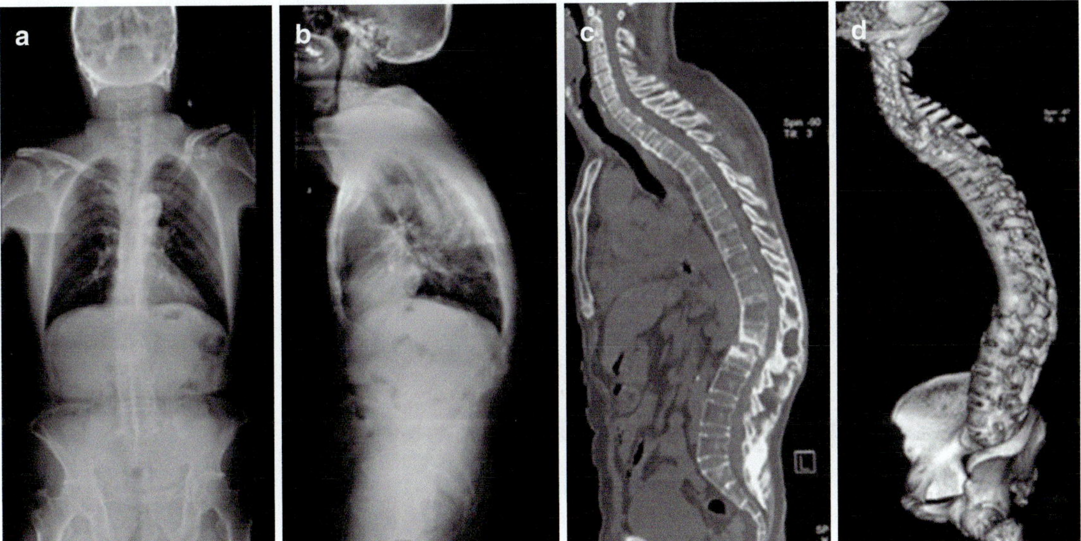

Fig. 14.6 A male patient (51 years old) suffered from Andersson lesion. (**a**, **b**) Preoperative X-ray demonstrated global kyphosis (54°) and regional kyphosis (31°) at L1/L2 level. (**c**, **d**) Sagittal 3D-CT image showed three-column fractures with irregular discovertebral osteolysis surrounded by reactive sclerosis. On both T1WI (**e**) and T2WI (**f**, **g**) images, hypointensity was shown at both endplates of the lesion site (sclerosis) with mixed signal changes in adjacent vertebral bodies. (**h**, **i**) Immediately after surgery, postoperative X-ray showed the regional kyphosis was corrected to 2° by transpedicular subtraction and disc resection osteotomy performed at L1/2. (**j**, **k**) 1.5 years after surgery, postoperative radiograph showed that the correction maintained. (**l–o**) The cosmetic deformity was corrected obviously. (Reprinted, with permission, from: Zhang, X., Wang, Y., Wu, B. et al. Eur SpineJ(2016)25:2587.https://doi.org/10.1007/s00586-015-4213-6)

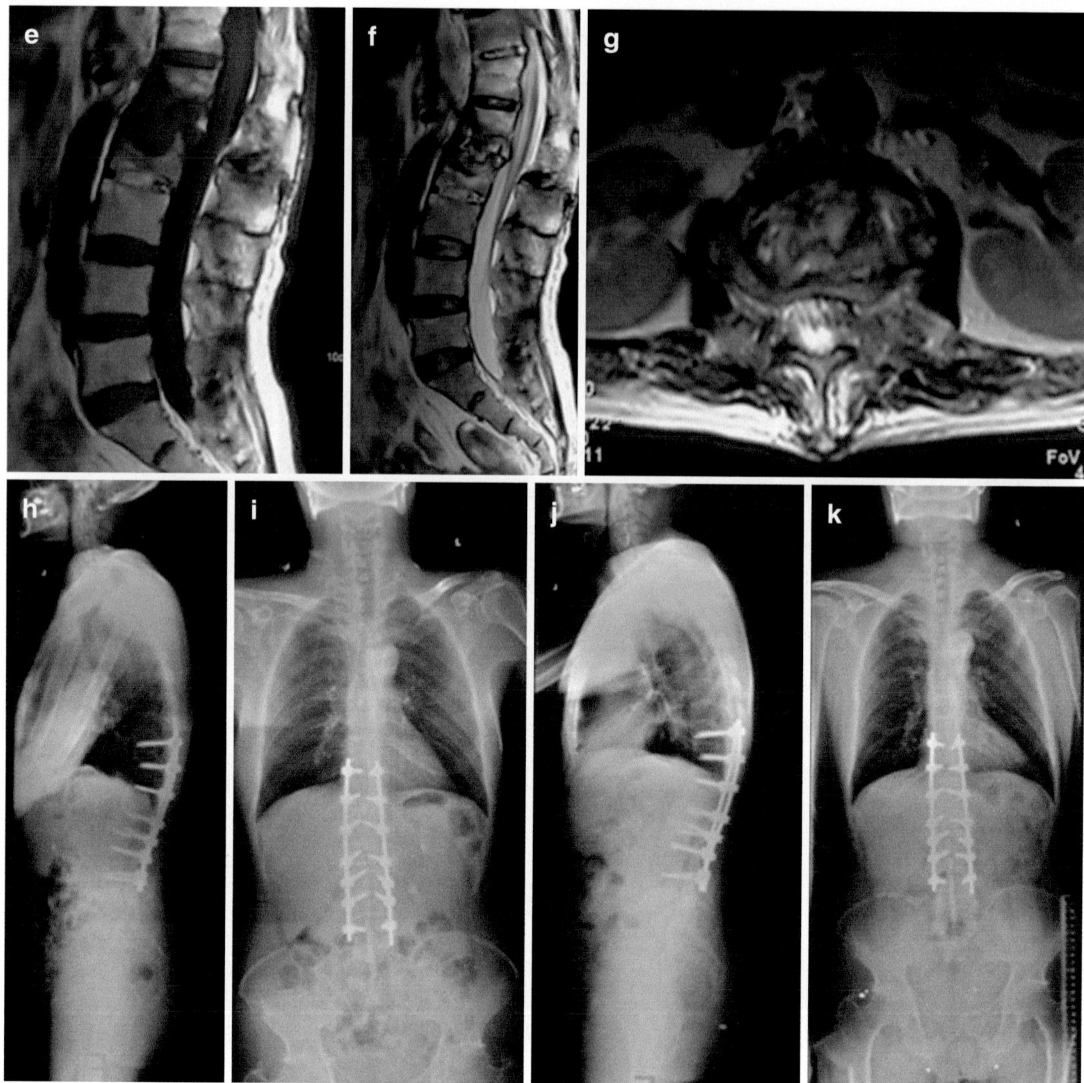

Fig.14.6 (continued)

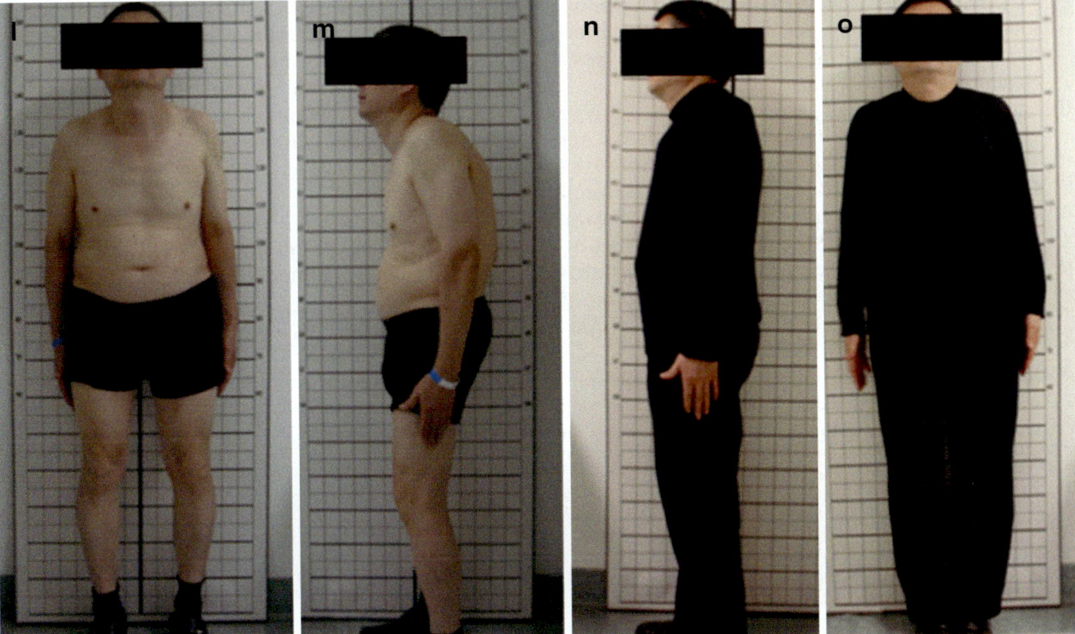

Fig.14.6 (continued)

References

1. Feldtkeller E, Vosse D, Geusens P, van der Linden S. Prevalence and annual incidence of vertebral fractures in patients with ankylosing spondylitis. Rheumatol Int. 2006;26:234–9.
2. Zhang X, Wang Y, Wu B, Hu W, Zhang Z, Wang Y. Treatment of Andersson lesion-complicating ankylosing spondylitis via transpedicular subtraction and disc resection osteotomy, a retrospective study. Eur Spine J. 2016;25:2587–95.
3. Peh WC, Luk KD. Pseudoarthrosis in ankylosing spondylitis. Ann Rheum Dis. 1994;53: 206–10.
4. Qian BP, Qiu Y, Wang B, Sun X, Zhu ZZ, Jiang J, Ji ML. Pedicle subtraction osteotomy through pseudarthrosis to correct thoracolumbar kyphotic deformity in advanced ankylosing spondylitis. Eur Spine J. 2012;21:711–8.
5. de Bron JL, Vries MK, Snieders MN, van der Horst-Bruinsma IE, van Royen BJ. Discovertebral (Andersson) lesions of the spine in ankylosing spondylitis revisited. Clin Rheumatol. 2009;28:883–92.
6. Fang D, Leong JC, Ho EK, Chan FL, Chow SP. Spinal pseudarthrosis in ankylosing spondylitis. Clinicopathological correlation and the results of anterior spinal fusion. J Bone Joint Surg. 1988;70:443–7.
7. Van Royen BJ, Kastelijns RC, Noske DP, Oner FC, Smit TH. Transpedicular wedge resection osteotomy for the treatment of a kyphotic Andersson lesion-complicating ankylosing spondylitis. Eur Spine J. 2006;15:246–52.
8. Andersson O. Röntgenbilden vid spondylarthritis ankylopoetica. Nord Med Tidskr. 1937;14:2000–2.
9. Shih TT, Chen PQ, Li YW, Hsu CY. Spinal fractures and pseudoarthrosis complicating ankylosing spondylitis: MRI manifestation and clinical significance. J Comput Assist Tomogr. 2001;25:164–70.
10. Arnold MH, Brooks PM, Ryan M, Francis H. A destructive discovertebral lesion: septic discitis, ankylosing spondylitis, or rheumatoid arthritis? Clin Rheumatol. 1989;8:277–81.
11. Kim KT, Lee SH, Suk KS, Lee JH, Im YJ. Spinal pseudarthrosis in advanced ankylosing spondylitis with sagittal plane deformity: clinical characteristics and outcome analysis. Spine. 2007;32:1641–7.
12. Cawley MI, Chalmers TM, Kellgren JH, Ball J. Destructive lesions of vertebral bodies in ankylosing spondylitis. Ann Rheum Dis. 1972;31(5):345–58.
13. Rasker JJ, Prevo RL, Lanting PJ. Spondylodiscitis in ankylosing spondylitis, inflammation or trauma? A description of six cases. Scand J Rheumatol. 1996;25:52–7.
14. Wholey MH, Pugh DG, Bickel WH. Localized destructive lesions in rheumatoid spondylitis. Radiology. 1960;74:54–6.

15. Park YS, Kim JH, Ryu JA, Kim TH. The Andersson lesion in ankylosing spondylitis: distinguishing between the inflammatory and traumatic subtypes. J Bone Joint Surg. 2011;93:961–6.
16. Chan FL, Ho EK, Fang D, Hsu LC, Leong JC, Ngan H. Spinal pseudarthrosis in ankylosing spondylitis. Acta Radiol (Stockholm: Sweden). 1987;1987(28):383–8.
17. Dihlmann W, Delling G. Disco-vertebral destructive lesions (So-called Andersson Lesions) associated with ankylosing spondylitis. Skelet Radiol. 1978;3:10–6.
18. Chan FL, Ho EK, Chau EM. Spinal pseudarthrosis complicating ankylosing spondylitis: comparison of CT and conventional tomography. AJR Am J Roentgenol. 1988;150:611–4.
19. Sakaura H, Hosono N, Mukai Y, Fujii R, Yoshikawa H. Paraparesis due to exacerbation of preexisting spinal pseudoarthrosis following infliximab therapy for advanced ankylosing spondylitis. Spine J. 2006;6:325–9.
20. Wang G, Sun J, Jiang Z, Cui X. The surgical treatment of Andersson lesions associated with ankylosing spondylitis. Orthopedics. 2011;34:e302–6.
21. Chang KW, Tu MY, Huang HH, Chen HC, Chen YY, Lin CC. Posterior correction and fixation without anterior fusion for pseudoarthrosis with kyphotic deformity in ankylosing spondylitis. Spine. 2006;31:E408–13.
22. Chen LH, Kao FC, Niu CC, Lai PL, Fu TS, Chen WJ. Surgical treatment of spinal pseudoarthrosis in ankylosing spondylitis. Chang Gung Med J. 2005;28:621–8.
23. Zheng GQ, Song K, Zhang YG, Wang Y, Huang P, Zhang XS, Wang Z, Mao KY, Cui G. Two-level spinal osteotomy for severe thoracolumbar kyphosis in ankylosing spondylitis. Experience with 48 patients. Spine. 2014;39:1055–8.

15 The Management and Prevention of Complications

Tianhao Wang, Geng Cui, and Guoquan Zheng

Spinal osteotomy for kyphotic deformity of ankylosing spondylitis (AS) has high risk due to large trauma, long operation time, and high difficulty of operation. It has been reported the incidence of complications is up to 40% [1, 2]. To manage and prevent complications is also crucial to the success of surgery. The complications are divided into intraoperative complications and postoperative complications. The former includes pedicle screw misplacement, blood loss, dura laceration/cerebrospinal fluid leakage, neurovascular injury, blindness, and sagittal translation [2–4]. The latter includes internal fixation failure, infection, pseudarthrosis, loss of correction, proximal junctional kyphosis/failure, and complications caused by changes in the volume of thoracic and abdominal cavity [3, 5–7]. With enhancement of ideas and techniques of spinal osteotomy, the effect of surgical correction for spinal kyphosis of AS has been greatly improved. The incidence of complications of pseudarthrosis and loss of correction is decreasing gradually. Instead, the reports for nerve injury and blood loss are increasing. Foreseeing the complications and comprehending how to prevent them can make the surgeons more confident, resulting in a better consequence for the patients [8].

T. Wang · G. Cui · G. Zheng (✉)
Department of Orthopaedics, General Hospital of Chinese PLA, Beijing, China

1 Neurological Complications

1.1 Mechanism of Occurrence

The incidence of neurological complications is reported to be 4–15% [9, 10]. The major causes are the translation of the vertebral body, excessive dural kinks, and spine canal compromise (Fig. 15.1). Besides, the improper operation during surgery can also lead to nerve injury. Furthermore, the inadequate laminectomy and latent decompression also contribute to neurologic deficit. The injury of the nerve root and spinal cord leads to lower limb pain, numbness, or decreased muscle strength.

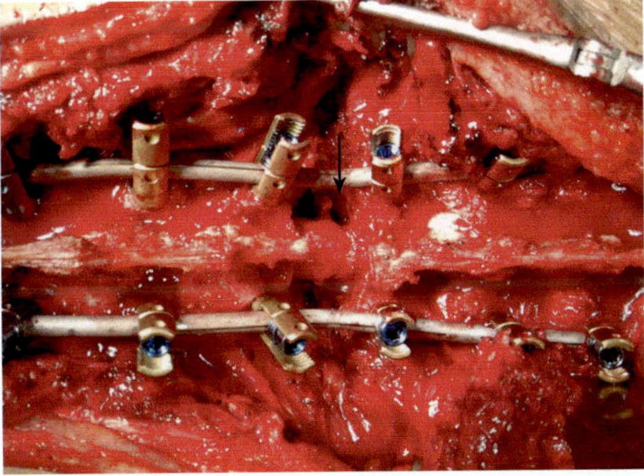

Fig. 15.1 The dural kinks were caused by inadequate decompression of the laminae

Y. Wang (ed.), *Surgical Treatment of Ankylosing Spondylitis Deformity*,
https://doi.org/10.1007/978-981-13-6427-3_15

1.2 Prevention

The osteotomy level should not be located at spinal cord area. A complete resection of the bone mass around the nerve root should be performed to avoid compression of the dura and nerve roots during reduction [9]. The procedure of reduction and closure of the osteotomy vertebra should be performed under direct view. Avoiding violent operation will prevent the injury of nerve. We think that the monitoring of neurologic function is important during operation. When SEP or MEP prompted a neurologic deficit, closing the osteotomy space should be stopped, and thorough decompression should be performed [11].

2 Dura Laceration/CSFL

2.1 Mechanism of Occurrence

CSFL is one of the common complications during spine surgery with an incidence of 10–30% [12–14]. In patients with AS, the dura is often extremely thin due to the surrounding chronic inflammation, especially in the midline [8, 9]. Also, there may be dura ossifications in some patients. Therefore, dura laceration is likely to happen during the operation and mainly occurs in the lamina resection.

2.2 Prevention

The decompressions should be performed carefully, avoiding excessive damage to the dura mater and unintended injury to the neural elements. When dura laceration occurs, it should be repaired with a waterproof suture. An artificial biofilm or a slice of muscle is also an alternative for helping reparation. After surgery, the incision drainage should be prolonged. Most of the patients are free of continuous leakage of cerebrospinal fluid and also do not suffer from delayed healing of surgical wounds.

3 Sagittal Translation (ST)

3.1 Mechanism of Occurrence

ST is any measurable displacement more than 2 mm between the posterior inferior edge of the cranial vertebral body and the posterior superior edge of the caudal body at the osteotomy level [15]. A majority of scholars regard ST as a kind of complication of AS. Some scholars insist that ST plays a crucial role during close-open osteotomy. However, it is reported that ST significantly increased the incidence of neurologic deficits with the incidence of 25% [9].

After spinal osteotomy in AS patients, the kyphotic spine changes to lordosis with apex at osteotomized vertebrae. The spinal cord (cauda nerve) and dural sac flex secondarily and conform to the shape of the spinal canal. Besides, the osteotomy results in shortening of middle and posterior columns. Consequently, the spinal cord (cauda nerve) and dural sac crinkle in the vertebral canal and close to the posterior wall of the vertebral body. The spinal cord is vulnerable to injury of bone steps caused by ST.

There are three probable reasons for ST: [1] inconsistency of the depth of proximal and distal pedicle screws beside the level of osteotomy, [2] mismatch between rod hinge and osteotomy hinge, and [3] unequal length of the upper and lower sides of the sagittal triangle of osteotomy (Fig. 15.2).

3.2 Prevention

Decompression range of laminae should be enlarged to avoid compression of the spinal cord (cauda nerve) and nerve root. Appropriate depth of pedicle screws and rod placement are also significant for avoiding ST occurrence. Furthermore, during a long follow-up of ST patients, we observe spontaneous bone reconstruction in middle and posterior column, and the spinal canal is remodeled. This phenomenon is described in burst vertebrae fracture either. The degree of ST is decreased during this procedure (Fig. 15.3).

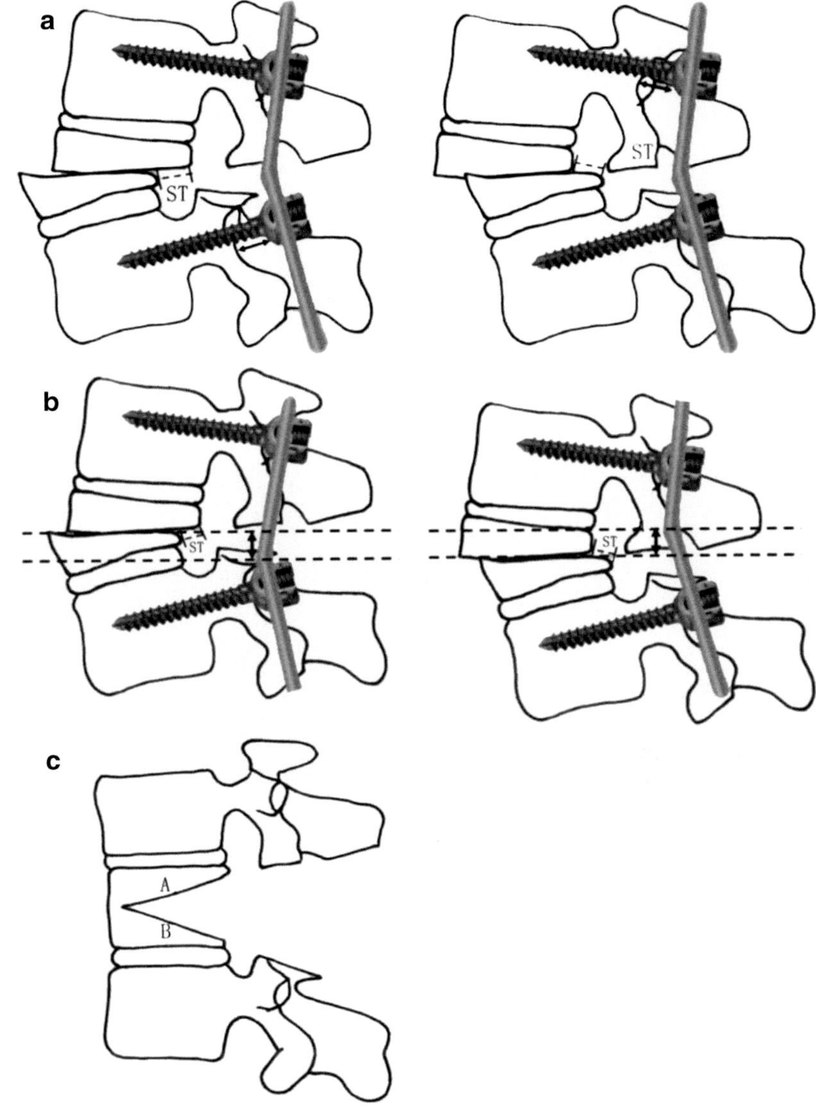

Fig. 15.2 (**a**) Inconsistency of the depth of proximal and distal pedicle screws beside the level of osteotomy. (**b**) Mismatch between rod hinge and osteotomy hinge. (**c**) Unequal length of the upper and lower sides of the sagittal triangle of osteotomy, a ≠ b

4 Vascular Complications and Blood Loss

4.1 Mechanism of Occurrence

The main vascular complications were anterior vertebral vascular injury, intraspinal venous plexus rupture bleeding, deep venous thrombosis, etc. The major vessels injury is mainly due to the sharp anterior edge of osteotomized vertebrae which may pierce elongated and tight blood vessels in open-wedge osteotomy [16]. But the technique of open-wedge osteotomy is currently less applied on correcting severe kyphotic deformity, and there are few reports on the injury of the anterior vertebral artery.

Perioperative bleeding of spinal osteotomy in AS patients is up to 1200–2400 ml [17–19]. Because of long-term bone and joint deformities, ankylosis, and lack of exercise, the blood vessel

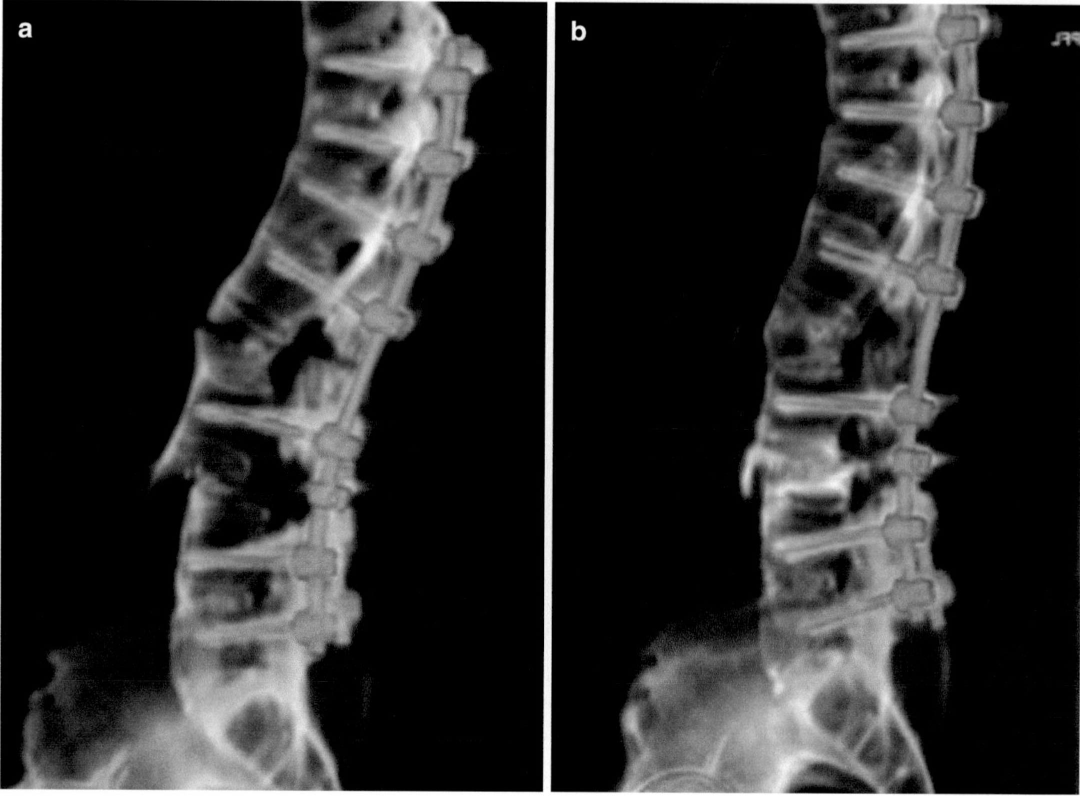

Fig. 15.3 (**a**) Postoperative sagittal computed tomography of ST level showed ST and the huge bony step occurred at the osteotomy level of L3 clearly. (**b**) In sagittal computed tomography of ST level at 18-month follow-up, ideal fusion was obtained and the streamline of the spinal canal was restored

wall lacks elasticity and is not easy to shrink and close. No matter intraoperative or postoperative, AS patients usually suffer more blood loss than ordinary patients.

4.2 Prevention

PSO, VCD, and closing wedge osteotomy techniques are suggested because they are effective in reduction of the risk of anterior vertebral vascular injury. The anterior cortical bone should be drilled as thin as much as possible to avoid injury of anterior vertebral artery by the cortex.

Improving the efficiency of operation and closing of the osteotomy surface as soon as possible are the most effective ways to reduce intraspinal venous plexus hemorrhage. General measures include abdominal vacant in the prone position, and controlled hypotension can reduce bleeding.

The main portion of blood loss occurs during osteotomy. Therefore, the surgeon should be skilled to make this period shorter. Furthermore, the use of Gelfoam or Surgiflo is helpful to decrease blood loss. Prophylactic use of large doses of tranexamic acid is an effective and safe way of reducing blood loss [20]. High-dose aprotinin is reported to have a better effect on reducing blood loss than tranexamic acid [21].

5 Abdominal Complications

5.1 Mechanism of Occurrence

As a result of correction, the status of the abdomen changed suddenly, which can result in abdominal complications. The abdominal complications after spinal deformity correction are rare, but some severe complications can cause even death and other potential risks [6]. The complications mainly are abdominal distension, superior mesenteric artery syndrome, paralytic ileus, stress ulcer, and tensive blisters of the skin [7]. It is especially common in patients with a long history of kyphosis and paravertebral soft tissue contracture [3] (Fig. 15.4).

5.2 Prevention

These complications are caused by abdominal volume change after surgery. So it is hard to prevent during operation. A lateral position is conducive to reduce the extrusion to duodenum by superior mesenteric artery. By means of abrosia, gastrointestinal decompression, and application of gastric mucosal protective agent, the symptoms disappeared gradually. As for the treatment of tensive blisters and skin lesion, hydropathic compress of magnesium sulfate is suggested.

6 Internal Fixation Complications

6.1 Mechanism of Occurrence

The pedicle screws and rods system have achieved satisfactory results in the correction of severe spinal deformity, and the complications such as screw loosening, prolapse, fracture, loss of correction, and pseudoarthrosis have been gradually reduced. As long as AS patients have strong bone fusion ability and there is a stable internal fixation, delayed fusion or non-fusion is rarely occurring [3, 22].

However, in most patients AS is always accompanied by osteoporosis. It may cause pedicle screw cutting or pulling out during the procedure of reduction [23]. The insufficiency of correction is

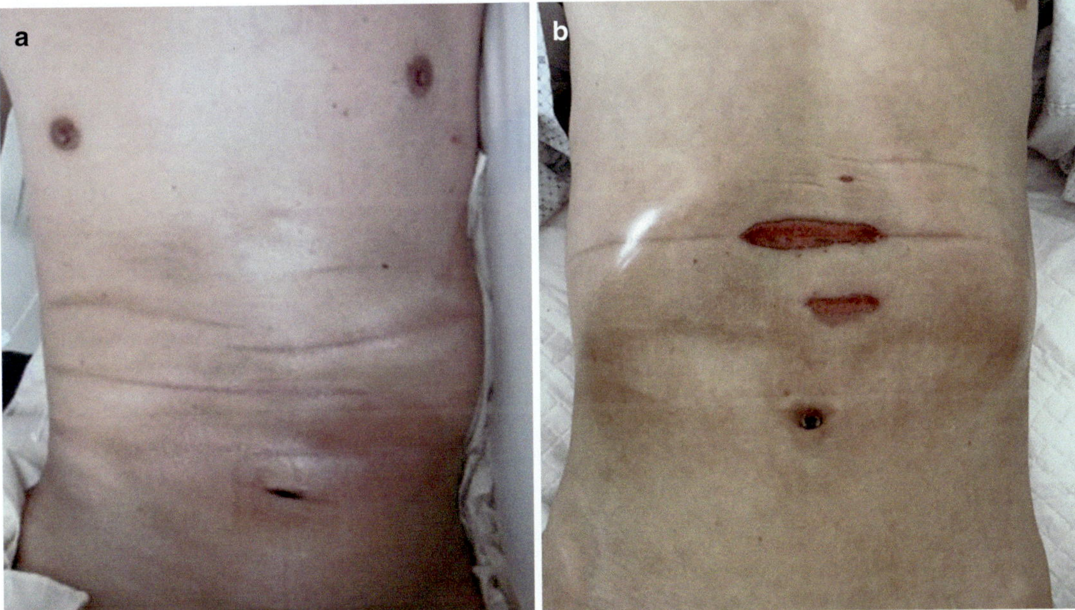

Fig. 15.4 (**a**) Postoperative abdominal tension. (**b**) Skin lesions due to excessive abdominal tension

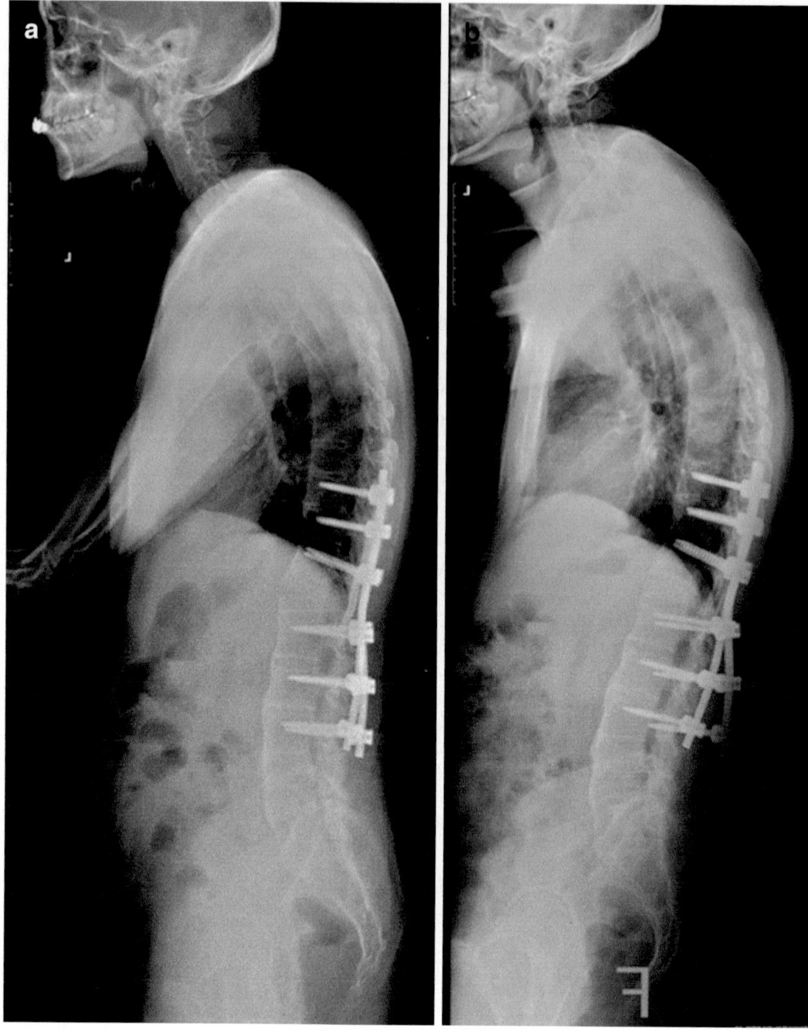

Fig. 15.5 (**a**) 40-year-old male with AS underwent vertebral column decancellation for correcting thoracolumbar kyphosis. (**b**) 5 months after surgery, it was found that pedicle screw pulled out at L2 and L3

another risk factor. In this group of patients, the gravity center is still located in front of the spine. So the fixed segments suffer greater stress. The risk of fixation failure and delayed fusion or pseudarthrosis is increased consequently (Fig. 15.5).

6.2 Prevention

Lengthening the internal fixation segment and placing transverse connecting rod are helpful in reducing stress concentration on screws. The larger diameter and length of the pedicle screw can also be selected to increase the holding force of the screw. The pedicle screws augmented by bone cement are reported to increase pullout strength [24]. An excellent bone-screw interface and fixation strength can also be achieved by using multiaxial expandable pedicle screws [25]. Besides, the application of external fixator brace is suggested postoperatively.

7 Proximal Junctional Kyphosis (PJK)

7.1 Mechanism of Occurrence

PJK is an important complication after long-segment spinal fusion in adolescent idiopathic scoliosis and adult spinal deformity. The

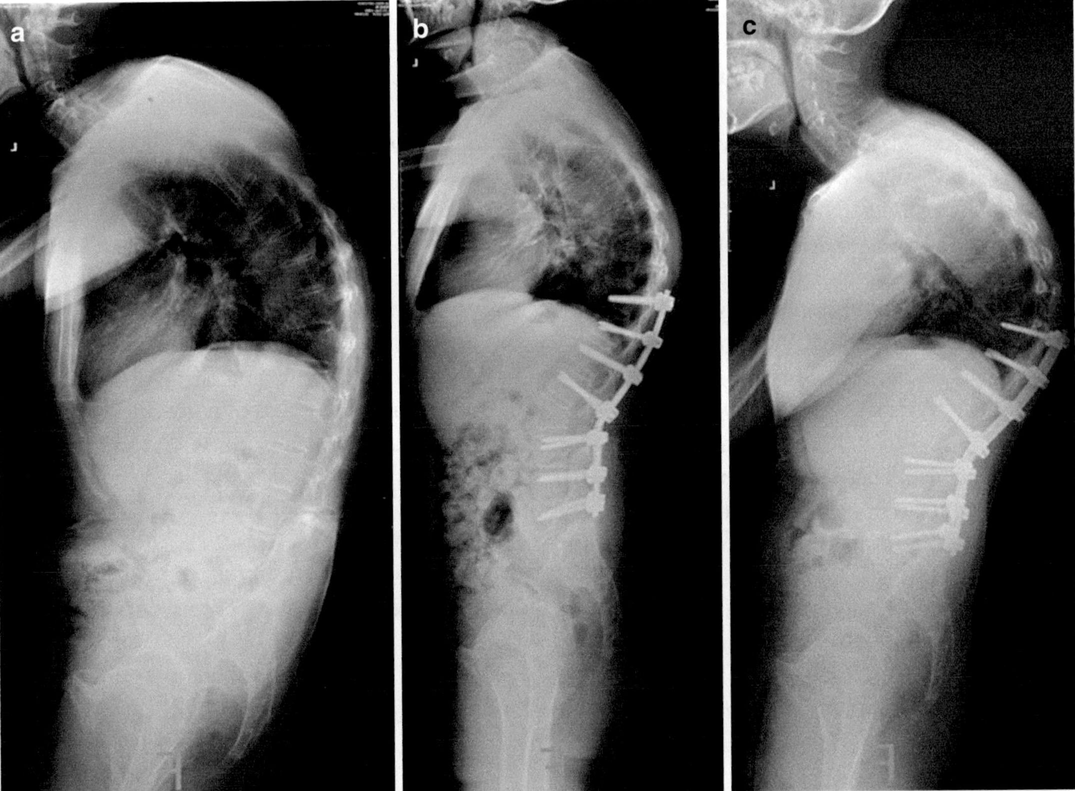

Fig. 15.6 A 34-year-old male with ankylosing spondylitis treated with posterior osteotomy and instrumented fusion (T10-L5). (**a**) Preoperative PJA was 22°; TK was 79°; SVA was 140 mm. (**b**) Three months postoperative PJA was 24°; TK was 72°; SVA was 84 mm. (**c**) Two years after operation, PJA was 35°; TK was 83°; SVA was 67 mm

increasing degree of proximal junctional area could lead to back pain, screw pullout, fracture, and sagittal imbalance. In recent years, several studies have reported some cases indicating that PJK occurred in AS patient with an incidence of 6–15% [3, 14, 26] (Fig. 15.6). The three aspects will affect the incidence of PJK: [1] greater preoperative sagittal imbalance, [2] greater local kyphosis at proximal junctional area, and [3] greater curvature correction [26]. In rigid spine of AS patient, a larger sagittal angle of proximal junctional segments leads to stress concentration, which may lead to PJK aggravation or even proximal junctional failure.

The recent research indicates that the AS patients with PJK do not suffer from more additional pain than the patients without PJK, and even none of them experienced proximal junctional failure during the follow-up [26]. But we still need to give special attention to its occurrence because it may progress during longer follow-up.

7.2 Prevention

A better surgical planning is vital to reconstruct sagittal balance and avoid PJK occurrence. Reducing osteotomy angle in some severe cases will not only ensure patients' normal visual field but also decrease risk of PJK. It is suggested that extending the fusion to a higher level when patient had pre-existing PJK decreases the risk of PJK. The inflammatory markers should also be monitored to prevent disease progression [14].

8 Loss of Correction

8.1 Mechanism of Occurrence

Satisfactory surgical correction could be achieved in AS patients following spinal osteotomy and all radiographic parameters improved significantly after surgery. However, loss of correction has also been reported by several authors in the follow-up period, with manifestation of global kyphosis increasing and lumbar lordosis decreasing (Fig. 15.7) [14]. Loss of correction is less likely to occur in the operated segments due to the solid spinal fusion. But it is mainly ascribed to non-fused segments. There are two probable mechanisms leading to loss of correction. Firstly, the increased kyphotic angle of proximal non-fused segments and distal intervertebral disc wedging were mostly associated with the deformation of proximal and distal structure, respectively [27]. Secondly, the mobility of non-fused segments adjacent to the operated levels may lead to the change of proximal or distal non-instrumented segments, resulting in the loss of correction [27].

8.2 Prevention

For postoperative care, examination of ESR and CRP level should be emphasized to evaluate underlying inflammation [14]. Application of anti-inflammation medication should be regularly performed for AS patients without fully ossified bridging syndesmophytes during the follow-up period to prevent the loss of correction and is also beneficial for avoidance of hip joint dysfunction.

9 Infection

9.1 Mechanism of Occurrence

Because of the characteristics of autoimmune diseases of ankylosing spondylitis, it is usually

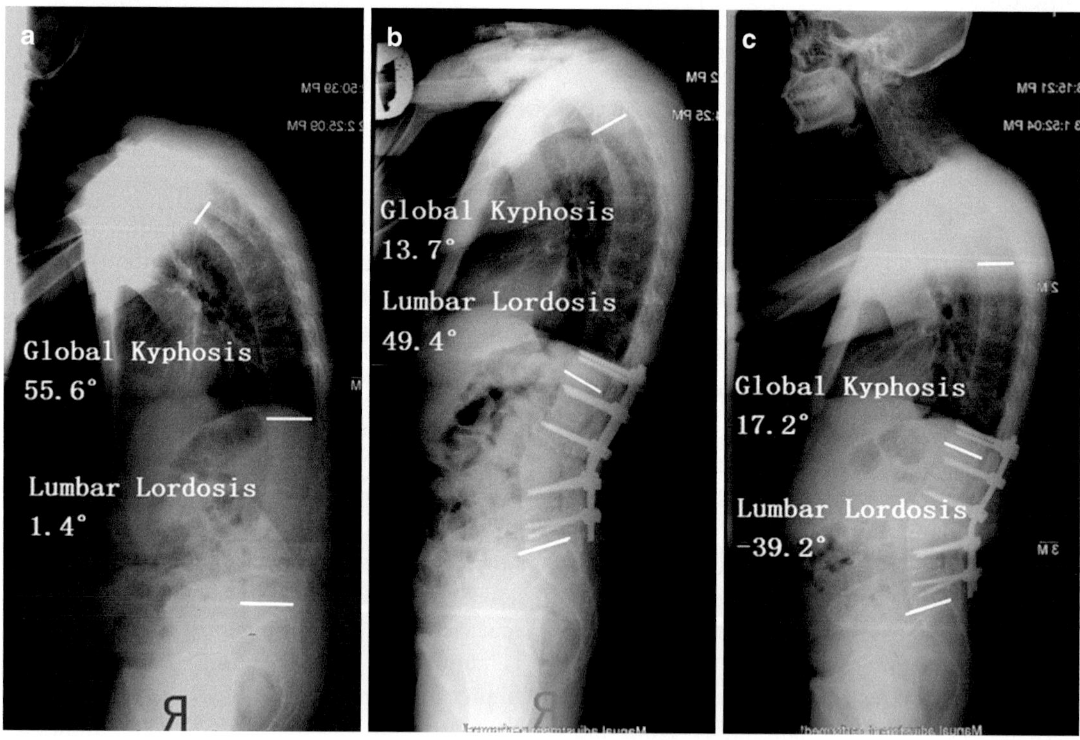

Fig. 15.7 A 46-year-old male AS patient with thoracolumbar kyphosis (**a**) underwent L3 PSO (**b**). (**c**) A worsening global kyphosis combined with decreased lumbar kyphosis was found 6 months after surgery. A mild loss of correction was identified

accompanied by higher complication and a relatively large age in patients undergoing orthopedic surgery, which can lead to a higher incidence of postoperative infection (24.6%) [4]. Superficial or deep infection of the incision, pulmonary infection, urinary tract infection, and meningitis are reported. Deep infection of the incision is considered to be related to the heavy weight of the patient or the late start of standing exercise. Subarachnoid infection and meningitis are caused by secondary cerebrospinal fluid leakage.

With the improvement of anesthetic monitoring and method of irrigating the wound in the operation, autologous blood transfusion, and development of internal fixation, the patient is able to stand and walk as soon as possible, making the postoperative infection rate decrease to 2.6% [4].

9.2 Prevention

All surgeries have to be performed using aseptic techniques. Complete flushing of the wound and reducing the input of allogeneic blood could decrease the risk of infection. Early functional exercise also contributes to avoid infection. Almost all infected patients can be cured after debridement, soft tissue repair, and antibiotic treatment.

References

1. Mundwiler ML, Siddique K, Dym JM, Perri B, Johnson JP, Weisman MH. Complications of the spine in ankylosing spondylitis with a focus on deformity correction. Neurosurg Focus. 2008;24:E6.
2. Yang BP, Ondra SL, Chen LA, Jung HS, Koski TR, Salehi SA. Clinical and radiographic outcomes of thoracic and lumbar pedicle subtraction osteotomy for fixed sagittal imbalance. J Neurosurg Spine. 2006;5:9–17.
3. Chang KW, Chen YY, Lin CC, Hsu HL, Pai KC. Closing wedge osteotomy versus opening wedge osteotomy in ankylosing spondylitis with thoracolumbar kyphotic deformity. Spine (Phila Pa 1976). 2005;30:1584–93.
4. Willems KF, Slot GH, Anderson PG, Pavlov PW, de Kleuver M. Spinal osteotomy in patients with ankylosing spondylitis: complications during first postoperative year. Spine (Phila Pa 1976). 2005;30:101–7.
5. Fu J, Song K, Zhang YG, Zheng GQ, Zhang GY, Liu C, et al. Changes in cardiac function after pedicle subtraction osteotomy in patients with a kyphosis due to ankylosing spondylitis. Bone Joint J. 2015;97-B:1405–10.
6. Liu C, Song K, Zhang Y, Fu J, Zheng G, Tang X, et al. Changes of the abdomen in patients with ankylosing spondylitis kyphosis. Spine (Phila Pa 1976). 2015;40:E43–8.
7. Sugrue PA, O'Shaughnessy BA, Nasr F, Koski TR, Ondra SL. Abdominal complications following kyphosis correction in ankylosing spondylitis. J Neurosurg Spine. 2009;10:154–9.
8. Zhao Y, Wang Y, Wang Z, Zhang X, Mao K, Zhang Y. Effect and strategy of one-stage interrupted two-level transpedicular wedge osteotomy for correcting severe kyphotic deformities in ankylosing spondylitis. Clin Spine Surg. 2016;30(4):E454–9.
9. Buchowski JM, Bridwell KH, Lenke LG, Kuhns CA, Lehman RA, Kim YJ, et al. Neurologic complications of lumbar pedicle subtraction osteotomy: a 10-year assessment. Spine (Phila Pa 1976). 2007;32:2245–52.
10. Van Royen BJ, De Gast A. Lumbar osteotomy for correction of thoracolumbar kyphotic deformity in ankylosing spondylitis. A structured review of three methods of treatment. Ann Rheum Dis. 1999;58:399–406.
11. Wang Y, Zhang Y, Mao K, Zhang X, Wang Z, Zheng G, et al. Transpedicular bivertebrae wedge osteotomy and discectomy in lumbar spine for severe ankylosing spondylitis. J Spinal Disord Tech. 2010;23:186–91.
12. Zhang X, Zhang Z, Wang J, Lu M, Hu W, Wang Y, et al. Vertebral column decancellation: a new spinal osteotomy technique for correcting rigid thoracolumbar kyphosis in patients with ankylosing spondylitis. Bone Joint J. 2016;98-B:672–8.
13. Zheng GQ, Song K, Zhang YG, Wang Y, Huang P, Zhang XS, et al. Two-level spinal osteotomy for severe thoracolumbar kyphosis in ankylosing spondylitis. Experience with 48 patients. Spine (Phila Pa 1976). 2014;39:1055–8.
14. Zhu Z, Wang X, Qian B, Wang B, Yu Y, Zhao Q, et al. Loss of correction in the treatment of thoracolumbar kyphosis secondary to ankylosing spondylitis: a comparison between Smith-Petersen osteotomies and pedicle subtraction osteotomy. J Spinal Disord Tech. 2012;25:383–90.
15. Chang KW, Chen HC, Chen YY, Lin CC, Hsu HL, Cai YH. Sagittal translation in opening wedge osteotomy for the correction of thoracolumbar kyphotic deformity in ankylosing spondylitis. Spine (Phila Pa 1976). 2006;31:1137–42.
16. Arun R, Dabke HV, Mehdian H. Comparison of three types of lumbar osteotomy for ankylosing spondylitis: a case series and evolution of a safe technique for instrumented reduction. Eur Spine J. 2011;20:2252–60.
17. Chiffolot X, Lemaire JP, Bogorin I, Steib JP. Pedicle closing-wedge osteotomy for the treatment of fixed sagittal imbalance. Rev Chir Orthop Reparatrice Appar Mot. 2006;92:257–65.

18. Cho KJ, Bridwell KH, Lenke LG, Berra A, Baldus C. Comparison of Smith-Petersen versus pedicle subtraction osteotomy for the correction of fixed sagittal imbalance. Spine (Phila Pa 1976). 2005;30:2030–7. discussion 2038.
19. Murrey DB, Brigham CD, Kiebzak GM, Finger F, Chewning SJ. Transpedicular decompression and pedicle subtraction osteotomy (eggshell procedure): a retrospective review of 59 patients. Spine (Phila Pa 1976). 2002;27:2338–45.
20. Elwatidy S, Jamjoom Z, Elgamal E, Zakaria A, Turkistani A, El-Dawlatly A. Efficacy and safety of prophylactic large dose of tranexamic acid in spine surgery: a prospective, randomized, double-blind, placebo-controlled study. Spine (Phila Pa 1976). 2008;33:2577–80.
21. Baldus CR, Bridwell KH, Lenke LG, Okubadejo GO. Can we safely reduce blood loss during lumbar pedicle subtraction osteotomy procedures using tranexamic acid or aprotinin? A comparative study with controls. Spine (Phila Pa 1976). 2010;35:235–9.
22. Chang KW, Tu MY, Huang HH, Chen HC, Chen YY, Lin CC. Posterior correction and fixation without anterior fusion for pseudoarthrosis with kyphotic deformity in ankylosing spondylitis. Spine (Phila Pa 1976). 2006;31:E408–13.
23. Kiaer T, Gehrchen M. Transpedicular closed wedge osteotomy in ankylosing spondylitis: results of surgical treatment and prospective outcome analysis. Eur Spine J. 2010;19:57–64.
24. Paré PE, Chappuis JL, Rampersaud R, Agarwala AO, Perra JH, Erkan S, et al. Biomechanical evaluation of a novel fenestrated pedicle screw augmented with bone cement in osteoporotic spines. Spine (Phila Pa 1976). 2011;36:E1210–4.
25. Wu ZX, Cui G, Lei W, Fan Y, Wan SY, Ma ZS, et al. Application of an expandable pedicle screw in the severe osteoporotic spine: a preliminary study. Clin Invest Med. 2010;33:E368–74.
26. Wang T, Zhao Y, Liang Y, Zhang H, Wang Z, Wang Y. Risk factor analysis of proximal junctional kyphosis after posterior osteotomy in patients with ankylosing spondylitis. J Neurosurg Spine. 2018;29:75–80.
27. Qiao M, Qian BP, Mao SH, Qiu Y, Wang B. The patterns of loss of correction after posterior wedge osteotomy in ankylosing spondylitis-related thoracolumbar kyphosis: a minimum of five-year follow-up. BMC Musculoskelet Disord. 2017;18:465.

Part V

AS Kyphosis with Hip Joints Involvement

Spinal Osteotomy and Total Hip Replacement for Ankylosing Spondylitis: Which Prior to Perform

16

Guoquan Zheng, Diyu Song, Zhijun Xin, and Yan Wang

Ankylosing spondylitis (AS) is a common inflammatory rheumatic disease involving primarily the sacroiliac joints, axial skeleton, hips, and, less commonly, knee joints [1–3]. About 18.5% to 20% of patients with AS have radiographic evidence of spinal fusion [4]. A thoracic hyperkyphosis combined with a flattening of the lumbar lordosis may be the characteristic spinal deformity in the later stages of AS, which results in structural and functional impairments and even causes the patient's forward gaze to be affected. The most common spinal deformity which can lead to sagittal imbalance is a rigid thoracolumbar kyphosis (TLK).

In approximately 30% to 50% of AS patients, the hip joints may be involved, and 90% of those patients with affected hips may present with bilateral hip ankylosis [5]. Hip involvement ranges from flexion contractures to complete ankylosis, often in a disabling flexed position [6]. Sagittal imbalance, such as loss of lumbar lordosis and severe thoracic or thoracolumbar kyphosis, and ankylosing hips can all contribute to the functionally disabled and stooped posture, which is the typical appearance of AS patients. For surgical treatment of these patients, the aim is to restore function and relieve pain [7, 8]. Total hip replacement (THR) and corrective spinal osteotomy are the most common and useful surgical intervention techniques [9–16].

Functionally, fixed thoracolumbar kyphosis combined with severe hip flexion contracture can significantly compromise ambulatory capacity in patients with advanced cases of the disease [16]. Therefore, the interrelationship between the hip and spine is essential in the evaluation and management of patients with sagittal spinal deformity coexisting with hip joint involvement. Those patients who have spinal flexion deformity combined with affected hips may require two operations. So, the controversy is which one should be performed first: spinal realignment corrective osteotomy or THR.

Some authors recommend that the THR for fused hips should be performed before the correction of spinal deformities [13, 17–20]. In 1963, Lee [21] first reported that a THR should be carried out before a spinal osteotomy, and the author stated that the pain relief and the improvement in range of movement (ROM) of the hip may help assessing the residual sagittal spinal deformity of patients combined with severe hip flexion deformity more accurately. Disability caused by spinal deformity, which requires corrective operation, and site of osteotomy, as well as levels of osteotomy, are also better evaluated after the correction of the hip deformity [22]. Other authors hold the opposite opinion. Kubiak et al. confirmed that correction of spinal deformity should be carried

G. Zheng (✉) · D. Song · Z. Xin · Y. Wang
Chinese PLA General Hospital, Beijing, China

Y. Wang (ed.), *Surgical Treatment of Ankylosing Spondylitis Deformity*,
https://doi.org/10.1007/978-981-13-6427-3_16

out before THR in order to prevent malposition of future acetabular component in patients with both severe spinal deformity and fused hips [23]. Tang et al. [24] reported that the pelvis was extended when patients with AS stand up by using a stereolithographic model. Anterior dislocation of the prosthesis may be expected if an acetabular component is inserted anatomically. In 2007, they improved this technique through using three-dimensional computed tomography (CT) reconstructions and also demonstrated the extended pelvis [25].

In our opinion, determining surgical sequence should be based on patient circumstances. The following aspects should be considered before surgery decisions were made.

Firstly, for AS patients with a severe spinal kyphosis and hip deformity, they may have the potential risk of dislocation of the prosthesis after the THR, especially in the early stages (Fig. 16.1). It is essential that we should take the spine and hip deformities as a whole rather than a separate entity. Now it is well known that the spinal kyphotic deformity secondary to AS may cause the body's center of gravity to shift forward and downward, and subsequently retroversion of the pelvis, extension of the hips, flexion of the knees, and even plantar flexion of the ankles may be observed in order to compensate for the sagittal imbalance. So, the hip joints may be excessively hyperextended with the patient in an upright posture if THR was carried out prior to the corrective spinal osteotomy, and the ROM of hip was restored, which may explain the risk of dislocation. Tang [24] argued that AS patients are more inclined to have anterior dislocation while acetabular components are placed in their anatomic and normal position because the positions of hips may become relatively hyperextended after THA. It has been shown that compensatory mechanisms of the spine and pelvic are necessary for maintaining optimal sagittal balance and a well functional ROM in both the native and artificial hips. Therefore, the risk of complications following THA may increase without the compensation at the spinopelvic junction [26].

Secondly, it is difficult for a surgeon to decide the positions of acetabular component for AS patients who also have spinal deformity if they undergo THA first. Acetabular component positioning may be achieved with the use of pelvic parameters intraoperatively or by navigation referenced from the anterior pelvic plane. However these static measurements may not correlate with the true acetabular anteversion in functional positions of standing and sitting [27]. Furthermore its relevance has been questioned in several articles because of the wide variation in normal values in both the sitting and standing positions and the inability to correlate the anterior pelvic plane with other spinopelvic parameters [26, 28, 29]. As we have known, patients with spinopelvic malalignment have an increased preoperative spinopelvic tilt and accordingly have a high incidence of excessive anteversion of acetabular components. Bhan et al. [30] demonstrated that exceeding anteversion may lead to impingement of the prosthetic neck, or difficulties in the placement of the hip or reduction of the hip during operation, and may also cause anterior instability of the prosthesis subsequently. Buckland et al. [27] found that correction of sagittal spinal deformity following THR resulted in reduced acetabular anteversion. Sato et al. [31] recommended reducing the anteversion of the acetabular component; however, this may result in insufficient acetabular anteversion and resultant posterior dislocation after correction of spinal alignment and pelvic tilt [28]. Phan et al. [32] suggested that patients with rigid and unbalanced spine, who take THA firstly without a sagittal balance spine and subsequently undergo spinal corrective surgery, may require revision surgery of the acetabular component to adapt with the reorientated pelvic after spinal realignment if instability and impingement of the hip exist. Therefore, the placement of the acetabular component should depend on prior spinal surgery for those AS patients who have rigid spinal imbalance.

Thirdly, the ideal corrective angle of spinal osteotomy is independent of acetabular anteversion

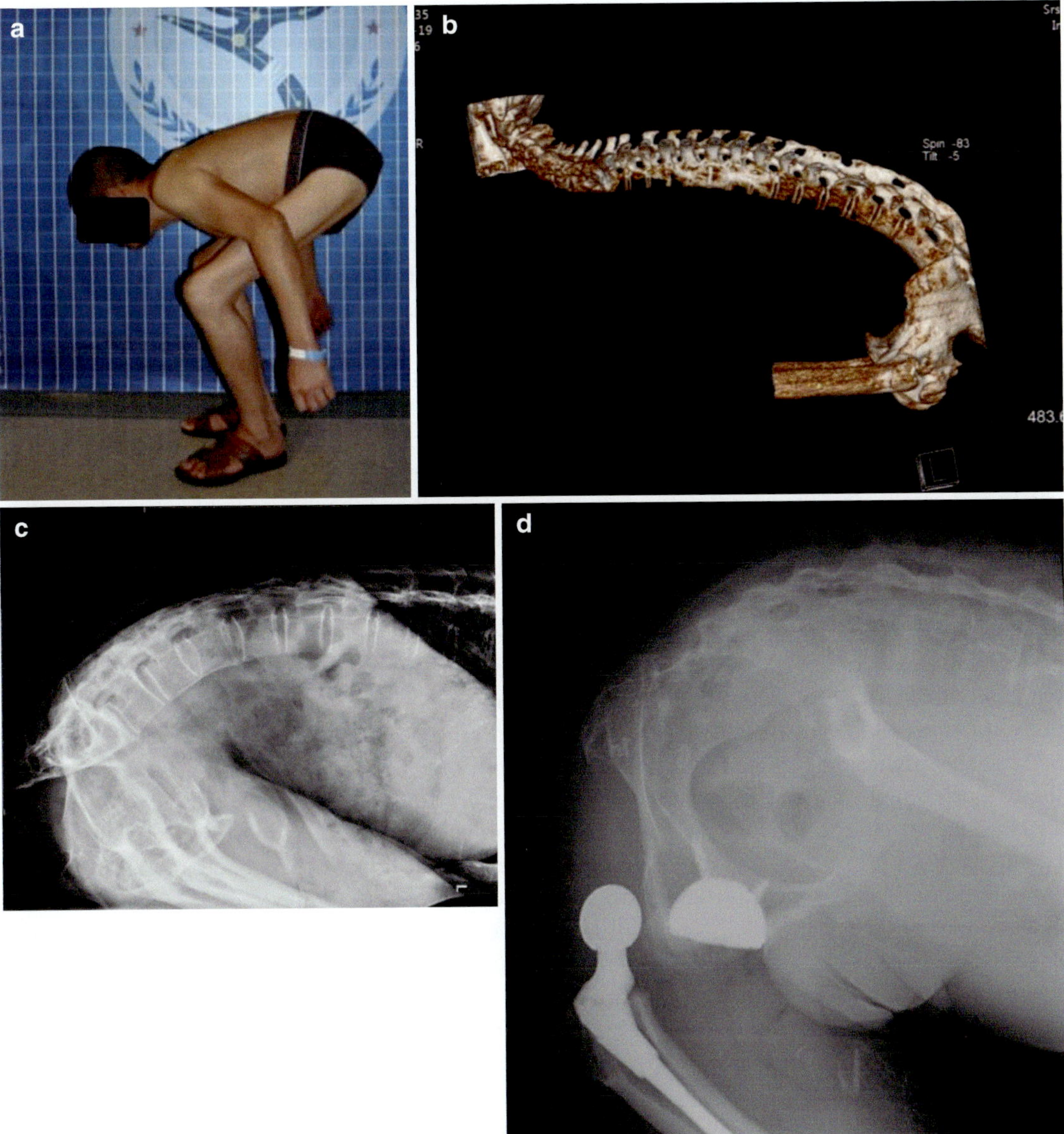

Fig. 16.1 The photos show a male patient who was 53 years old and had a spinal kyphotic deformity and ankylosed hip resulting from AS. Besides the pain in the hips and back, the main problem was the deformity which restricted his normal daily activities. The prone position on the operating table could not be achieved, so a THA was performed firstly. (**a**) The clinical photograph before THA; (**b** and **c**) The CT reconstruction and X-ray show severe kyphotic spine and hip flexion contracture; (**d**) Posterior dislocation of the component was founded 3 days after THA surgery

and can be calculated according to the pelvic incidence (PI), which is an anatomical parameter and remains invariable after realignment of the spine [33–35]. Following spinal osteotomy, a relatively normal sagittal alignment between the spine and pelvis can be acquired, which may help guiding the position of the acetabular component. Song [33] and Van Royen [34, 35], respectively, presented a mathematical and biomechanical method which can be used for calculating the deformity and correction angle of osteotomies in sagittal plane before surgery. In order to visualize the planning procedure of spinal osteotomies, Van Royen also developed a new program based on computer [35]. Our method was that firstly the theoretical value of postoperative pelvic tilt (PT) of an individual patient was calculated according to preoperative PI and then the plumb line redefined through the hip axis [36] and finally the angle for shifting the center of trunk was required, which was just the corrective osteotomy angle required for the spine [33].

Finally, the nursing management of AS patients during perioperative period of THR and rehabilitation after THR can be carried out more easily and safely after the spinal deformity was corrected previously (Fig. 16.2). Because the spine of AS patient is kyphotic and fragile, some serious operative complications, such as paraplegia, can occur during the process of THR. Some authors [37, 38] had reported patients with AS might usually have vertebral body fractures and traumatic paraplegia during bed transfers in hospital or due to falls; however these injuries might also occur during process of TRH due to the surgical position [39]. Hyperextension of the rigid and immobile spine was the possible mechanism [40]. Besides, the osteoporosis of the spine, which is usually present in AS patients [41], increased the risk of vertebral body fractures and resultant spinal cord injury [42]. In AS patients, the shearing fractures of the intervertebral discs were more common than those of the vertebral bodies [43]. So, the management and nursing in perioperative period of THR may be achieved more safely and conveniently, if the correction of spinal deformity was previously performed.

However, for few AS patients with severe hip joint flexion contractures and spinal kyphosis deformity, whose intraoperative positioning cannot be undertaken, a spinal corrective osteotomy should not be performed prior to THR. In the setting of spinal osteotomy, the surgical procedure is performed with the patient in prone position. Sometimes the deformity is so severe that the head and trunk of AS patient almost come into contact with the legs at the ankylosing condition, and putting the patients in prone position on the operating table for spine surgery becomes impossible.

For these patients, there may be two possible choices for treatment. The first option would be to perform THR and subsequently spinal osteotomy because the total hip arthroplasty procedure can be performed with lateral position (Fig. 16.3). After THR, the ROM of hip joints can be improved, which makes the prone position on operating stable possible. Nevertheless, we should bear in mind that THR first may increase the risk of prosthetic dislocation. Therefore, when performing total hip replacement prior to spinal corrective osteotomy, it is crucial that the pelvic tilt and the influence of subsequent spinal correction on pelvic tilt should be comprehended during the planning of acetabular orientation [29]; and it is also important that before THR surgery the relationship and matching between the spine and the pelvis should be evaluated so that the malposition of acetabular component can be prevented. The second one would be to proceed with resection of the femoral neck first and then spinal osteotomy. And the THR would be performed lastly. The purpose of resection of the femoral neck is to change the ankylosing condition of joints and improve ROM of the hip. Then the patients can lie in prone position for spine operation. The benefit of this treatment pathway is that spinal osteotomy can be ensured before THR. However, patients with resection of the femoral neck may feel more uncomfortable, such as pain in the hip, in the early periods after surgery and also have inconvenience in rehabilitation after spinal osteotomy due to inability to stand or walk.

In a word, we recommend that a spinal corrective osteotomy surgery should be performed prior to a THR for the AS patients with coexisting spine and hip deformity, except that the intraoperative positioning cannot be achieved due to the severe deformity. Of course, the quality of life is very low in the period of time between spinal osteotomy and THR, because the patients cannot move if the sagittal plane deformity was corrected while the bilateral hip joints were still ankylosed.

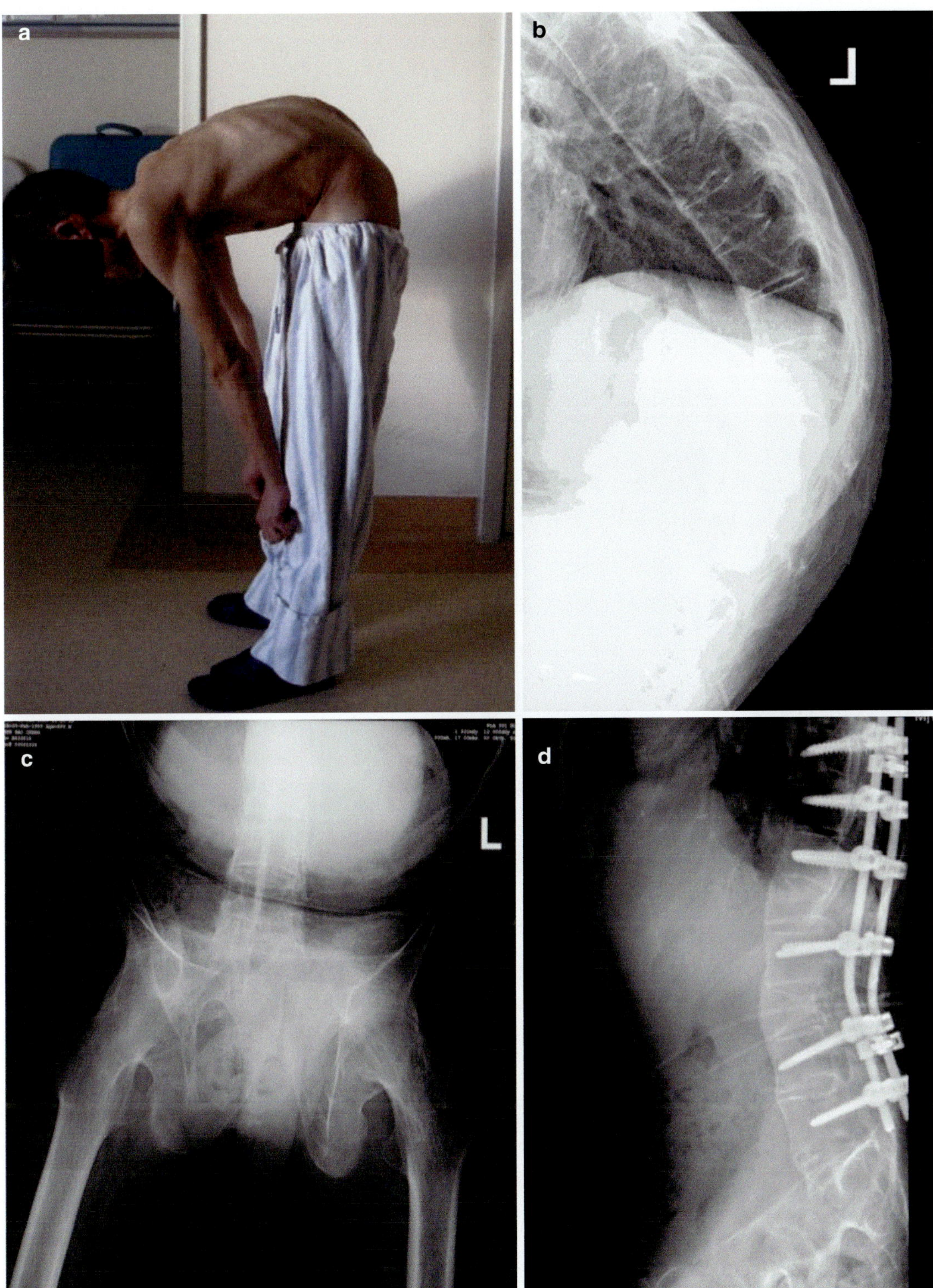

Fig. 16.2 The photos show a 48-year-old man resulting from AS. (**a**) The clinical picture before spinal osteotomy; (**b** and **c**) Preoperative X-ray shows kyphotic spine coexisting with hip deformity; (**d**) Postoperative X-ray shows that the alignment of the spine is good; (**e**) The patient could stand erectly and acquired full correction of the spinal deformity after the spinal osteotomy

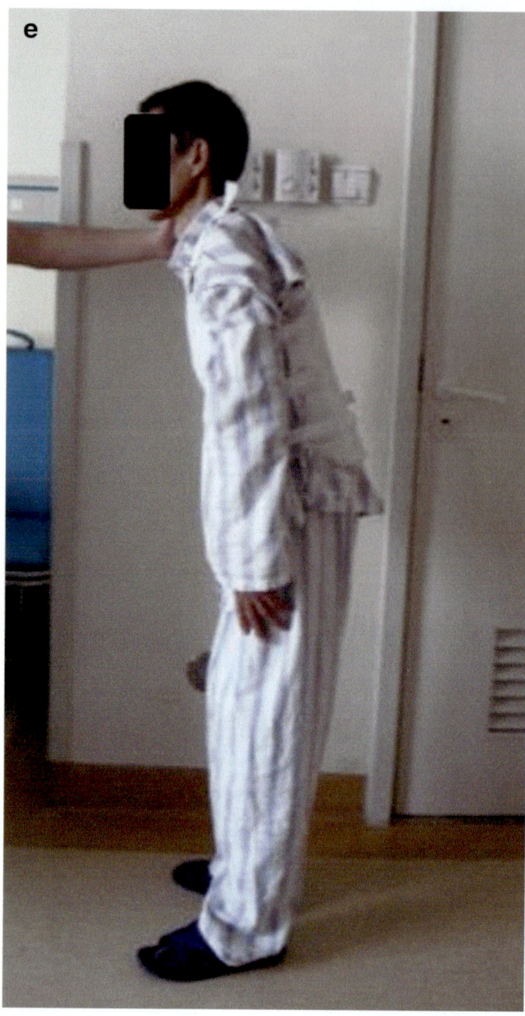

Fig. 16.2 (continued)

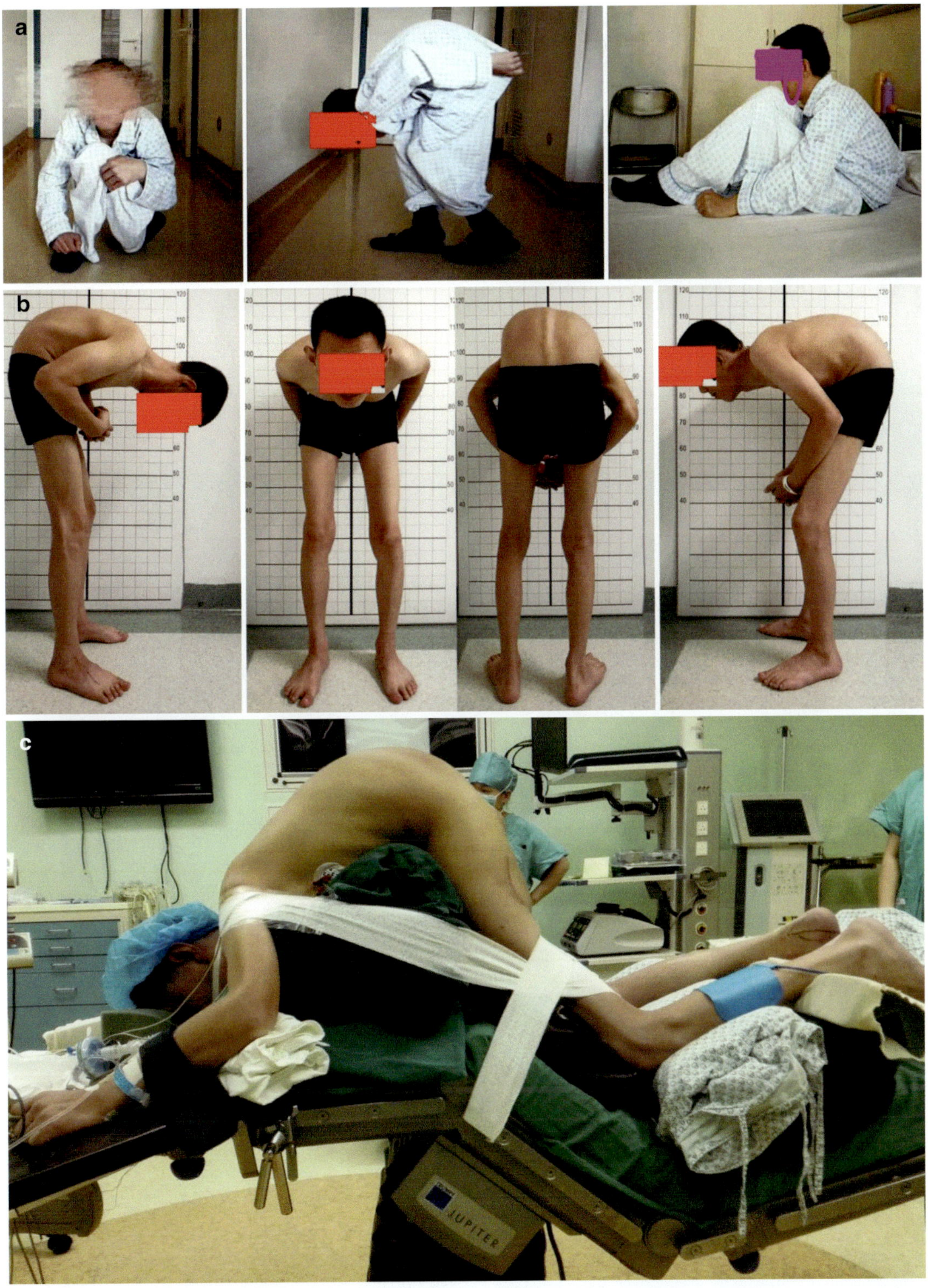

Fig. 16.3 The photos show a 36-year-old man resulting from AS whose spine and bilateral hip joints were involved. (**a**) The clinical picture before any surgery shows that the patient cannot stand erectly and cannot lie straight on the bed, and he must sit on the posterior malleolar for face-to-face communication; (**b**) Bilateral THR was performed before spinal osteotomy because the intraoperative positioning of the patient could not be performed due to the severe overall deformity. After the THR, there was a space between the chest and the thigh; (**c**) Intraoperative position; (**d**) Postoperative X-ray shows that the alignment of the spine is good; (**e**) The patient can lie straight on the bed, stand erectly, and sat on the bed after the spinal osteotomy

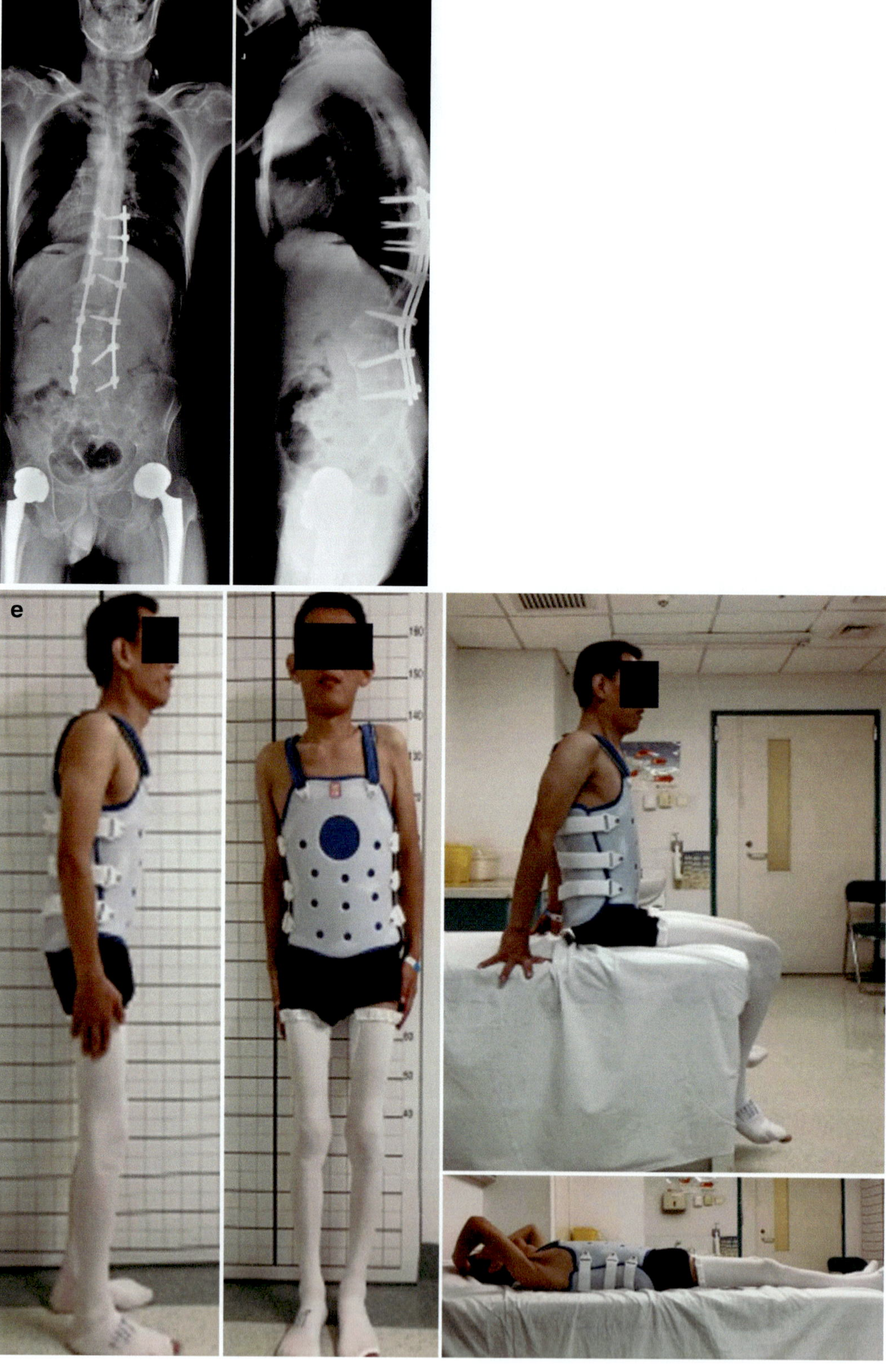

Fig. 16.3 (continued)

All the patients involved in this chapter have signed the informed consent form to publish details in these cases.

References

1. Braun J, Sieper J. Ankylosing spondylitis. Lancet. 2007;369:1379–90.
2. Dagfinrud H, Mengshoel AM, Hagen KB, et al. Health status of patients with ankylosing spondylitis: a comparison with the general population. Ann Rheum Dis. 2004;63:1605–10.
3. Weinstein PR, Karpman RR, Gall EP, Pitt M. Spinal cord injury, spinal fracture, and spinal stenosis in ankylosing spondylitis. J Neurosurg. 1982;57:609–16.
4. Chen HA, Chen CH, Liao HT, et al. Factors associated with radiographic spinal involvement and hip involvement in ankylosing spondylitis. Semin Arthritis Rheum. 2011;40(6):552–8.
5. Joshi AB, Markovic L, Hardinge K, Murphy JCM. Total hip arthroplasty in ankylosing spondylitis: an analysis of 181 hips. J Arthroplasty. 2002;17:427–33.
6. Kubiak EN, Moskovich R, Errico TJ, et al. Orthopaedic management of ankylosing spondylitis. J Am Acad Orthop Surg. 2005;13(4):267.
7. Brinker MR, Rosenberg AG, Kull L, Cox DD. Primary noncemented total hip arthroplasty in patients with ankylosing spondylitis: clinical and radiographic results at an average follow-up period of 6 years. J Arthroplasty. 1996;11:802–12.
8. Iorio R, Healy WL. Heterotopic ossification after hip and knee arthroplasty: risk factors, prevention, and treatment. J Am Acad Orthop Surg. 2002;10:409–16.
9. Li J, Xu W, Xu L, et al. Hip resurfacing arthroplasty for ankylosing spondylitis. J Arthroplasty. 2009;24:1285–91.
10. Joshi AB, Markovic L, Hardinge K, et al. Total hip arthroplasty in ankylosing spondylitis: an analysis of 181 hips. J Arthroplasty. 2002;17:427–33.
11. Sweeney S, Gupta R, Taylor G, et al. Total hip arthroplasty in ankylosing spondylitis: outcome in 340 patients. J Rheumatol. 2001;28:1862–6.
12. Gerscovich EO, Greenspan A, Montesano PX. Treatment of kyphotic deformity in ankylosing spondylitis. Orthopedics. 1994;17:335–42.
13. McMaster MJ. A technique for lumbar spinal osteotomy in ankylosing spondylitis. J Bone Joint Surg Br. 1985;67:204–10.
14. Hehne HJ, Zielke K, Bohm H. Polysegmental lumbar osteotomies and transpedicled fixation for correction of long-curved kyphotic deformity in ankylosing spondylitis: report on 177 cases. Clin Orthop. 1990;258:49–55.
15. Kilgus DJ, Namba RS, Gorek JE, et al. Total hip replacement for patients who have ankylosing spondylitis: the importance of formation of heterotopic bone and of the durability of fixation of cemented components. J Bone Joint Surg. 1990;72A:834.
16. Walker LG, Sledge CB. Total hip arthroplasty in ankylosing spondylitis. J Rheumatol. 1991;29(6):198–204.
17. McMaster MJ. Osteotomy of the cervical spine in ankylosing spondylitis. J Bone Joint Surg Br. 1997;79:197–203.
18. Weale AE, Marsh CH, Yeoman PM. Secure fixation of lumbar osteotomy. Surgical experience with 50 patients. Clin Orthop Relat Res. 1995;321:216–22.
19. Bisla RS, Ranawat CS, Inglis AE. Total hip replacement in patients with ankylosing spondylitis with involvement of the hip. J Bone Joint Surg Am. 1976;58:233–8.
20. Camargo FP, Cordeiro EN, Napoli MM. Corrective osteotomy of the spine in ankylosing spondylitis: experience with 66 cases. Clin Orthop Relat Res. 1986;208:157–67.
21. Lee ML. Orthopaedic problems in ankylosing spondylitis. Rheumatism. 1963;19:79–82.
22. Mahesh BH, Jayaswal A, Bhan S. Fracture dislocation of the spine after total hip arthroplasty in a patient with ankylosing spondylitis with early pseudoarthrosis. Spine J. 2008;8(3):529–33.
23. Kubiak EN, Moskovich R, Errico TJ, et al. Orthopaedic management of ankylosing spondylitis. J Am Acad Orthop Surg. 2005;13(4):267.
24. Tang WM, Chiu KY. Primary total hip arthroplasty in patients with ankylosing spondylitis. J Arthroplasty. 2000;15:52–8.
25. Tang WM, Chiu KY, Kwan MF. Sagittal pelvic mal-rotation and positioning of the acetabular component in total hip arthroplasty: three-dimensional computer model analysis. J Orthop Res. 2007;25:766–71.
26. Lazennec JY, Brusson A, Rousseau MA. Lumbar-pelvic-femoral balance on sitting and standing lateral radiographs. Orthop Traumatol Surg Res. 2013;99(1 Suppl):S87–S103.
27. Buckland AJ, Vigdorchik J, Schwab FJ, et al. Acetabular anteversion changes due to spinal deformity correction: bridging the gap between hip and spine surgeons. J Bone Joint Surg Am. 2015;97(23):1913.
28. Rousseau MA, Lazennec JY, Boyer P, Mora N, Gorin M, Catonné Y. Optimization of total hip arthroplasty implantation: is the anterior pelvic plane concept valid? J Arthroplasty. 2009;24(1):22–6.
29. Eddine TA, Migaud H, Chantelot C, et al. Variations of pelvic anteversion in the lying and standing positions: analysis of 24 control subjects and implications for CT measurement of position of a prosthetic cup. Surg Radiol Anat. 2001;23(2):105–10.
30. Bhan S, Eachempati KK, Malhotra R. Primary cementless total hip arthroplasty for bony ankylosis in patients with ankylosing spondylitis. J Arthroplasty. 2008;23:859–66.

31. Sato T, Nakashima Y, Matsushita A, Fujii M, Iwamoto Y. Effects of posterior pelvic tilt on anterior instability in total hip arthroplasty: a parametric experimental modeling evaluation. Clin Biomech (Bristol, Avon). 2013;28(2):178–81.
32. Phan D, Bederman SS, Schwarzkopf R. The influence of sagittal spinal deformity on anteversion of the acetabular component in total hip arthroplasty. Bone Joint J. 2015;97-B(8):1017.
33. Song K, Zheng G, Zhang Y, et al. A new method for calculating the exact angle required for spinal osteotomy. Spine (Phila Pa 1976). 2013;38: E616–20.
34. Van Royen BJ, De Gast A, Smit TH. Deformity planning for sagittal plane corrective osteotomies of the spine in ankylosing spondylitis. Eur Spine J. 2000;9:492–8.
35. van Royen BJ, Scheerder FJ, Jansen E. ASKypho plan: a program for deformity planning in ankylosing spondylitis. Eur Spine J. 2007;16:1445–9.
36. Vialle R, Levassor N, Rillardon L, et al. Radiographic analysis of the sagittal alignment and balance of the spine in asymptomatic subjects. J Bone Joint Surg Am. 2005;87:260–7.
37. Fox MW, Onofrio BM, Kilgore JE. Neurological complications of ankylosing spondylitis. J Neurosurg. 1993;78:871–8.
38. Hitchon PW, From AM, Brenton MD, et al. Fractures of the thoracolumbar spine complicating ankylosing spondylitis. J Neurosurg. 2002;97(2 Suppl):218–22.
39. Danish SF, Wilden JA, Sschuster J. Iatrogenic paraplegia in 2 morbidly obese patients with ankylosing spondylitis undergoing total hip arthroplasty: report of 2 cases. J Neurosurg Spine. 2008;8:80–3.
40. Murray GC, Persellin RH. Cervical fracture complicating ankylosing spondylitis: a report of eight cases and review of the literature. Am J Med. 1981;70:1033–40.
41. El MA, Borderie D, Cherruau B, et al. Osteoporosis, body composition, and bone turnover in ankylosing spondylitis. J Rheumatol. 1999;26(10):2205–9.
42. Ticó N, Ramon S, Garcia-Ortun F, Ramirez L, Castelló T, Garcia-Fernández L, Lience E. Traumatic spinal cord injury complicating ankylosing spondylitis. Spinal Cord. 1998;36:349–52.
43. Trent G, Armstrong G, O'Neil J. Thoracolumbar fractures in ankylosing spondylitis. High-risk injuries. Clin Orthop Relat Res. 1988;227:61–6.

Part VI

Hip Involvement in Ankylosing Spondylitis

17 Hip Involvement in Ankylosing Spondylitis

Ming Ni, Bo Wu, Hao Liu, Peng Ren, Haiwen Peng, Qingyuan Zheng, Jingyang Sun, Wei Chai, Guoqiang Zhang, and Yan Wang

Ankylosing spondylitis (AS) is a chronic inflammatory disease which primarily affects axial skeleton including the sacroiliac joints and spine but also involves other joints. Some patients, however, are mainly affected in the peripheral joints such as the hip and, less commonly, the knee joints. Hip joint accounts for 25–50% in peripheral involvement of AS, 50–90% patients of which have bilateral diseases, leading to stiff hip and loss of joint function. AS was once believed to mainly affect females, but recent studies tend to reveal similar prevalence between males and females. Male patients generally have more progressive spine and hip deformities, whereas females have more peripheral involvement with milder symptoms and thus higher rate of misdiagnosis and underdiagnoses. Young age at onset is a risk factor for severe disease. Loss of hip function and severe pain often lead to remarkable disability.

1 Basic Pathological Changes

The major pathological change of AS in the involved axial skeleton is known as enthesopathy, which coexists with synovitis in the AS hip joint. Femoral head becomes bigger in size as fibrosis and/or ossification progresses. In contrast with rheumatoid arthritis (RA), osteogenesis prevails over osteoclastic process in AS and thus leads to significant osteophyte formation.

AS will directly cause bony ankylosis of the spine and kyphotic deformity. The center of gravity would move downward and forward, resulting in spinal sagittal imbalance. As a result, the body would entail compensatory posterior pelvic tilt, external pelvic rotation, and flexion of the knee. All these secondary changes would, however, decompensate when hip joints become ankylosed, especially with bony fusion. Various hip deformities then begin to develop for pain relief, with or without severe spine deformities. Ankylosed hip itself would naturally cause progressively more severe disuse atrophy of surrounding muscles. AS patients, in addition, may develop osteoporosis and flexion deformity of the knee joint.

2 Clinical Presentation

The typical signs and symptoms of AS often appear gradually and present as a recurrent chronic dull pain or stiffness in the gluteal region or lower back, exacerbated by longtime standing or sedentary lifestyle. Individuals often experience pain and stiffness in the early morning hours or when standing up after a long time sitting but may improve with physical

M. Ni · B. Wu · H. Liu · P. Ren · H. Peng · Q. Zheng · J. Sun · W. Chai · G. Zhang (✉) · Y. Wang
Chinese PLA General Hospital, Beijing, China

Y. Wang (ed.), *Surgical Treatment of Ankylosing Spondylitis Deformity*,
https://doi.org/10.1007/978-981-13-6427-3_17

activity. Hip involvement may be ignored at early stage, which could present as intermittent pain, although some may experience severe radiating pain. In the beginning, pain may be unilateral and occasional but gradually becomes constant and bilateral. Patients are forced to sustain certain positions for pain relief, which could eventually cause ankylosis and loss of hip function. Spine will also develop segmental kyphotic deformity to varying degrees.

3 Radiographic Features

The earliest and most common changes in the hip involvement of AS are focal joint space narrowing (JSN). Demonstrable by plain X-ray include JSN and, as disease progresses, erosions and disappearance of joint space and eventually bony ankylosis. Some patients can present on X-ray with bone destruction and acetabular protrusion, rather than JSN and ankylosis.

Pelvic hyperextension leads to flattening of true pelvis and upper shift of obturator foramen.

Osteoporotic changes are commonly seen in the proximity of AS hips. The early- and middle-stage radiographic signs include focal or scattered decreased trabecular bone, with surrounding circular and stripped sclerotic medulla. After entering the later stage, trabecular bone further reduces with mixed radiolucency and radiopacity of various shapes inside. As ankylosing spondylitis progresses with recurrent disease activity, the medulla experiences process of constant damage and reconstruction, resulting in coexistent osteoporotic and sclerotic bone, the latter of which serves as a strong support for femoral head. As such, femoral head collapse is rarely developed despite common periarticular osteoporosis of the hip joint. The femoral medullary cavity often takes the form of Dorr type B or C, known as stove-pipe canal (Fig. 17.1).

3.1 BASRI-Hip

Radiographic hip score in AS is graded 0–5, with grade 0 being normal and 5 most severe [1]. Hip involvement in AS is defined as those above grade 2 according to BASRI-hip (see Table 17.1).

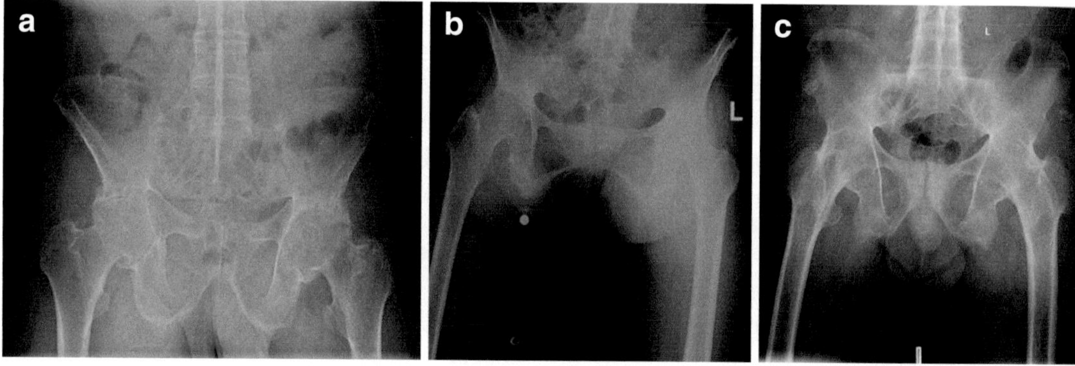

Fig. 17.1 Ankylosing spondylitis of the hip joint affected by different stages of X-ray. The pelvis presented a retrograde sign, the small pelvic ring became flattened, and the obturator transverse ellipse became a longitudinal ellipse. Osteoporosis around the hip joint. (**a**) the hip gap narrowed and the acetabulum was slightly insinuated. (**b**) the space between the hip joint was obviously narrow and blurred, and the clinical examination showed that there was no activity in the bilateral hip joint, which was characterized by the fiber rigidity sign. (**c**) the two sides of the hip joint disappeared, replacing the bone trabecula with the femoral head and the acetabulum

Table 17.1 Classification of Hip Involvement in Ankylosing Spondylitis

Grade		Description
0	Normal	No change
1	Suspicious	Possible focal joint space narrowing
2	Minimal	Definite narrowing, leaving a circumferential joint space >2 mm
3	Moderate	Narrowing but with circumferential joint space ≤2 mm or bone-on-bone apposition of <2 cm
4	Severe	Bone deformity or bone-on-bone apposition >2 cm or total hip replacement

Acknowledgements This study was conducted with approval from the Ethics Committee of Chinese PLA General Hospital, and all patients provided informed consent for their participation in this study. All figures in this chapter were recorded and edited by authors.

Reference

1. MacKay K, Brophy S, Mack C, et al. The development and validation of a radiographic grading system for the hip in ankylosing spondylitis: the bath ankylosing spondylitis radiology hip index. J Rheumatol. 2000;27(12):2866–72.

18 Hip Replacement in Patients with Ankylosing Spondylitis

Ming Ni, Bo Wu, Hao Liu, Peng Ren, Haiwen Peng, Qingyuan Zheng, Jingyang Sun, Wei Chai, Guoqiang Zhang, and Yan Wang

Total hip arthroplasty (THA) has become the golden standard treatment for end-stage hip disorders. THA has been increasingly a mature surgery when it comes to surgical techniques, prosthesis design, product materials, and manufacturing process after half a century of development. Hip involvement in AS is one of the most complex end-stage hip diseases and poses great challenges for THA surgical techniques. All relevant information including joint anatomy, periarticular soft tissues, and adjacent spine and knee functional status should be taken into consideration for a complete surgical plan.

1 Surgical Indications

For hip disorders other than AS, THA is reserved for those with severe functional impairment and pain with significant joint destruction. By contrast, surgical indications for hip involvement of AS are somewhat different. Some younger AS patients suffer from rapid progression with remarkable hip joint and periarticular tendon and ligaments involvement, which greatly adds to the complexity of the joint replacement procedure and thus negatively influences the surgical outcome. Therefore, these patients may need a more aggressive treatment, e.g., THA to better relieve pain and enhance function for them. Meanwhile, early THA could avoid disuse atrophy of soft tissues which is beneficial for postoperative recovery and patients' quality of life. To postpone surgical treatment means constant nonfunctional status of the hip joint, stiffness, and muscle dystrophy and disuse osteoporosis, all of which would complicate the THA procedure and be detrimental for postoperative rehabilitation. Joint ankylosis leads to poor postoperative recovery, and proper surgical timing means everything for symptom relief and recovery of the hip involvement of AS patients.

The surgical indications for the hip involvement of AS patients include severe bone destruction on X-ray; intolerable and recurrent pain that standard conservative treatment has little efficacy on; functional impairment of the hip, e.g., stiff hip and flexion contracture; and young patients with mature bone and rapid disease progression and significant pain. It should be noted that elevated ESR and disease activity do not constitute surgical contraindications.

2 Surgical Contraindications

Recent systemic or local infections, absent hip abductors, severe fibrosis, or major quadriceps strength deficiency.

M. Ni · B. Wu · H. Liu · P. Ren · H. Peng · Q. Zheng · J. Sun · W. Chai · G. Zhang (✉) · Y. Wang
Chinese PLA General Hospital, Beijing, China

Y. Wang (ed.), *Surgical Treatment of Ankylosing Spondylitis Deformity*,
https://doi.org/10.1007/978-981-13-6427-3_18

3 Preoperative Evaluation of the Patient and Surgical Plan

Most AS patients are chronically ill with anemia, malnutrition, and poor overall health status; therefore, multidisciplinary evaluation of the patients for their surgical tolerability, nutritional status, autoimmune status, major organ function, and airway difficulty is a must. Meanwhile, the orthopedic surgeon should ensure the best possible overall health status and operational security of the patients by working alongside with other relevant departments.

For patients using immunosuppressants and glucocorticoids, our experience is as follows: discontinuation of immunosuppressants 2 weeks before the operation, but continuation of original steroids until perioperative period when they are switched to preoperative and intraoperative 40 mg methylprednisolone, respectively, on the day of operation. The patients would receive methylprednisolone for another 3 days postoperatively, and then they will return to original steroid therapy regimens.

Unlike other THA candidates, AS patients would generally develop complex bone destruction, deformities, joint fusion, and osteoporosis to different levels in their hip joints at the same time. Therefore, attending surgeons must carefully assess the involved hips to guarantee right prosthesis selection, proper surgical plan, and satisfactory treatment outcome. Apart from the hip joint itself, a thorough evaluation of spinal, sacroiliac, and pelvic status is also necessary for a successful THA in such patients.

Full-length anteroposterior and lateral spinal, flexion-extension spinal, and pelvic and femoral X-rays should all be taken. Spinal and joint surgeons should cooperate to evaluate the spinal, sacroiliac, and pelvic joint status and severities in order to determine whether and how much additional spinal correction is needed, all of which will further map how THA should be performed, especially the orientation of the acetabular cup (shown later).

Anesthesia for AS patients poses a great challenge, for it is simply unfeasible to perform spinal or epidural anesthesia in such patients. Instead, general anesthesia is usually the only option under such condition (see Fig. 18.1). Furthermore, ossification and ankylosis of the cervical spine commonly exists, which makes traditional oropharyngeal tracheal intubation very difficult and easily leads to cervical fractures. It is therefore a must to evaluate the range of motion and flexibility of the patients' cervical spine beforehand. During intubation process, the anesthesiologist should use gentle techniques and avoid violent cervical extension and possible iatrogenic fractures and spinal cord injuries. Nasotracheal intubation should be performed under such circumstance.

4 Patient Positioning and Surgical Disinfection

Joint ankylosis usually exists in the hips and several spine segments of AS patients, which brings challenges for standard patient positioning. For those patients with insignificant spine deformity, it may still be feasible to perform THA using standard lateral decubitus position and posterior approach. However, when severe kyphosis develops, the patient's head, cervical spine, and upper body would leave the surgical bed and make stable positioning impossible. Therefore, it is strongly advisable to first securely position the head, cervical spine, upper body, and limbs of the patient onto the surgical bed, and carefully assess the pelvic ring and lower lumbar spine, and try to use external assisting device to help with pelvic and lower lumbar locating and referencing.

For those patients with ankylosed hips, especially adducted hips, traditional standard disinfection and draping are a great challenge. Under this condition, the patients should receive an enlarged area of surgical disinfection with the assistance of another person helping flex and extend the knee joints for inner thigh disinfection and proper draping. During the process, the assistant should take extra care not to overextend and fracture the lower limbs of the patients.

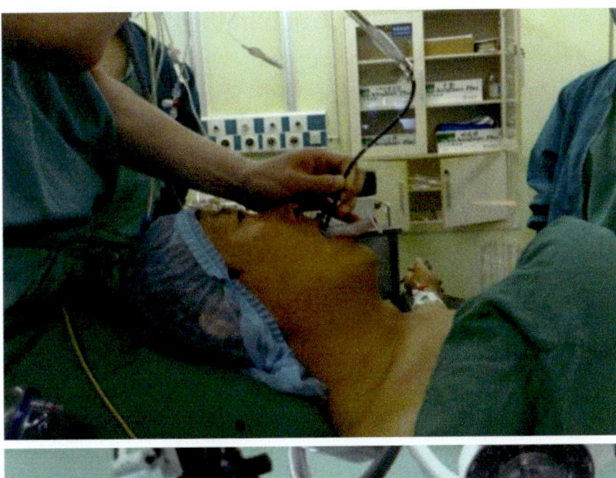

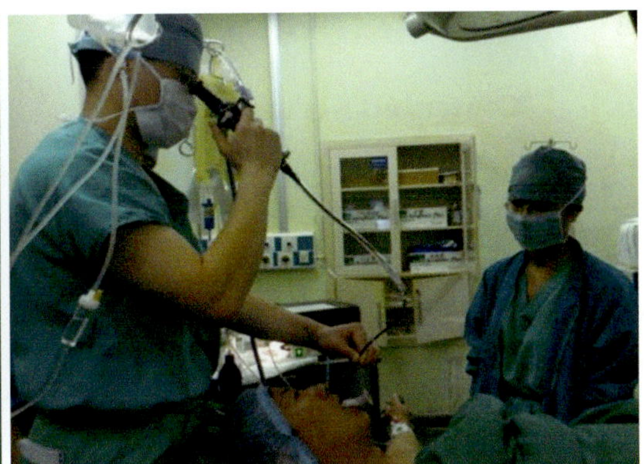

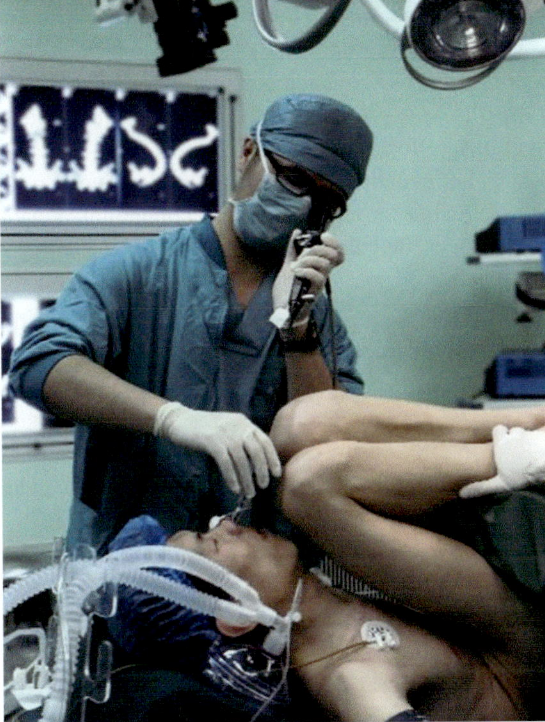

Fig. 18.1 While epidural anesthesia is difficult for cervical spondylosis, fiberoptic bronchoscopy assisted intubation and general anesthesia

5 Prosthesis Selection for Total Hip Arthroplasty

The bone quality around the hip is often poor with varying degrees of osteoporosis in ankylosing spondylitis. Bone absorption, destruction and reconstruction, concomitant or alternation, will lead to the hip anatomy variation during the process of ankylosing spondylitis involving the hip joint. At this time the selection of the appropriate prosthesis for joint anatomical reconstruction and reliable initial stability is particularly important. With the continuous development of the design concept and prosthesis materials, both cemented fixation and cementless fixation prostheses have excellent prosthesis type to be selected.

6 Cemented Hip Prosthesis

6.1 Cemented Acetabular Components

Cemented acetabular components were thick-walled polyethylene cups. Vertical and horizontal grooves often were added to the external surface to increase stability within the cement mantle, and wire markers were embedded in the plastic to allow better assessment of inclination and inclination of the components on postoperative radiographs. The external surface of the prosthesis has a small bump with a height of 3 mm, to ensure the formation of 3 mm thick continuous cement mantle, avoid the phenomenon of "bottoming out," which results in a thin or discontinuous cement mantle. Most prostheses have high-edge design to prevent dislocation. A flange at the rim of the component aids in pressurization of the cement as the cup is pressed into position in some prostheses. Although implant design and cement technology have been improved, the long-term survivorship of cemented acetabular components has not substantially improved. At present, the high cross-linked polyethylene cemented acetabular cup is used to match the fourth generation of ceramic femoral head, which is expected to prolong the long-term survivorship of cemented acetabular components in the future.

6.2 Cemented Femoral Components

Most cemented femoral components were fabricated of cobalt-chrome alloy, which can increase the cobalt-chrome alloy and reduce the stresses within the proximal cement mantle. The cross section of the stem should have a broad medial border, and the angular roundness is designed to reduce the deformation and prevent the sharp edges from cutting the cement mantle. The current popular design of the femoral stem is taper slip type construct and composite beam philosophy, the former is represented by Exeter stem, which is smooth taper shank with no collar. The surface of the prosthesis is not combined with the cement, which can subside in the cement mantle. The prosthesis converts the axial stress to compressive forces during the subsidence process, which can be stabilized again after subsidence. The latter is represented by the Lubinus SpII stem, which has a collar, cobalt-chrome alloy, with anatomic shape, surface grooves, and matte surface structure. The design concept of this prosthesis is to form a solid combination of bone cement and prosthetic surface, so that the prosthesis and bone cement can be integrated to eliminate the micromotion between the prosthesis and cement shell. The long-term results of the SPII are excellent in Europe. The prosthesis has been used for nearly 20 years in our department. Clinical results have proved that the prosthesis has a good clinical effect (see Figs. 18.2 and 18.3).

The cemented prosthesis for patients with ankylosing spondylitis has a congenital advantage over the cementless prosthesis.

1. Ankylosing spondylitis patients are mostly accompanied by osteoporosis, with poor bone, and some patients achieve the degree of severe osteoporosis. Therefore, it is difficult to obtain reliable elastic compression with cementless prosthesis, and cemented prosthesis can achieve immediate fixation.
2. The risk of infection in ankylosing spondylitis is higher than that in other hip replacement patients. When cement is fixed, it can be mixed with antibiotics to reduce the risk of infection.
3. The femoral medullary cavity of the patients with ankylosing spondylitis is often chimney, and most of the cementless prosthesis is difficult to match.

7 Cementless Hip Prosthesis

The cementless (biological fixation) hip prosthesis has become the mainstream type of prosthesis. According to the latest statistics, about 90% of acetabular prostheses in the United States are biological, and the majority of Chinese doctors choose cementless hip prosthesis in the primary hip replacement and so do our department.

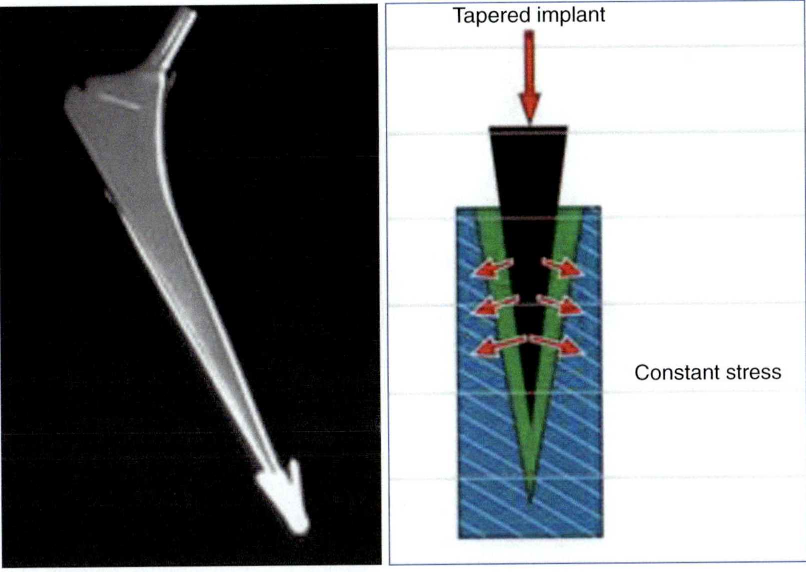

Fig. 18.2 Taper slip type construct design concept of femoral handle

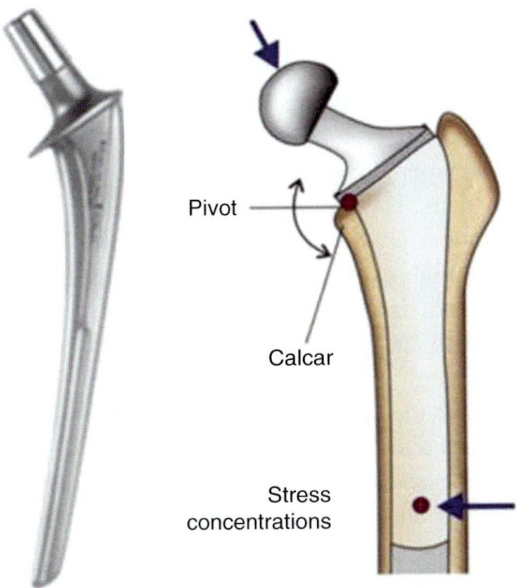

Fig. 18.3 Composite beam type construct design concept of femoral handle

7.1 Cementless Acetabular Components

In view of the characteristics of acetabular bone in ankylosing spondylitis patient, how to obtain reliable elastic compression fixation and long-term biological fixation are the main factors for the selection of cementless acetabular cup. With the improvement of metal materials and the design process, a new generation of porous-coated hemispherical prosthesis has gradually become the mainstream. More roughened surface provides a more reliable initial stability for the prosthesis implantation, and the pore size between 100 and 400 μm and the porosity of 70% are more conducive to bone growth, which provides a basis for long-term biological fixation. The new generation of porous metal coating and metal matrix is also the overall metal structure, with certain strength, so the coating can be made thicker, reaching 1.5 mm. Its advantages include reducing the modulus of elasticity while maintaining the strength of the cup, increasing the space of bone growth, and increasing the surface roughness and friction of the prosthesis to increase the stability of prosthesis implantation. Based on the above porous metal materials, various companies have developed the corresponding porous metal coating acetabular prosthesis. The new generation of acetabular cup is more suitable for ankylosing spondylitis and other poor bone conditions (see Fig. 18.4).

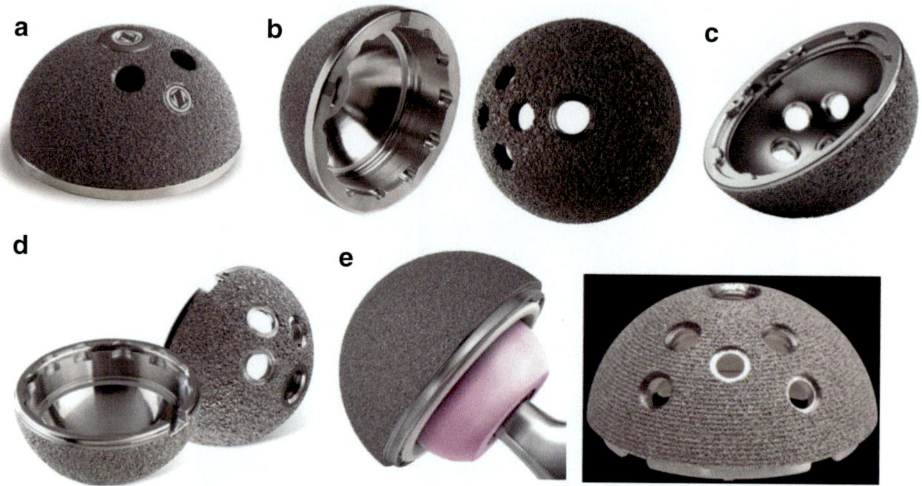

Fig. 18.4 A porous metal coating made by various major manufacturers: (**a**) Zimmer Continuum; (**b**) Biomet Regenerex; (**c**) Stryker Tritanium; (**d**) Smith & Nephew R3; (**e**) Johnson & Johnson Pinnacle gription

7.2 Cementless Femoral Components

Similar with the cementless acetabular prosthesis, the cementless femoral prosthesis also needs to consider how to obtain a firm initial fixation (initial stability); how to achieve strong bone union (permanent stability); how to promote bone growth; and how to avoid stress shielding, bone resorption, and thigh pain and other factors. For ankylosing spondylitis, it is important to choose the appropriate femoral stem because of the variation of the medullary cavity and the osteoporosis.

The current mainstream design of the femoral stem is the tapered stem, which can obtain initial stability through fit and fill/without fill. At present, there are many kinds of taper design options. The advantages of tapered stem include:

The tapered stem was better able to obtain press fit and initial stability, and it uses a three-point stem fixation to obtain immediate stability. Because the tapered stem is closely contacted with the cortex inside and outside, the three fixed points are medial calcar femorale (point 1), lateral cortex (point 2), and distal prosthesis (point 3).

The tapered stem can reduce stress shielding and bone resorption. Stress shielding is the result of too much stress in the prosthesis resulting in too little bone force. The use of cobalt-chrome alloy or shape design for anatomical and cylindrical will increase the role of stress shielding. The tapered stem is usually made of titanium alloy, tapered design to reduce the cross-sectional area of the prosthesis, and short stem and bony ingrowth that is limited to the proximal stem; these design factors will reduce the role of stress shielding.

The tapered stem can reduce the incidence of thigh pain. The incidence of thigh pain in early cementless prostheses was as high as 40%, with severe thigh pain reaching 4%. The incidence of thigh pain in cementless prostheses is closely related to the design factors of the prosthesis, such as high elastic modulus, large size, fixed to the backbone, and distal overfilling. The tapered stem can avoid the above factors in the design, and it can reduce the occurrence of thigh pain by using low elastic modulus metal, reducing cross-sectional area, only fixed to the metaphysis with a short stem.

It is more convenient to implantation, and most tapered stem requires only proximal formation without the need for distal reaming and alignment of the backbone area, making surgical procedures easier and operation time shorter.

Acknowledgements This study was conducted with approval from the Ethics Committee of Chinses PLA General Hospital, and all patients provided informed consent for their participation in this study. All figures are recorded by authors.

19 The Clinical Classification and Surgical Techniques of Ankylosing Spondylitis (AS)

Guoqiang Zhang, Ming Ni, Bo Wu, Hao Liu, Peng Ren, Haiwen Peng, Qingyuan Zheng, Jingyang Sun, Wei Chai, and Yan Wang

Different levels of pathological changes in the involved hip of ankylosing spondylitis patients result in different function damages and varying joint deformities, which can influence the surgical decision of hip replacement. Whether these patients have spinal deformity, the location or severity of spinal deformity also can influence the surgical decision. Therefore, based on the severity of spinal deformity, we made a new classification system of hip involvement with or without spinal deformity, which would benefit us to make the preoperative plan and select surgical techniques.

Principle of the Classification [1]

1. Based on the range of motion (ROM) of the involved hip, they are grouped into stiff hip with limited ROM and fibrous and bony ankylosed hip with no ROM.
2. Based on the sagittal deformity, they are grouped into Type A (<30° of flexion contracture) and Type B (more than 30° of flexion contracture).
3. Major spine deformities affecting the pelvis positioning belong to the joint hip-spine deformity.

Type			Characteristic		
Type I	Joint stiffness		Joint space stenoses, usually have arthrokatadysis	Damage of articular surface	Severe pain with limited ROM
Type II	Fibrous ankylosis	IIA (flexion contracture <30°)	Joint space blurred or severe narrow	Fibrous union	Without ROM
		IIB (flexion contracture ≥30°)			
Type III	Bony ankylosis	IIIA (flexion contracture <30°)	Joint space disappeared, and the bone trabecula passed through the joint interface	Osseous union	Without ROM
		IIIB (flexion contracture ≥30°)			
Type IV	Hip-spine deformity	IVA (cervicothoracic spinal deformity)	Hip joint lesions with all kinds of spinal deformity or sacroiliac deformity		
		IVB (lumbosacral spinal deformity)			

G. Zhang · M. Ni · B. Wu · H. Liu · P. Ren · H. Peng · Q. Zheng · J. Sun · W. Chai · Y. Wang (✉)
Chinese PLA General Hospital, Beijing, China

Y. Wang (ed.), *Surgical Treatment of Ankylosing Spondylitis Deformity*,
https://doi.org/10.1007/978-981-13-6427-3_19

1 Type I Joint Stiffness

1.1 Characteristic

In this type, ankylosing spondylitis with hip involvement patients usually have different levels of joint pain, gradually decreasing ROM, and functional limitation. The X-ray show hip joint space with stenoses in varied degrees; the acetabulum presents varying degrees of bone destruction and arthrokatadysis, sometimes it can break through the Kohler line. Usually the femoral medullary cavity morphology appears normal, and the majority of it is Dorr Type A. There is a different degree of osteoporosis in the surrounding bone of the hip joint. The sacroiliac joint mostly already got osseous union. There are different degrees of spinal deformity, and it most commonly appears as lumbar lordosis reduced or even disappeared.

1.2 Surgical Technique

Varying surgical approaches could be propitious for this type of joint replacement, so the choice mainly depends on the surgeon's preference. We routinely use the posterolateral approach.

The lateral position is routinely used for THA in author's hospital, because the involved hips usually remain in different degrees of ROM in such patients. Lumbosacral spinal deformity and sacroiliac joint lesions generally do not intervene the placement of normal lateral position.

Use the posterolateral approach to expose the articular cavity. But for the patients with severe acetabular protrusion or osteophyte of posterior acetabular wall, the first thing we probably see is not the neck of femur but the posterior acetabular wall or osteophyte. In order to identify the source of finding the bone on posterior hip joint, we can move the operating leg. Femoral neck will move with leg movement, while the posterior acetabular wall or osteophyte could not move. If the acetabulum bone covers the femoral neck, we need to cut off the osteophyte or a little bone of posterior acetabular to expose the femoral neck. Until now we can dislocate the hip joint. We should avoid the violent dislocation motion which could cause the fracture of acetabulum (Fig. 19.1).

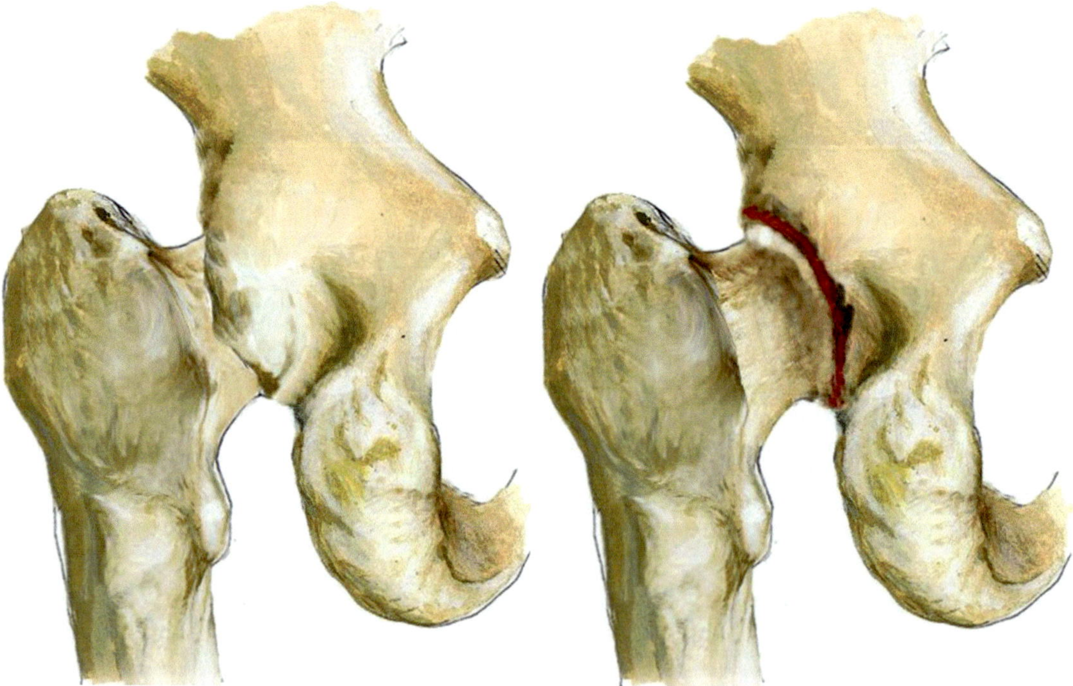

Fig. 19.1 Cut off the osteophyte or partial posterior acetabular to expose the femoral neck

1.3 The Preparation of Acetabulum [2]

The acetabular fossa of this type has a different degree of protrusion, so we should not perform routine acetabulum grinding procedure that gradually increases the diameter of reamers from the minimum size. The initial diameter of reamer should approximate to the diameter of osseous acetabulum. Make the acetabular component fit the acetabular periphery, and there may be a cavity at the bottom of the acetabulum due to acetabular protrusion. Use the femoral head to make autogenous bone granules (Size: 0.8 * 0.8 * 0.8 cm) and implant it in the bottom cavity in order to place the acetabular component in the anatomic rotation center (Fig. 19.2).

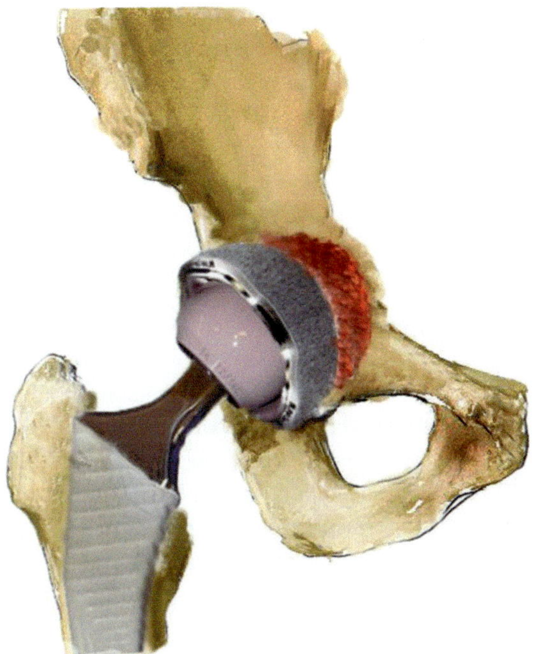

Fig. 19.2 Implant some autogenous bone granules in the bottom cavity in order to place the acetabular component in the anatomic rotation center

1.4 The Decision of Acetabular Component Implant Angles [3, 4]

The ankylosing spondylitis patient with hip involved usually has lumbosacral spinal deformity and sacroiliac joint lesions which may change the position of the pelvis. When the patient is naturally standing, the pelvis tends to be in retroversion (Fig. 19.3), and the angle of acetabular will change accordingly which could be calculated by relevant lumbosacral-pelvic parameters.

1.5 Spinal-Pelvic Relevant Parameters [4] (Fig. 19.4)

1.5.1 Pelvic Incidence (PI)

PI is defined as the angle between the line orthogonal to the inclination of the S1 endplate

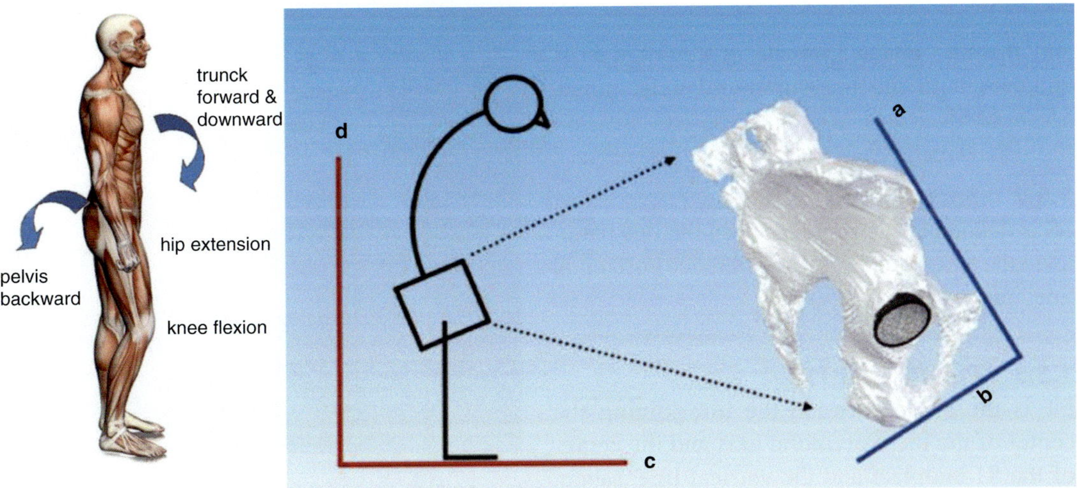

Fig. 19.3 The pelvis of ankylosing spondylitis patient tends to be in retroversion

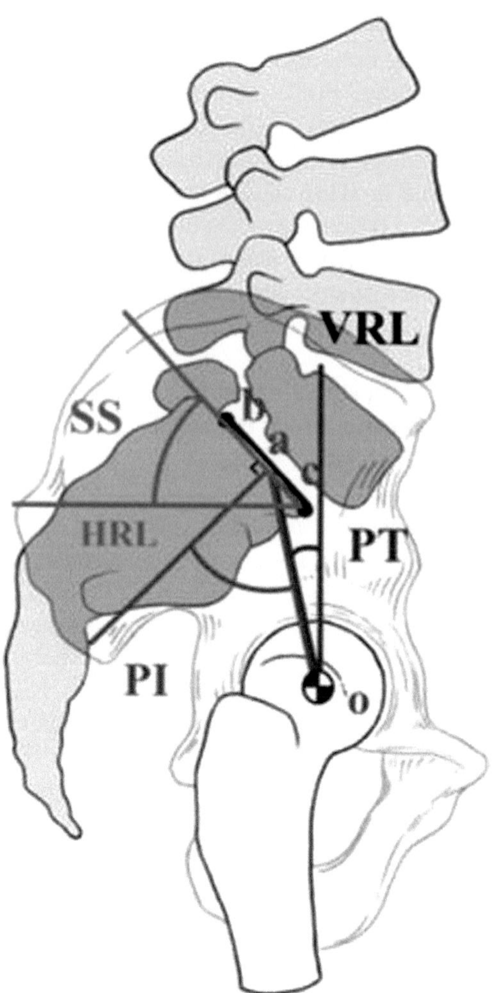

Fig. 19.4 Spinal-Pelvic Relevant Parameters

and the line connecting the center of the S1 endplate with the bicoxofemoral axis, range, 55° ± 10.6°.

1.5.2 Sacral Slope (SS)

SS is defined as the angle between the line parallel to the S1 endplate and the reference horizontal line, range, 41° ± 8.4°.

1.5.3 Pelvic Tilt (PT)

PT is the angle between the line joining the center of the bicoxofemoral axis and the center of the S1 endplate and the vertical line, range, 13° ± 6°.

1.6 The Relationship Between Pelvis Position and Acetabulum Angle in the Spontaneous Standing Posture

Posterior tilt of the pelvis → SS↓, PT↑, acetabular anteversion (AA)↑; PT increase 1°, AA increase 0.6°, and acetabular abduction angle increase 0.8. In conclusion, the changing AA value is △ PT × 0.6°, and the changing acetabular abduction angle is △ PT × 0.8°. Based on the above relationship, we can decrease the AA angle and acetabular abduction angle when implanted the acetabular component.

1.7 Typical Cases (Fig. 19.5)

Both cementless and cemented acetabulum cups are available in this type of patients, and we prefer the cementless acetabulum component. The best option of acetabular cup is the latest generation of hemispherical microporous-coated implant with screw fixation. The material of acetabular insert can choose delta ceramic or high cross-linked polyethylene.

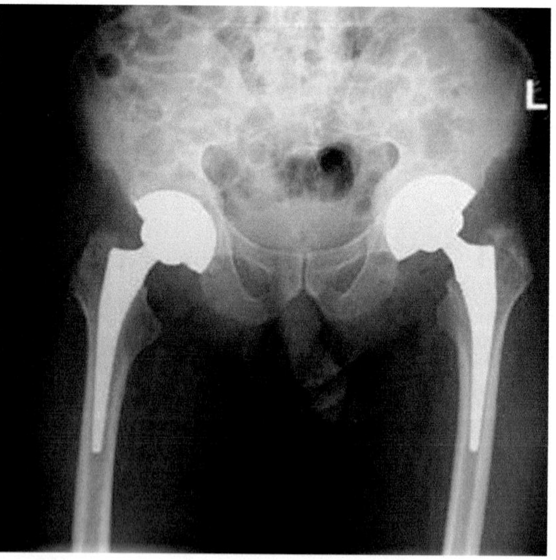

Fig. 19.5 THA for bilateral hips affected by ankylosing spondylitis

The reaming of femur medullary cavity can be routinely prepared and accomplished. Both cementless and cemented femoral components are available, and we prefer the cementless type. Because ankylosing spondylitis patients usually have poor bone quality, we should pay more attention to avoid the periprosthetic fracture when we are reaming the femur medullary cavity, implanting the prosthesis, relocating the hip joint, and releasing periarticular soft tissue.

2 Type 2 Fibrous Ankylosis

2.1 Characteristic

This type can be regarded as the intermediate type of ankylosing spondylitis with hip involvement patients. Their involved hips usually have severe narrow joint space and stable fibrous union (Fig. 19.6). The stable fibrous union fixes the involved hip on one posture, and the involved hip usually has no ROM or function. Even though the fibrous ankylosis of involved hip can relieve the pain, it also reduces the hip function which decreases the ability of daily living, especially in the nonfunction position. The X-ray shows that the pelvic is at hyperextension position; the joint space of involved hip is severe narrow and blurred; and the position of involved hip is abnormal, including flexion-extension malposition and rotation malposition.

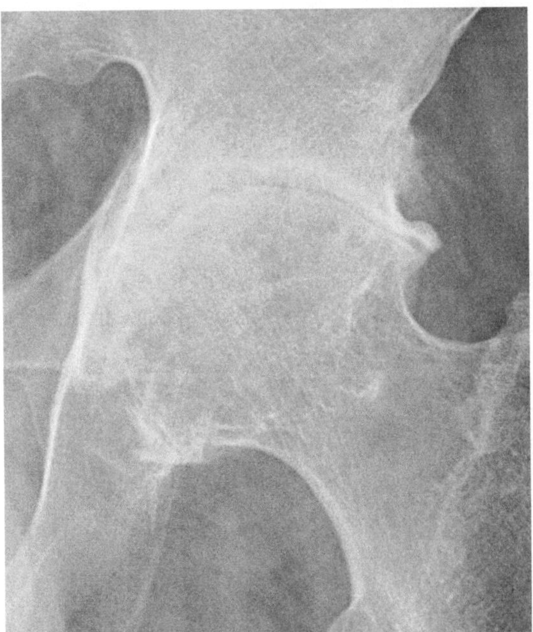

Fig. 19.6 A hip of fibrous ankylosis

The acetabulum has slight protrusion, but it seldom or never breaks through the Kohler line. Usually the femoral medullary cavity morphology appears as stovepipe type, and the majority of it is Dorr Type B/C. There is severe osteoporosis around the hip joint. Based on the sagittal deformity, they are grouped into Type A (<30° of flexion contracture) and Type B (more than 30° of flexion contracture). The sacroiliac joint mostly already got osseous union. There are different degrees of spinal deformity, and it most commonly appears as lumbar lordosis reduced or even disappeared, thoracolumbar kyphosis, and cervical bony ankylosis.

2.2 Surgical Technique

Use the posterolateral approach and anterolateral approach can finish joint replacement surgery of all the type of fibrous ankylosis hip. The anterior approach is not suitable for the fibrous ankylosis hip with severe flexion contracture. We commonly prefer the posterolateral approach.

The lateral position is routinely used in our joint replacement. Because the involved hips usually are bony ankylosis in varying posture and the spine has different degrees or segments of spinal deformity, it is difficult to position patients to the normal lateral posture. Therefore we need the assistive device to locate the pelvic and lower lumbar spine during the surgery.

Use the posterolateral approach to expose the articular cavity. After the full exposure of the femoral neck, postero-trochanteric region, and posterior acetabular wall, we can use in situ osteotomy technique to achieve the femoral neck osteotomy.

2.3 In Situ Osteotomy

This technique is mainly applicable to the hip that is hard to dislocate due to various reasons.

More specifically, we need to adequately expose the femoral neck, postero-trochanteric region, and posterior acetabular wall, and then use acetabular retractor to fully retract the posterior soft tissues of incision, especially the sciatic nerve along with posterior incision. Next, cut the femoral neck at the area close to the greater trochanter, and be careful not to damage the acetabular anterior wall. The femoral neck should better not be entirely cut off by goose saw. Retain a little anterior bone of the femoral neck, and break it manually to avoid goose saw hurting the important anterior soft tissue. If the hip is fixed in external rotation position that would lessen the posterior operating space, we can use reciprocal saw to finish the femoral neck osteotomy. Firstly, we can cut off a wedge-shaped bone block from the femoral neck near the posterosuperior area of the greater trochanter so that we can have sufficient space to bend coxa. Then flex and internal rotate the thigh, expose the femoral neck, and cut off the needless residual bone of the femoral neck according to regular procedure (Fig. 19.7).

2.4 The Preparation of Acetabulum

It is difficult to distinguish the boundary between the femoral head and acetabulum in the osteotomy area, and also it is hard to remove the femoral head from acetabulum directly. So at the first, we can use the smallest reamer to grind the residual femoral head adhered to acetabulum and remove a part of the inner cancellous material of the femoral head. Second we can use bone chisel or curette to seek the boundary between the femoral head and acetabulum (Fig. 19.8). We will expose the osseous acetabulum after removing all the residual femoral head. The initial diameter of reamer should approximate to the diameter of osseous acetabulum. Implant the autogenous bone granules in the bottom cavity due to severe acetabular protrusion. In patients with severe osteoporosis, it is better to use the press-fit hemispheric microporous-coated cementless implant with additional screws to improve the initial stability. The material of acetabular insert can choose delta ceramic or high cross-linked polyethylene.

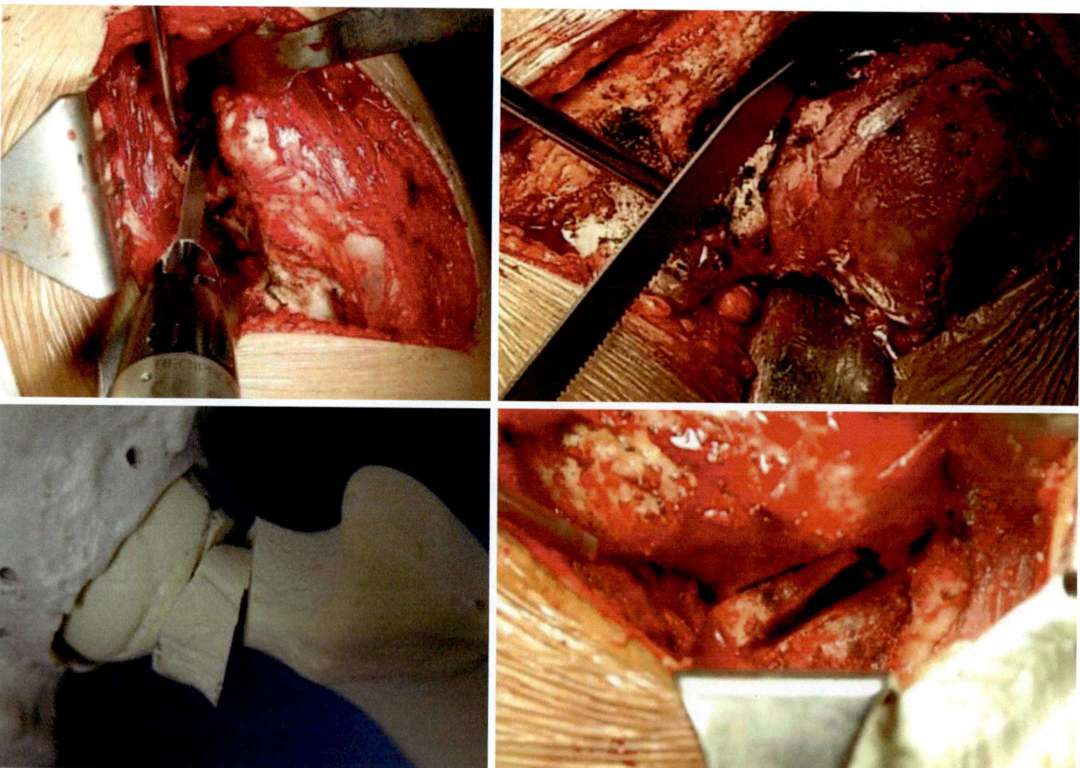

Fig. 19.7 Cut off a wedge-shaped bone block from the femoral neck near the posterosuperior area of the greater trochanter

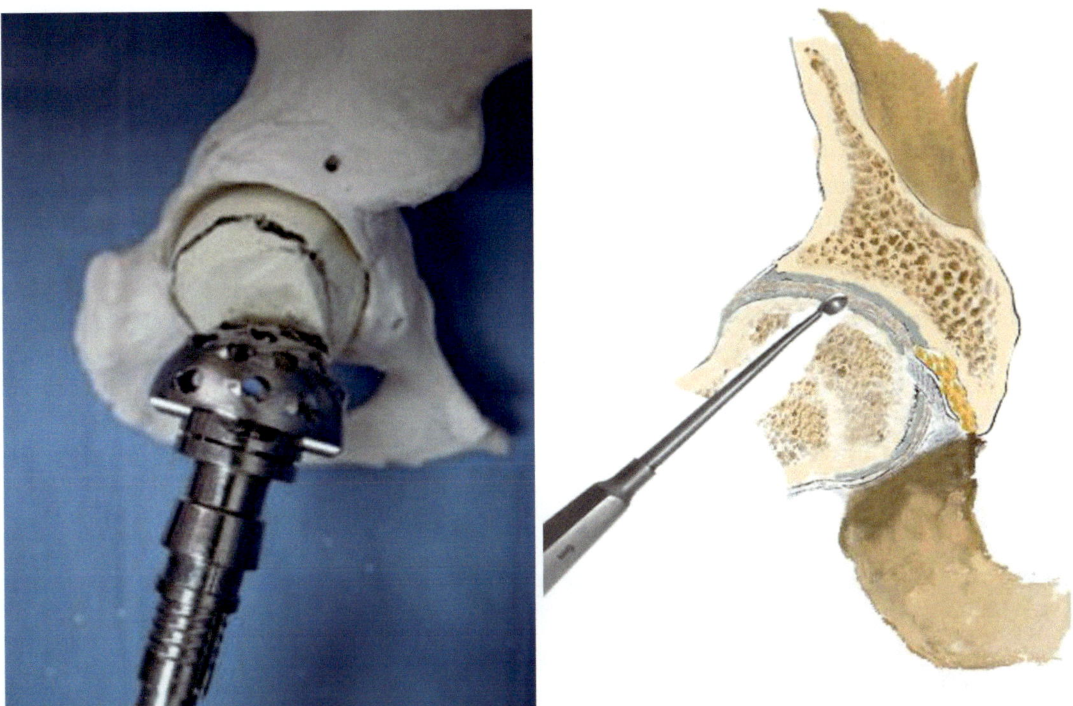

Fig. 19.8 Use the smallest reamer to grind the residual femoral head adhered to acetabulum. Seek the boundary between the femoral head and acetabulum

Usually the femoral medullary cavity morphology appears as stovepipe type, and we should assess it carefully to select the appropriate femoral stem prosthesis. It is difficult to obtain a standard anteroposterior (AP) or lateral X-ray due to hip deformity, so the accurate preoperative templating is hard to achieve. In this, flat tapered or 2D tapered cementless femoral stem prosthesis may be the best option. The front and back shape of femoral stem prosthesis are flat, and the medial and lateral side of it are wedge shaped. The initial stability of femoral stem mainly depends on the three-point fixation and the locking between cortical bone and prosthesis on the medial and lateral side. Commonly the femoral stem prosthesis is collarless and proximal porous-coated cementless implant. The porous-coated region is restricted to the proximal 1/3 to 5/8 of femoral stem prosthesis. The medial and lateral dimensions increase with the size of femoral component, but the front and back size remains unchanged. The implanting of this proximal porous-coated prosthesis needs the preparation of proximal femoral medullary cavity, usually it does not need to expand the distal femoral medullary cavity. This proximal porous-coated prosthesis suits to the femoral medullary cavity morphology of Dorr Type B/C. The typical prosthesis includes Taperloc (Biomet, Warsaw, IN), Tri-Lock (DePuy, Warsaw, IN), ML taper (Zimmer, Warsaw, IN), Accolade (Stryker), Corail (DePuy, Warsaw, IN), LCU (LINK, German), and so on. Most of these prostheses are HA-coated tapered stems, and they are suitable to the femoral medullary cavity morphology of Dorr Type B/C due to the cancellous bone press-fit design, especially accompany with serious osteoporosis. Because ankylosing spondylitis patients usually have poor bone quality, we should pay more attention to avoid the periprosthetic fracture when we are reaming the femur medullary cavity, implanting the prosthesis, relocating the hip joint, and releasing periarticular soft tissue. Periprosthetic fracture usually occurs around the trochanteric area at the time of hitting down metal rasps or femoral stem prosthesis; therefore sometimes we need bind several wires around the trochanteric area to prevent the occurrence of periprosthetic fracture.

2.5 Soft Tissue Balance Technique

Ankylosing spondylitis disease not only affects the bones but also affects soft tissues including muscles, tendons, and ligaments. The elasticity of involved soft tissues usually has different degrees of decline. If the hip is fixed in any particular position, due to the contracture and toughness of involved soft tissues, it is difficult to correct the deformity completely even after the joint replacement. Therefore we need appropriate releasing of soft tissues to correct the deformity.

We defined the flexion contracture as the involved hip fixed in the flexion angle beyond 30°. In these patients we need to release the anterior soft tissues of the hip to obtain full extension. The structures which are relevant to flexion contracture deformity include anterior osteophytes (femoral side and acetabulum side), anterior joint capsule, iliopsoas muscle, anterior tensor fasciae latae, anterior contracture band of rectus femoris, and so on. According to the above sequence, we should release the anterior soft tissues of the hip with checking the extension of the hip every time. As to mild-moderate flexion contracture, we can use the pie-crust technique to release anterior tensor fasciae latae. As to severe flexion contracture, we can transect the anterior tensor fasciae latae until muscular structure (Fig. 19.9). The overall density of the hip also could affect the ROM, and we suggest that it is rather mild lax than tight to these patients.

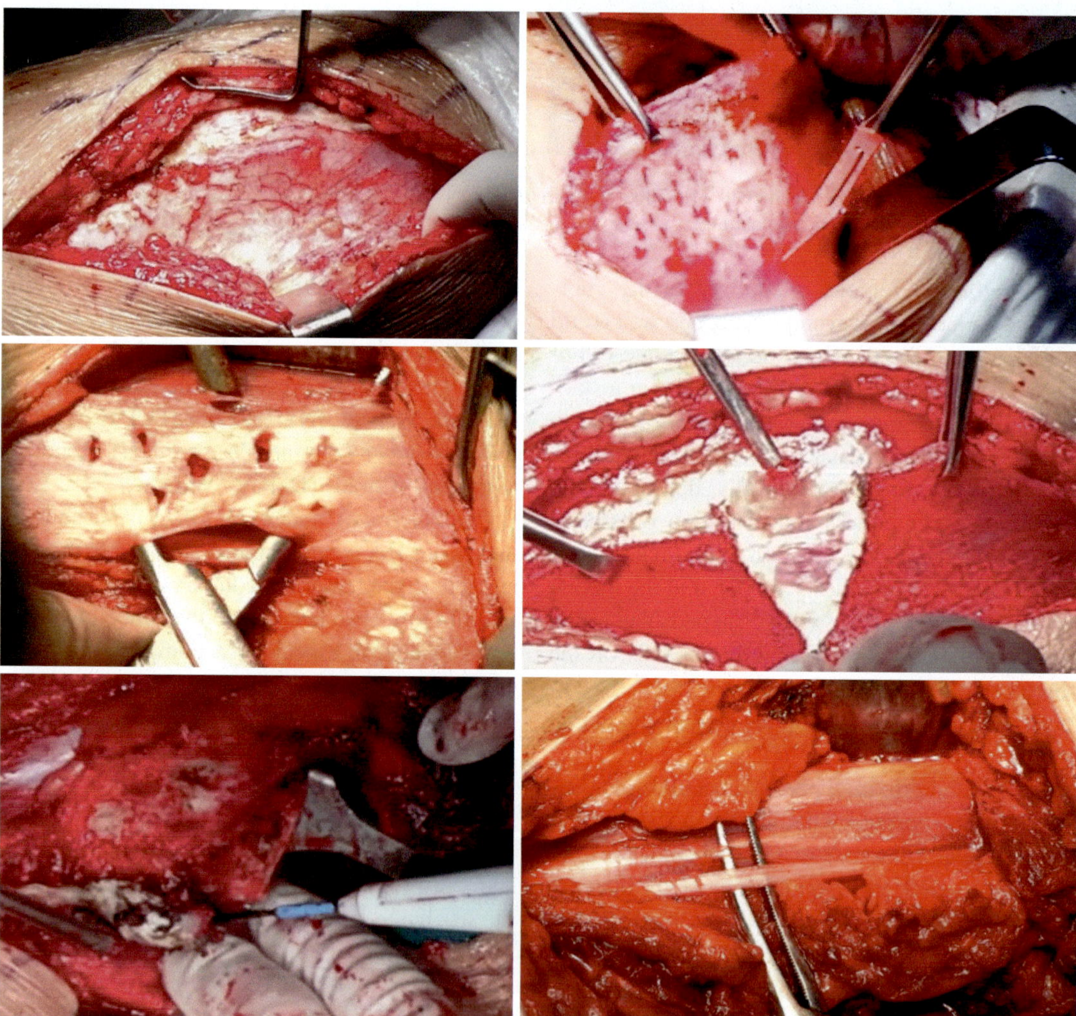

Fig. 19.9 Release of the anterior soft tissue

2.6 Typical Cases (Fig. 19.10)

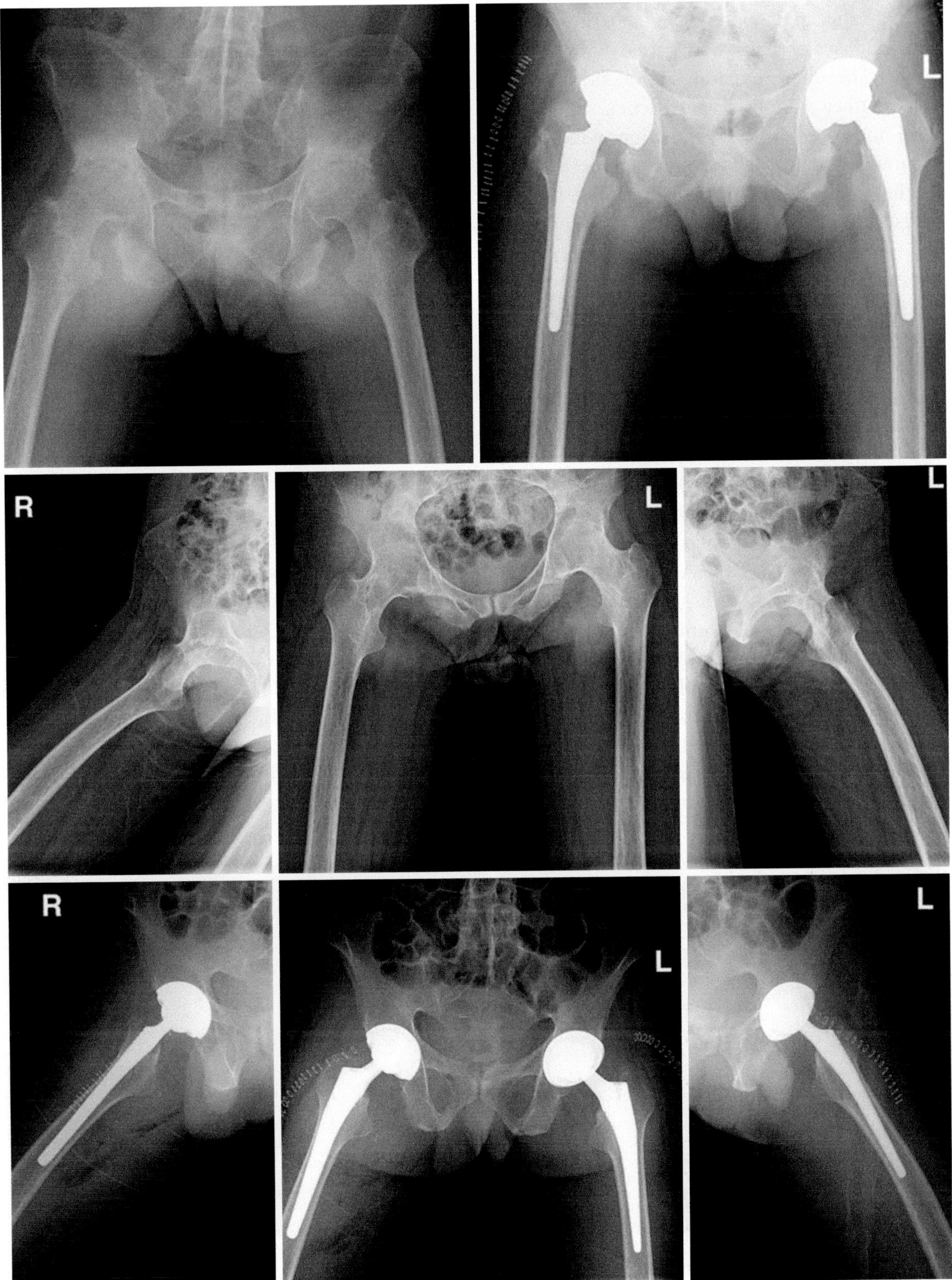

Fig. 19.10 X-rays images before and after THA

3 Type 3 Bone Rigidity

The hip joint gap in the patients with bony ankylosis disappeared completely, and the femoral head and acetabulum were fused with osseous tissue. The clinical manifestation is similar to that of fiber rigidity. The patient's hip joint is rigid in a certain body position without any motion and function. There is no obvious pain in the hip joint, but the loss of the joint function leads to a gradual limitation in daily living ability, especially when the hip joint is stiff at the nonfunctional position. The muscles around the hip joints are easy to fatigue. The X-ray showed the hyperextension of the pelvis. The joint space of the involved hip disappeared completely, and trabecula structure in femoral head and the acetabulum were sparse. The hip joint was in abnormal position including abnormal flexion or extension and abnormal rotation. The shape of the lateral medullary cavity of the femur is mostly chimney type, and the bone cortex is often Dorr B/C, but it also has Dorr A. There are obvious osteoporosis around the hip joint. According to the differences of the sagittal deformity of the hip, two subtypes were divided into II A (flexion deformity <30°) and II B (flexion malformation >30°). The sacroiliac joint has a state of bone fusion. There are often different degrees of formity in the spine, often manifested in the reduction and disappearance of the lumbar lordosis, the deformity of the thoracic and lumbar kyphosis, and the cervical spine osseous rigidity. CT scan showed the bone fusion of the hip joint, and the interface of the femoral head and acetabulum disappeared completely. However, the oval fossa has already existed, which is also an anatomical location marker for finding the true molars during the operation (Fig. 19.11).

3.1 Surgical Technique

All osseous ankylosis hips can be dealt with by posterior approach and anterolateral approach. The anterior lateral approach is difficult to complete the flexion-type osseous ankylosis. We routinely use the posterior approach to perform the operation.

We choose the conventional lateral position due to hip rigidity and ankylosing in different positions, and spinal deformity of different levels and segments exists. Therefore, it is difficult to put these patients in standard lateral recumbent position.

After exposure of the articular cavity, the femoral neck, the trochanteric region, and the posterior wall of the acetabulum were fully exposed. The osteotomy of the femoral neck was performed in situ.

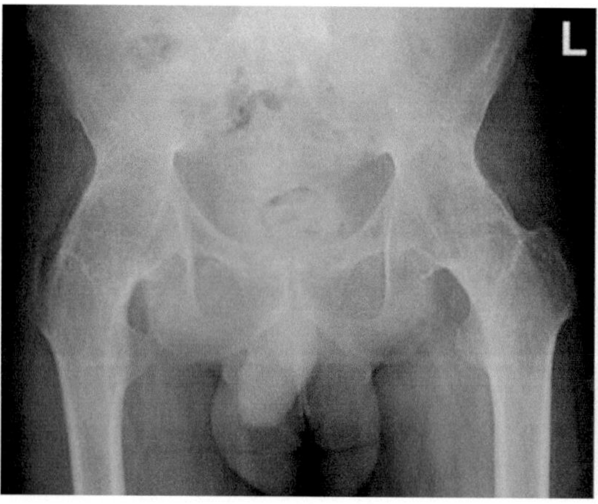

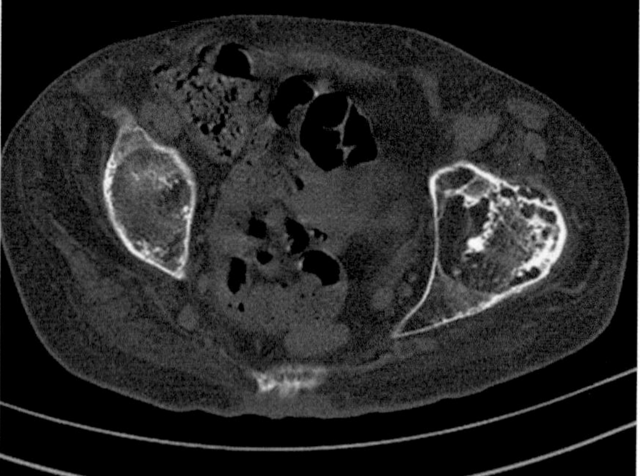

Fig. 19.11 X-ray and CT scan showed the bone fusion of the hip joint

3.2 Acetabulum Preparation

Because the interface of the femoral head and the acetabulum is completely bony fusion, the femoral head and neck cannot be completely removed. In the preparation of the acetabulum, first with acetabulum file the trumpet at the femoral neck osteotomy of the femoral head and neck along the direction of grinding, the initial formation of the acetabular fossa, and then lower the acetabular fossa with an osteotome or curette for soft tissue in the bone, soft tissue found in here is the soft tissue of acetabulum oval fossa. As a marker of acetabular acetabulum, the acetabulum can be grind into the acetabulum. If the bone is loose, the file can be worn in the last file, and the acetabulum can be expanded by compacting cancellous bone to increase the bony supporting force of the acetabulum. Residual femoral neck can be sawn off, but of course, part of the femoral neck cortical bone can be retained as part of the acetabular rim to enhance the supporting force and initial stability of the acetabular acetabulum (Fig. 19.12). The initial stability is strengthened with a screw with a hemispherical microporous coated cup. The delta ceramic liner or high cross-linked polyethylene liner can be selected.

The selection and preparation of the femoral side prosthesis can be referred to the sections of the fibrous ankylosis. But for a few femur of Dorr C type, the bone cortex is very thin, the osteoporotic patients, the bone cement prosthesis may be more reasonable choice. The 2 mm bone cement shell should be retained when the third generation of bone cement was used to implant the prosthesis. Similarly, due to poor quality of the bone in ankylosing spondylitis patients, we should avoid periprosthetic fractures when preparing pulp cavity, implant prosthesis, reduction of joint, and balance of soft tissue around the hip joint. Periprosthetic fractures are most commonly seen in the tuberosity area. They often occur when pressing the pulp cavity files and implant prosthesis. Sometimes, we need to bind the wires in this area to prevent fracture. The soft tissue balance technique for flexion and extension deformity can be referred in the section of fibrous osseous ankylosis.

3.3 Typical Cases (Fig. 19.13)

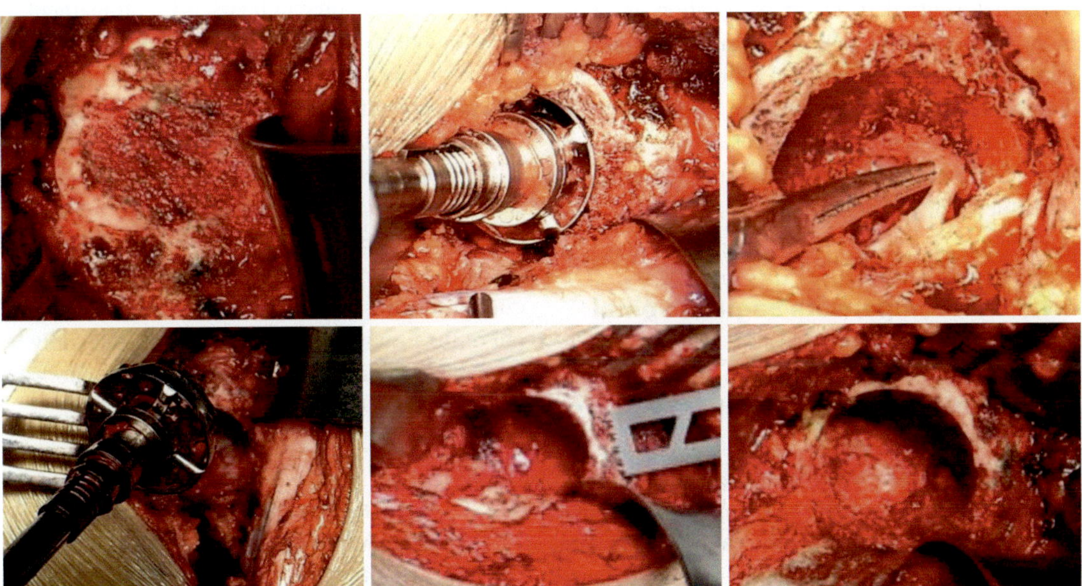

Fig. 19.12 The preparation for the acetabulum

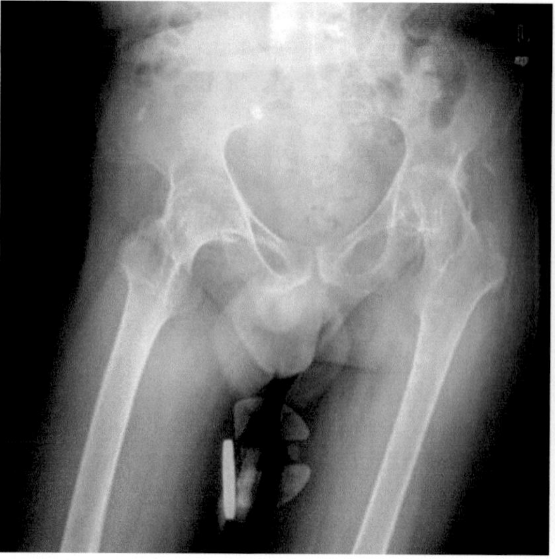
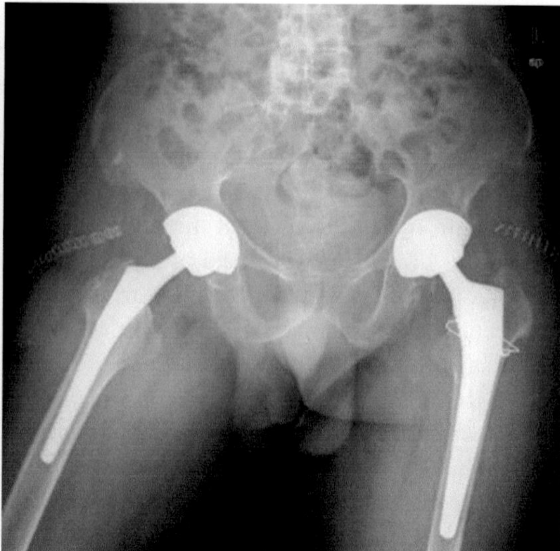

Fig. 19.13 X-ray image before and after surgery

4 Type 4 Combined Hip-Spine Deformity

This type of deformity is characterized with mostly bilateral, bony ankylosed hips and severe spinal deformity. Spinal kyphosis is dominant and may lead trunk forward and sagittal imbalance which needs surgical correction. The impact on THA of spinal deformity depends on its location, with the more adjacent to the pelvis, the greater impact on joint replacement of the hip. Two subtypes are divided according to the location of spinal deformity: (a) those with mainly cervicothoracic spinal deformity and (b) those with mainly lumbosacral spinal deformity (Fig. 19.14).

4.1 Decompensate Sagittal Spinal Deformity

4.1.1 The Impact on Total Hip Arthroplasty

Pelvic retroversion and hip hyperextension may be enrolled to compensate spinal kyphotic deformity. If these mechanisms cannot fully compensate severe spinal kyphosis, trunk imbalance may be present, and the spinal osteotomy procedure may be needed. THA for these patients is technique demanding for its twisted spinal-pelvic configuration due to both original deformity and spinal osteotomy procedure. In this situation, we drew a line that represents sagittal pelvis, which is the line of the anterior pelvic plane project on the sagittal plane. Another line we drew represents the vertical line after spinal osteotomy. The angle (called α Angle) between these two lines can be considered to be the deviation of the pelvis from the gravity line and can be used for adjustment of the acetabular cup anterversion (Fig. 19.15).

According to the aforementioned formula, theoretical acetabular anterversion = $20° - \alpha * 0.6°$ and theoretical acetabular abduction = $40 - \alpha * 0.8°$. If the calculated theoretical angles are within the Lewinnek safe zone of anterversion15 ± 10°, and abduction 40 ± 10°, the cup will be implanted according to these theoretical angles. In the circumstance of the calculated theoretical angles out of the Lewinnek safe zone, the cup can only be implanted within this classical safe zone, choosing the upper or lower bound of its range.

4.2 Spinal Osteotomy and Total Hip Arthroplasty, Which One First

For patients with ankylosing spondylitis with both hip involvement and severe spinal deformity,

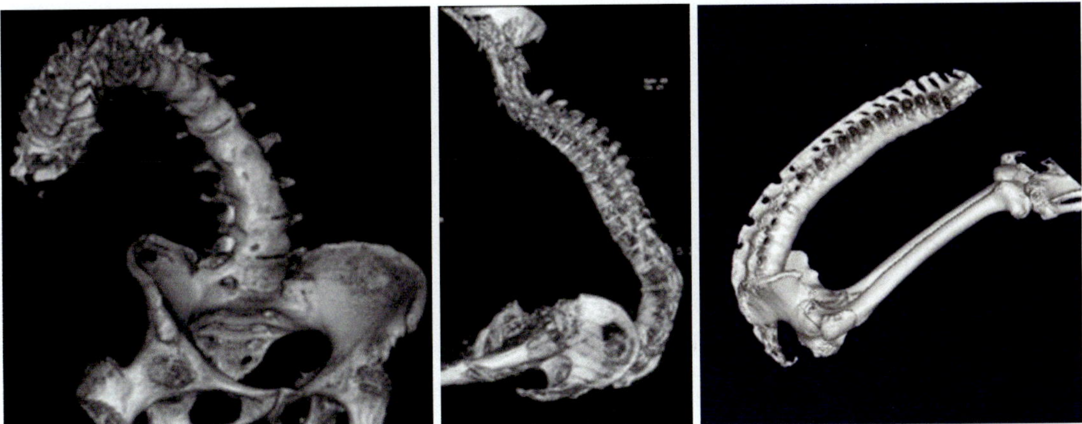

Fig. 19.14 Bony ankylosed hips with severe spinal deformity

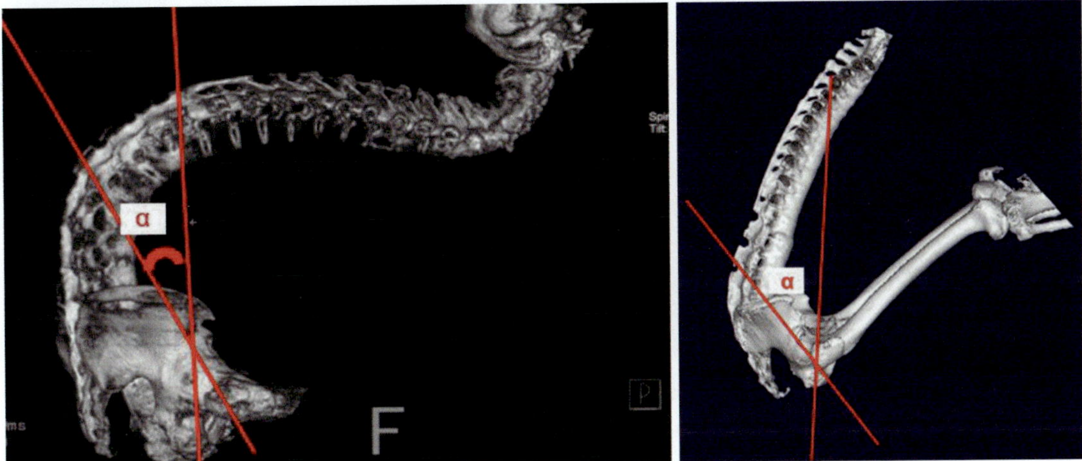

Fig. 19.15 α angle

it has always been controversial that spine osteotomy or hip replacement should be done first [5–7].

As early as 1963, Lee ML proposed that THA should be done before spine correction. He believed that more accurate assessment of the spine deformity could be achieved with improvement of hip ROM and pain alleviation after THA. Tang et al. found the pelvis was retroverted when patient was standing from a stereolithographic model, and if the acetabular cup orientation was in accordance with the anatomical acetabulum, the risk of anterior dislocation would increase. Our clinical experience showed that whether spine surgery or THA priority had its advantages and disadvantages. Hip surgeons preferred that spine surgery be done before THA, because spinal deformity, especially kyphotic deformity mainly involved in the lumbar spine, may significantly influence the orientation of the pelvis, thus affecting the accuracy of cup implantation. Risk of hip dislocation would increase if THA done before spine surgery (Fig. 19.16).

Spinal osteotomy procedure first makes it more convenient for hip surgeons to comprehensively make surgical plane.

The relative "normal" spine-pelvis alinement after spinal osteotomy procedure makes the patient's position more comfortable and cup orientation more precise during operation, thus reducing the difficulty and risk of the hip surgery.

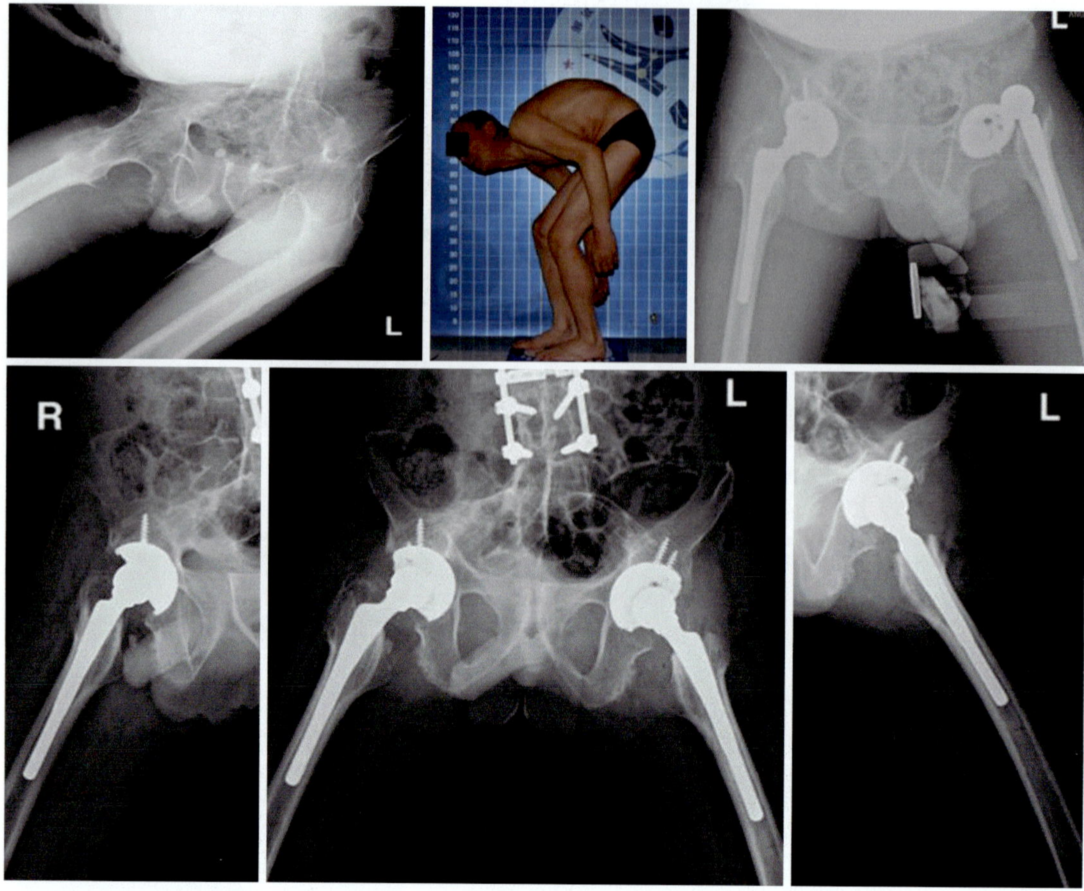

Fig. 19.16 Our case of hip dislocation when THA was done before spine surgery

4.3 Extremely Severe Combined Hip-Spine Deformity

Spine surgery before THA is impractical in patient with extremely severe combined hip-spine deformity due to the difficulty of putting patients in proper position; so hip surgery must be done first to correct hip flexion contracture deformity. Thus, it can facilitate an acceptable prone position for the following spine osteotomy. Hip surgeon and spine surgeon need collaboration to make a detailed preoperative plan, including location and how much degrees of spinal osteotomy, the possible location and degrees of residual deformity after spinal osteotomy, the impact of residual spinal deformity on the pelvis and acetabulum orientation, and the ideal acetabular shell anterversion and abduction.

4.3.1 Preoperative Plan

X-rays of the whole spine, pelvis, and bilateral hips are the most important images for preoperative plan. CT scan with 3D reconstruction of both the spine and lower limbs can provide more detailed information. The location, how much degrees, and the residual deformity of spinal osteotomy need to be determined (see Fig. 19.17).

4.3.2 Preoperative Preparation

It's difficult to keep patient in a satisfied position on the operation table because of the extremely severe combined hip-spine deformity. Standard decubitus position is always impossible (Fig. 19.18).

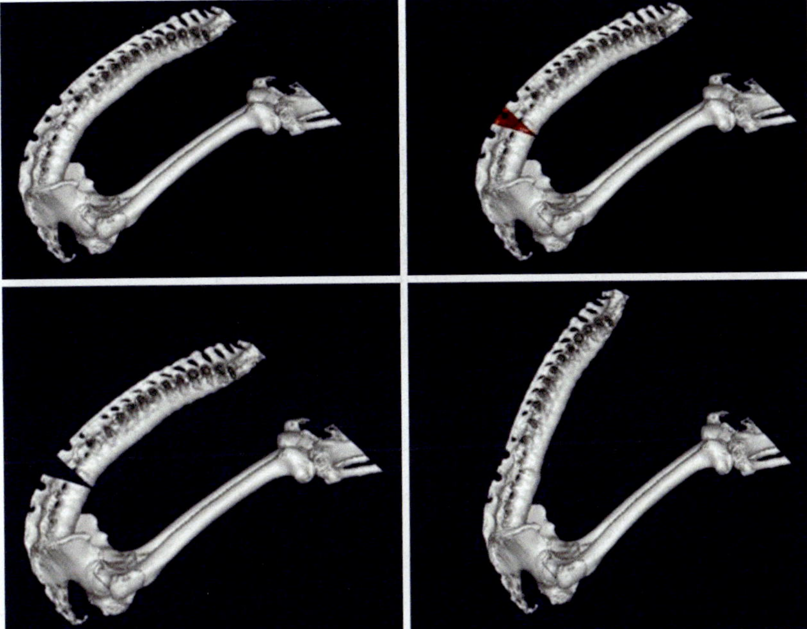

Fig. 19.17 A preoperative plan for the spinal osteotomy

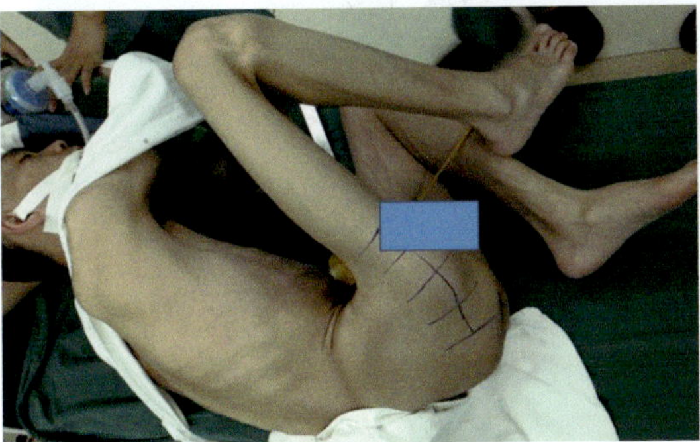

Fig. 19.18 Patient's position on the operation table

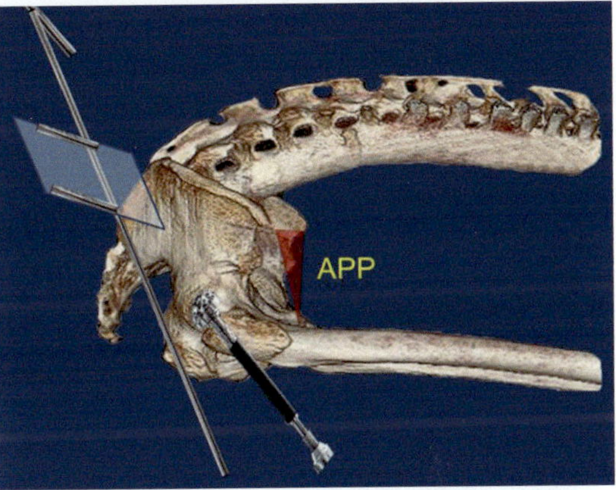

Fig. 19.19 The guide plate is installed on the operating bed, which is parallel to the front surface of the pelvis (APP). The guide plate can be used for accurate acetabular preparation and acetabular implantation in the operation

4.4 Sterilization and Draping

Skin sterilization area needs to be enlarged to prevent contamination during draping. Transnasal tracheal intubation with flexible bronchofiberscope is applied if needed.

4.4.1 Identification of the Pelvic Orientation

The severe hip-spine deformity and the unrestricted decubitus position hamper recognition of the pelvic orientation; assistive devices may be needed during operation to get a more accurate acetabular cup implantation (Fig. 19.19). Besides, intraoperative fluoroscopy is also helpful for guidance of cup implantation.

In addition to the application of assistive devices, intraoperative perspective is necessary to determine the accuracy of the placement of the acetabulum (Fig. 19.20).

4.5 Typical Cases (Figs. 19.21 and 19.22)

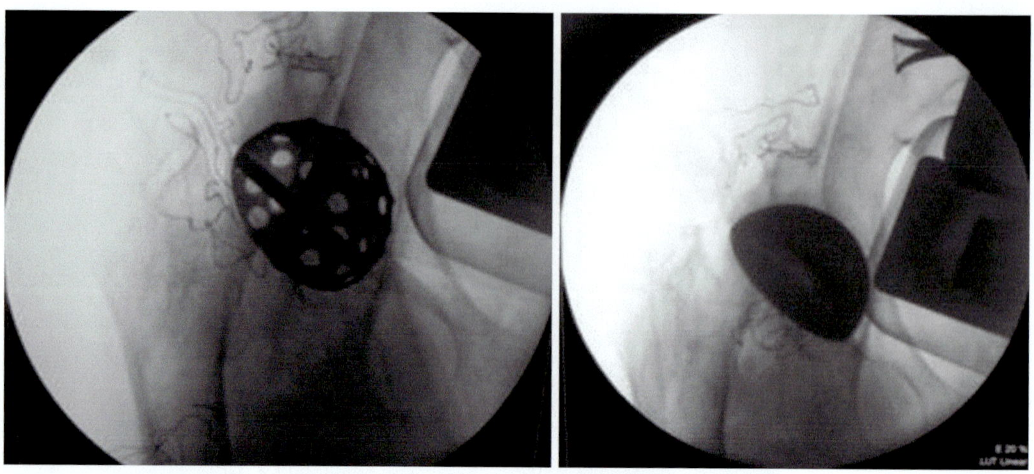

Fig. 19.20 Intraoperative perspective for the placement of the acetabulum

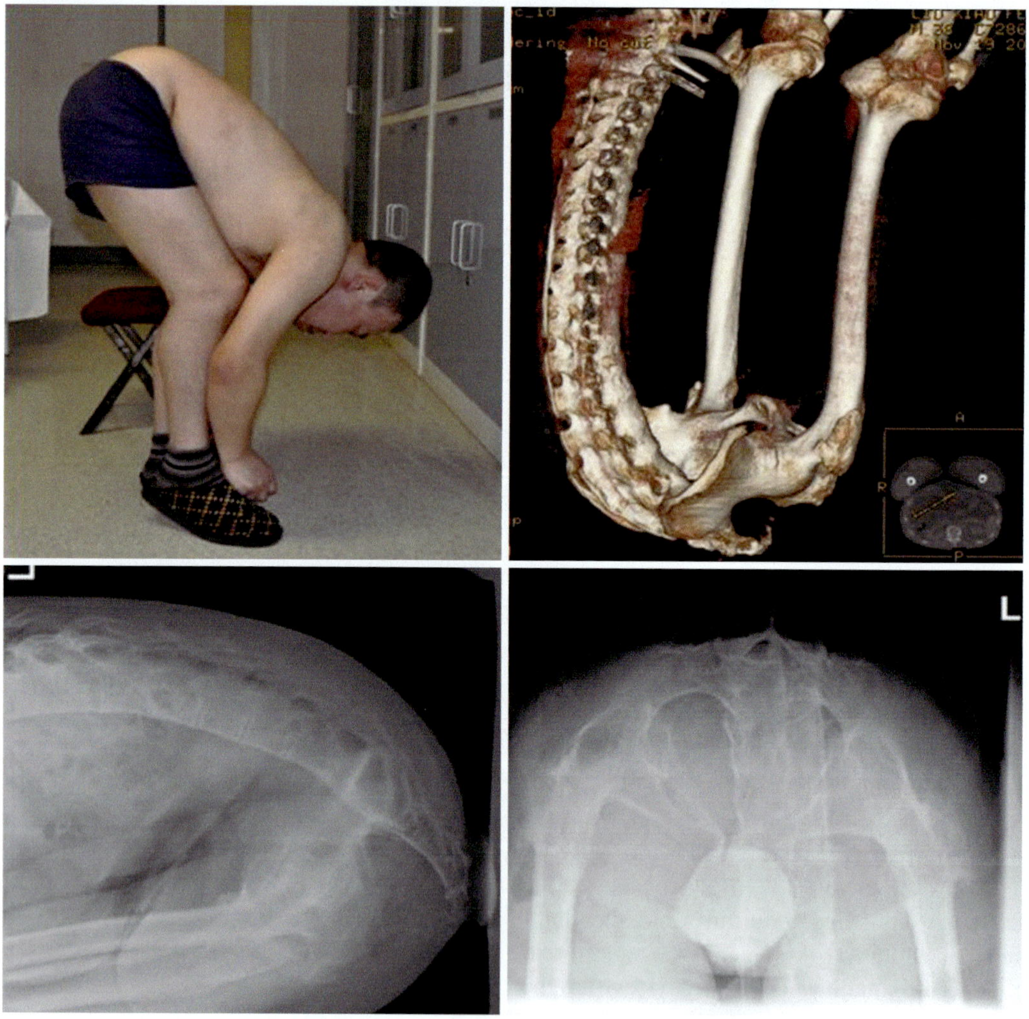

Fig. 19.21 Appearance, 3D CT reconstruction and X-ray images of a case

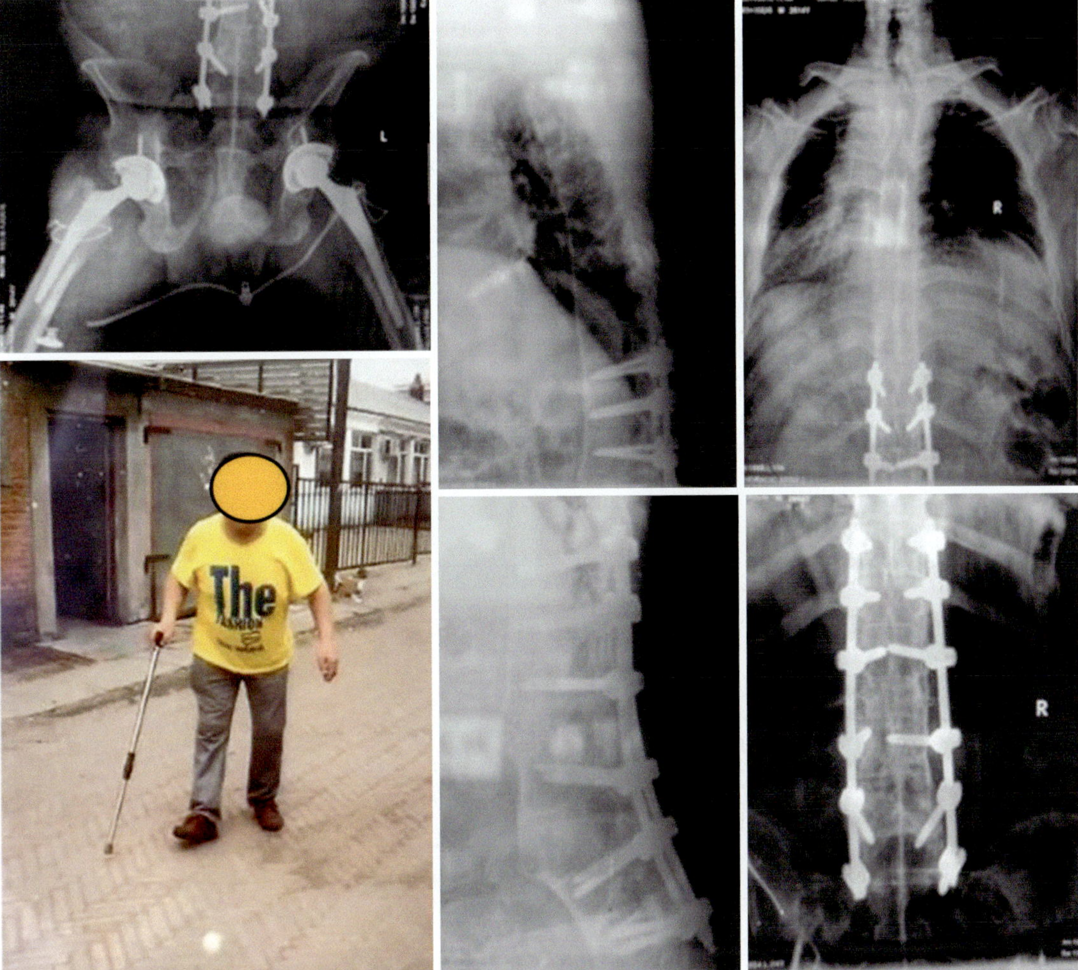

Fig. 19.22 Appearance and X-ray after surgery

Acknowledgements This study was conducted with approval from the Ethics Committee of Chinses PLA General Hospital, and all patients provided informed consent for their participation in this study. All figures are recorded by authors.

References

1. Wang Y, Zheng GQ, Zhang YG, et al. Proposal of a new treatment-oriented classification system for spinal deformity in ankylosing spondylitis. Spine Deform. 2018;6(4):366–72.
2. Gusis SE, Riopedre AM, Penise O, et al. Protrusio acetabuli in seronegative spondyloarthropathy. Semin Arthritis Rheum. 1993;23(3):155–60.
3. Saglam Y, Ozturk I, Cakmak MF, et al. Total hip arthroplasty in patients with ankylosing spondylitis: midterm radiologic and functional results. Acta Orthop Traumatol Turc. 2016;50(4):443–7.
4. Qian BP, Jiang J, Qiu Y, et al. The presence of a negative sacral slope in patients with ankylosing spondylitis with severe thoracolumbar kyphosis. J Bone Joint Surg (Am Vol). 2014;96(22):e188.
5. Mac-Thiong JM, Labelle H, Berthonnaud E, et al. Sagittal spinopelvic balance in normal children and adolescents. Eur Spine J. 2007;16(2):227–34.
6. Zhang X, Zhang Z, Wang J, et al. Vertebral column decancellation: a new spinal osteotomy technique for correcting rigid thoracolumbar kyphosis in patients with ankylosing spondylitis. Bone Joint J. 2016;98-B(5):672–8.
7. Zheng GQ, Zhang YG, Chen JY, et al. Decision making regarding spinal osteotomy and total hip replacement for ankylosing spondylitis: experience with 28 patients. Bone Joint J. 2014;96-B(3):360–5.

20 Ankylosing Spondylitis Involves Hip-Intraoperative and Postoperative Complications

Guoqiang Zhang, Ming Ni, Bo Wu, Hao Liu, Peng Ren, Haiwen Peng, Qingyuan Zheng, Jingyang Sun, Wei Chai, and Yan Wang

1 Intraoperative Complication

1.1 Neurovascular Injury

1.1.1 Sciatic Nerve Injury

The sciatic nerve of patients who have ankylosing spondylitis is often close to the posterior acetabular wall and femoral neck, which is in danger when performing THA in the posterior approach. Especially when the ankylosing hip joint requires in situ osteotomy, the operating space is too small to hurt the sciatic nerve by oscillating saw. Therefore, more extensive exposure of surrounding soft tissue, retracting the sciatic nerve fully and carefully, and use of the reciprocating saw, rather than the oscillating saw, are required in in situ femoral neck osteotomy. When the ankylosing hip is fused in the position of abduction and external rotation, the posterior operation space is small extremely, then the femoral neck osteotomy can be performed in front of the femoral neck under the same exposure or use the Hardinge approach.

G. Zhang · M. Ni · B. Wu · H. Liu · P. Ren · H. Peng · Q. Zheng · J. Sun · W. Chai · Y. Wang (✉)
Chinese PLA General Hospital, Beijing, China

1.1.2 Femoral Nerve Injury

The femoral nerve is often injured by releasing anterior contracture tissue with flexion fusion of the hip joint and the excessive stretching of the anterior soft tissue when extending the hip joint postoperatively. The femoral nerve is divided under the inguinal ligament, so few cases occur complete femoral nerve injury, most of which are characterized by decreased muscle strength of quadriceps femoris and local skin sensation, these symptoms will be recovered in a few months.

1.1.3 Femoral Artery Injury

During in situ osteotomy, if the front tissue is not protected or oscillating saw is not placed properly, it can also cause direct injury to the femoral nerve and femoral vessels. In author's hospital, one case had underwent artery injury while performing femoral neck osteotomy in posterior approach, which is repaired by urgent vascular surgery. Therefore, first, retractor should be inserted in front of the femoral neck. Second, the direction, length and good feel of oroscillating saw is very important. During in situ osteotomy, the direction of pendulum saw was strictly controlled. Length, good feel is very important. Once the anterior cortex of the femoral neck penetrates, the operator can have a sense of resistance decrease or resistance to the metal retractor. If not sure whether to cut through, leave the anterior thin-layer cortex, and choose osteotome.

Y. Wang (ed.), *Surgical Treatment of Ankylosing Spondylitis Deformity*,
https://doi.org/10.1007/978-981-13-6427-3_20

1.2 Intraoperative Fracture

1.2.1 Cervical Fracture

Cervical vertebrae fractures often occur during tracheal intubation and moving patients. The anesthesiologist must carefully evaluate the bone state of cervical vertebrae when intubating general anesthesia in patients with fused cervical vertebrae and perform nasal intubation under laryngoscope when necessary. Extension of the neck violently can lead to severe cervical fractures and quadriplegia and even be life-threatening. Special protection of the head and neck is required when moving patients and placing posture. We routinely wear neck brushes for these patients to avoid torsional fractures when torso and head-neck movements done incongruously.

1.2.2 Acetabular Fracture

Acetabular fractures often occur during in situ osteotomy and implantation of acetabular cups. If the position of the osteotomy is close to the acetabular side and the direction is wrong, the anterior acetabular wall is easily accidentally injured. Therefore, the tibia should be as close as possible to the trochanteric area when osteotomy of the femoral neck is performed. The direction of osteotomy should be parallel to the opening plane of the acetabulum. The implantation of the acetabular cup is another period of risk for acetabular fractures. The main reasons are weak elasticity and poor bone mass in patients with ankylosing spondylitis. It is easy to cause crack fracture or even burst fracture of acetabular wall when porous-coated acetabular cup is compacted. The operator should not be too careful to fully comprehend the characteristics of acetabular cup and bone quality and implant cup. Once the fractures occur, according to the fracture position, the corresponding scope and the initial stability of the prosthesis and some measures should be adopted, including immobility, delaying weight-bearing time postoperatively, and applying more acetabular cup screws and acetabular cup plates.

1.2.3 Femur Fracture

Femoral fractures are more likely to occur. It can be found in the procedure of surgical preparation, in situ osteotomy, prosthesis implantation, and soft tissue release. Since hip joints are always in the adducent or neutral position with stiffness and fusion, we disinfected and draping for lower limbs in the lateral position, and assistant to outreach excessively of lower limbs for more space to operate, but such strong abduction leads to fractures, and fractures occur in the femoral neck. Although most of the fractures have little effect on the implant and stability of the femoral prosthesis, they should be carefully avoided. When cutting the femoral neck bone in situ, We sometimes wrongly evaluate bone cutting depth. If there are bones not truncated ahead, strong rotation may cause here cleavage fracture of the lower limb, which then extends to the femoral calcar and femoral shaft. If the extension of cleavage site is shorter and prosthesis stability is not affected, the fracture may not be processed. However, once appeared from a chunk of the femoral calcar and femoral shaft fracture, you may need to have the corresponding fixed. Due to osteoporosis, or proximal femur dysplasia, the use of bone cement prosthesis, expanding pulp or femoral implant can lead to handle the femoral proximal or distal cleavage fracture when we are improper operation. A youth with bilateral hip osseous fusion in the author's hospital had spiral fracture (Vancouver B type) when he accepted the bilateral femoral enlarge pulp, and we have to use the bone plate and titanium bold to fix it. If there is too much violence, there may be a fracture of the femur in the treatment of the soft tissue and malformation of the hip joint. Once patients have fracture or suspicious fracture, we need to intraoperative fluoroscopy to judge the location, scope and influence to the stability of the prosthesis handle, and formulate the corresponding fracture treatment scheme, also may carry on the trauma doctor's advice of judgment and fracture treatment scheme.

1.3 Damage of Abduction Device

Ankylosing spondylitis itself involves the abductor and its tendinous attachment area, weak them. At the same time, long-term loss of muscle contraction due to hip joint stiffness leads to further muscular atrophy. Therefore, the traction and motion of joints in the operation are likely to injure the abduction device or even completely avulse it. The abduction device is an important factor for the recovery of hip function, so it is necessary to pay extra attention to avoid injury. In the case of the above damage, the continuity and stability of the outspread device should be reconstructed, such as abductor tendon suture and large rotor fixation.

1.4 Dislocation of the Hip Joint after Surgery

The factor which can mainly cause bad prosthesis position and postoperative hip dislocation in ankylosing spondylitis is the change of the function of the acetabulum due to the spine and pelvic deformity. The pelvis retroversion increases, and then the acetabulum anteversion increases meaning time, so the implantation of acetabular cup according to the normal position is easy to cause the acetabulum functional anteversion decreases and increase anterior dislocation risk. In addition, due to the presence spine deformity, especially in severe scoliosis, acetabulum components cannot be placed in the standard position during operation, so it is difficult to accurately place the acetabulum components. Therefore, if the patient has a kyphotic deformity requiring surgical correction, it is suggested to restore the sagittal balance to the anterior spinal surgery. At this time, the patient's pelvic SS/PT was fixed, the spine was basically restored to the upright state, and the artificial total hip arthroplasty could be operated with the reference of the sagittal function of the body at this time.

1.5 Heterotopic Ossification

The incidence of heterotopic ossification after THA is 11–43%, and the related genetic mechanism is still unclear. According to Sochart's studies, compared with the patients who accepted THA for other diseases, there was no increase regarding on occurrence of heterotopic ossification in patients with THA for AS.

1.6 Artificial Joint Infection

For patients with ankylosing spondylitis, the risk factors for infection include the following:

1. Lack of exercise due to long-term action inconvenience, unhealthy eating habits, poor nutrition intake.
2. Long-term use of drugs and continued intake of hormones or TNF inhibitors inhibiting the body's immunity.
3. The stiffness of the hip joint increases the difficulty of disinfection of the skin, and it is easy to be polluted when surgeons place the cup, especially in the adducent position.
4. The operation is difficult, operation time is prolonged, and more bleeding.

Part VII

The Joint Replacement of Ankylosing Knee in Ankylosing Spondylitis Patients

21 Clinical Characteristic

Ming Ni, Bo Wu, Hao Liu, Peng Ren, Haiwen Peng, Qingyuan Zheng, Jingyang Sun, Wei Chai, Guoqiang Zhang, and Yan Wang

The knee is one of the peripheral joints that usually have been involved by ankylosing spondylitis (AS). The clinical characteristics of involved joints usually are tendinitis and synovitis, and the knee is commonly covered with many tendons and synovium, so involved knee joints often have inflammation. The involved knees commonly have severe pain and loss of joint function, which present as joint stiffness or even ankylosis. The involved tendons and ligaments may be contractured, and the elasticity of involved soft tissues usually has different degrees of decline. As to patients with rapid progression or long duration, the muscles that surround the knee joint may have different degrees of amyotrophy, especially in the musculus quadriceps femoris. The ankylosing spondylitis patients with knee involved usually have hip lesions.

The clinical characteristics of ankylosing spondylitis patients with knee involved usually are similar to the patients with hip involved. Commonly there is stiffness or pain in the lumbosacral spine at the early stage, and then the lesion gradually invades to the knee joint which show joint swelling and pain. The range of motion (ROM) of the involved knee may be normal in the initial period and the involved knee usually tends to flex to alleviate pain. At the late stage, the ROM gradually decreases and mostly fix in flexion posture at last. The severe flexion deformity may show as "goose head" subluxation. At this stage, the patients usually could not walk and need assistive devices such as wheelchair to move.

The X-ray shows osteoporosis in the surrounding bone of the knee joint and narrow joint space. The joint space with knee ankylosis disappeared. Since the knee usually was in flexion posture, lateral view is a better choice to check the joint space.

M. Ni · B. Wu · H. Liu · P. Ren · H. Peng · Q. Zheng
J. Sun · W. Chai (✉) · G. Zhang · Y. Wang
Chinese PLA General Hospital, Beijing, China

Y. Wang (ed.), *Surgical Treatment of Ankylosing Spondylitis Deformity*,
https://doi.org/10.1007/978-981-13-6427-3_21

22 Surgical Technique of Total Knee Arthroplasty (TKA) for Ankylosing Spondylitis (AS)

Ming Ni, Bo Wu, Hao Liu, Peng Ren, Haiwen Peng, Qingyuan Zheng, Jingyang Sun, Wei Chai, Guoqiang Zhang, and Yan Wang

Total knee arthroplasty (TKA) is the first choice to restore the joint function of the ankylosing knee in ankylosing spondylitis (AS) patients. For patients who are not ankylotic, the surgery usually works very well. Even though the TKA surgery could improve the joint function greatly in the patients who are ankylotic, for the reason of decreased elasticity of involved soft tissues affected by ankylosing spondylitis, it usually could not restore knee kinematics as well as normal level. We should assess the joint status carefully and pre-estimate the operation result exactly, and an adequate preoperative conversation could make the patients understand the benefits and limitations of their surgeries.

1 Preoperative Plan and Assessment

We should carefully assess the condition of the skin, musculus quadriceps femoris, ROM, blood supply of legs, and neurological function before the TKA of involved knee in ankylosing spondylitis patients.

Use X-ray to assess the osteoporosis, joint dysplasia, joint space, and the location of the patella. In addition, we should check the posture and region of bony ankylosis for patients who are ankylotic.

2 Prosthesis Selection

There are different degrees of contracture in the involved soft tissues due to ankylosing spondylitis disease, and the posterior cruciate ligament usually is involved and non-functional, so it is better to use the posterior-stabilized (PS) prosthesis instead of the cruciate-retaining (CR) prosthesis. Involvement of the medial and lateral collateral ligament makes the mediolateral stability hard to maintain, the use of condylar-constrained prosthesis should be part of the preoperative plan. The condylar-constrained prosthesis has constraint column on PE insert and could couple with extension rods in both the tibial side and femoral side, which can improve the joint stability and protect the weak collateral ligaments. For patients who have severe flexion contracture deformity, it is better to use the rotating hinge prosthesis to deal with the severe flexion and extension imbalance.

3 Approach and Disclosure

We still choose the middle of the anterior knee and the medial patellar approach to open the joint. As the blood supply in front of the knee

M. Ni · B. Wu · H. Liu · P. Ren · H. Peng · Q. Zheng · J. Sun · W. Chai (✉) · G. Zhang · Y. Wang
Chinese PLA General Hospital, Beijing, China

Y. Wang (ed.), *Surgical Treatment of Ankylosing Spondylitis Deformity*,
https://doi.org/10.1007/978-981-13-6427-3_22

joint is supplied vertically from the branch of the deep fascia artery network, the thickness of the skin flap must reach the deep fasciae. The skin of patients with AS is thin; therefore, all thick skin flaps are required to be separated to open the joint cavity.

The blood supply of the knee joints depends on the vascular network that surrounds the knee. The artery network mainly issued by the deep femoral artery, lateral circumflex femoral artery, femoral artery, descending genicular artery, popliteal artery from the knee, anterior tibial artery and the upper end from the anterior tibial recurrent artery branch, occasionally in the branches of posterior tibial artery. The veins of the knee joint is the same as the arrangement of the veins in the other parts of the limbs, and are also divided into two groups: the shallow and the deep. The shallow group was subcutaneous, and the deep group was accompanied by the artery. The vein of the knee is formed around the patellar vein, which is remitted to the large saphenous vein in the rear of the knee joint, and the posterior part of the knee is inserted into the small saphenous vein.

Because of the osseous fusion of patellofemoral joint, the osteotomy of the patellofemoral fusion area should be taken first, and the patellar and the femur should be separated to remove the patella to the lateral. During the osteotomy, the patella and anterior condyle fusion area should be fully exposed, and four tendons and patellar tendons should be protected, and the fusion area should be slightly inclined to the anterior condyle of the femur. However, attention should not be paid to the horizontal bone in the anterior femoral cortex. For the deformity of the flexion contracture, the extensor device has enough subluxation to the side, so it is easy to get enough space for operation. However, for extension malformations or mild flexion deformity, there are contractures and difficult lateral subluxation in knee extension devices, so additional technical assistance is needed. These techniques mainly include quadriceps snip, V-Y quadricepsplasty, and tibial tubercle osteotomy.

4 Quadriceps Snip (QS)

The method of quadriceps snip, which Insall introduced in 1988, is on medial parapatellar approach, cut off the tendinous part of patellar tendon, along lateral inclination of 45° or muscle fiber direction, does not cut off the muscle fiber. When it is completed, patellar turndown can be achieved outward, and the patellar tendon on the tibial tuberosity attachment decreased significantly. When the incision was closed, the suture was rebuilt. The technique maintains the lateral femoral oblique muscle intact and does minimal effect on the function of the knee extension device, and there is no delay in knee extension. At the same time, the blood supply of the patella was less. Postoperative rehabilitation and routine were not changed. When the technology is not fully exposed, it can be directly converted to V-Y molding, or the tibial tubercle osteotomy is used to achieve better exposure.

5 V-Y Quadricepsplasty

For patients with ankylosing knees, tibial tubercle osteotomy should not be considered when the bone is too loose or blood supply of the skin is poor on the tibial tubercle. At this time, V-Y quadricepsplasty can prolong and protect the knee extension device. If the initial release and quadriceps snip cannot meet the purpose of oblique exposure, V-Y quadricepsplasty will be applied. During the process, we should use wet cotton pad to protect the distal patellar ligament terminal. We must use the nonabsorbable suture with large bearing capacity. The lateral loosening gap can be conserved in order to maintain a good patellar trajectory.

V-Y Quadricepsplasty Suture: In the proximal part of quadriceps, a V-shaped fascial flap was made, and the triangular flap was opened from the coronal plane. The front flap has 1/3 thickness of the whole flap, and the posterior flap has 2/3. The inverted V-shaped flap was tracked downward to the quadriceps tendon with interrupted sutures. Then the front flap is turned to the distal end and sutured. The open part of the posterior flap and the four tendons of the "V"-shaped tip of the femoral head were sutured. The knee should be in semi-flexion during suturing. It should be 35–45° in general. At the same time, we should record the flexion angle when the patellar tendon tension reached maximum. We use the same angle of knee brace after surgery so as to prevent ligament tear in excessive activity. Within 6 weeks after surgery, the knee flexing must be carried out under the protection of the fixed support and avoid the use of the CPM machine. In V-Y quadricepsplasty, the knee extension devices are involved, and blood accumulation of the joint cavity is serious. So a drainage tube must be placed.

V-Y quadricepsplasty can prolong and protect the knee extension device and increase the flexion angle of knee joint, but there are still some complications, such as hematoma, insufficient knee extension after operation, and patellar ischemia necrosis caused by blood flow. We suggest that this method would be the final choice.

6 Tibial Tubercle Osteotomy

The skin incision of the lower end extends downward to the distal tibial tubercle at 6–8 cm, to expose the tibial tubercle. Attention should be paid on the inside of the incision of the tibial tuberosity, should not directly cutting through the tibial tubercle; but on the upper edge of the tibial tubercle down at about 6–8 cm, using reciprocating saw, osteotomy incision is on a horizontal line, but not deep. And then, do trapezoidal osteotomy while protecting the tibial tubercle. The length of the whole osteotomy block was at least 8–10 cm, and a short osteotomy would significantly increase the risk of fracture of the tibial tubercle.

During the process of osteotomy, we must ensure the integrity of the soft tissue connected to the cutting block and the integrity of the lateral joint capsule and muscles. The integrity is conducive to maintaining the blood supply of the tibial tubercle and the patellar tendon and is of great help in postoperative healing.

In the reconstruction of the tibial tubercle, if the contracture of the knee extension device is serious and the patella is low, the osteotomy block can be moved up properly. Two or three steel wires or screws can be used to complete the fixed way. If the fixation is fixed, the passive extension of the knee after the operation can start early, but the active extension of the knee should be delayed. The osteotomy of the tibial tubercle is the best indication of a stiff or ankylosis knee with a low patellar bone.

7 Osteotomy and Soft Tissue Balance

For patients without ankylosis, after fully opening the joint, gently and slowly extend the knee joint, separate the fibrous adhesion between the femur and tibia, and clear the meniscus, anterior cruciate ligament, and fibrous hyperplasia tissue. The osteotomy of the proximal tibia at the proximal end of the tibia was dissected according to the 5-degree (or 6-degree) osteotomy of the distal femur. We prefer the hybrid technique of the PCA line, the Whiteside line, the proximal tibial osteotomy surface, and the external femoral circumflex. After fully opening the joint, gently and slowly extend the knee joint, separate the fibrous adhesion between the femur and tibia, and clear the meniscus, anterior cruciate ligament and fibrous hyperplasia tissue.

For the ankylosis of the knee, the fusion interface area of the femur and tibia is first found and marked after opening the joint during the operation. The tibial osteotomy guiding device was installed under the ankylosis, and the thickness of the osteotomy was set as 10 mm below the distance of the fusion interface. Then the osteotomy line and the two osteotomies at the upper 5 mm were performed to remove the osteotomy block. At this time, the joint cavity could be fully exposed, and the knee joint could be moved. Attention should be paid to protect the bilateral collateral ligaments, fully expose the distal femur, and remove the tibial bone in the fusion area. The distal femur osteotomy was located by routine intramedullary localization. Because of bone fusion, the bone of the posterior condyle may be partially destroyed, so the hybrid technique of the condyle line and the tibial osteotomy surface is used in the external rotation osteotomy.

The knee joint affected by AS, whether osseous ankylosis or not, is often not serious, and there is no need for a special loosening technique to balance. There is an obvious imbalance between the straightening gap and the flexion gap. For the deformity of the straight position, the limitation of flexion is mainly due to the shortening of the knee extension device. If the flexion angle of the knee is still not more than 40° at this time, a certain degree of buckling can be improved by the special exposure technique described above. For the flexion deformity, the posterior articular capsule, the internal and external head of the gastrocnemius muscle, and the distal femur with osteotomy can be straightened. If the flexion deformity is heavier, which is more than 40°, it often needs to release the knee posterior shortening of the hamstring tendon insertion and prosthesis flexion to obtain condylar limit equilibrium gap. If the severe flexion deformity and subluxation occur, it often indicates that the extensor and flexion space is extremely unbalanced and the collateral ligament is poorly developed. At this time, the distal femur and proximal tibial osteotomy should be added, and the hinge knee joint should be reconstructed. Unlike rheumatoid arthritis, the flexion contracture of the knee joint with ankylosing spondylitis requires the acquisition of passive extension during the operation.

8 Postoperative Treatment and Rehabilitation

For patients with ankylosing spondylitis, it is important to give effective analgesia after operation. Patients tend to show more severe pain than other causes of joint replacement, especially during the rehabilitation of joint function. So the use of more potent analgesic drugs and combined use of different analgesic methods for multimodal analgesia are more effective, including intraoperative analgesia and postoperative analgesic for cocktails and nonsteroidal anti-inflammatory drugs and physical pain or the postoperative femoral nerve block catheter or epidural catheter anesthesia analgesia. Sometimes the need to consult the rheumatologist jointly develops effective analgesia and strong column inflammation control scheme.

Active rehabilitation after operation is very important for better knee function and prevents loss of motion during operation. For those with malformed extension, the goal of rehabilitation exercise is to maximize the joint flexion and strengthen the four muscle strengths of the femoris to eliminate or reduce the extension of the knee. For the patients with V-Y lengthening, the maximum flexion of the joint must be controlled after operation, which is usually limited to about 45° and gradually increased 7–10 days after the operation. In the meantime, it is recommended to use a knee joint with a locking angle to ensure the protection of the ligaments. After the operation, it is very important to exercise the muscle strength of the four head muscles of the femoral head. It is suggested that the standard strength rehabilitation training should be carried out under the guidance of the rehabilitative physician. In addition, the effect of the hematoma of the joint cavity on the rehabilitation exercise should be paid attention to because of the extensive four head muscle relaxants during the operation.

For the cases with the tibial tubercle osteotomy, if it can be firmly fixed, early passive knee exercise after operation should be applied, but active knee extension training, would be recommended while the X-ray showing bone healing 6 weeks after surgery. Pay attention to the skin incision, and prevent skin incision nonunion or infection.

The goal of rehabilitative exercise for the flexion deformities is to achieve the complete straightening of the knee joint and the strength of the four head muscles of the femoris. The severe knee flexion deformity, although passively straightened in surgery, is very easy flexion contracture again postoperative. For this kind of serious cases, the knee is fixed with conventional straight leg plaster for 3–6 weeks. In the first 2 weeks, the knee has been fixed with plaster both day and night. 2 weeks later, plaster was fixed only at night, and patient has the knee extension and flexion, and quadriceps strength training during day time. The protection after 2 weeks during the day after removal of plaster in the family or therapist's practice walking. 3 months later, any voluntary exercise will not increase the activity of the knee, but 1 months after the operation, four femoral head exercises and knee joint pressing exercises should be emphasized. Only in this way can we ensure that the ankylosis knee joint has enough extension and flexion function. Two months after the operation, the degree of knee flexion is increased, and manipulation can be used.

No matter how severe the deformity of ankylosing knees is, the decision for the replacement of the knee must be very carefully considered and the preoperative plan must be communicated with the patient in detail. Surgeons should also keep in mind that the purpose of surgery is not to reconstruct a new normal knee joint but to restore the joint function as much as possible and improve the quality of life of patients.

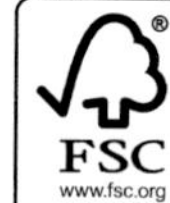

MIX
Papier aus verantwortungsvollen Quellen
Paper from responsible sources
FSC® C105338

If you have any concerns about our products, you can contact us on
ProductSafety@springernature.com

In case Publisher is established outside the EU, the EU authorized representative is:
Springer Nature Customer Service Center GmbH
Europaplatz 3, 69115 Heidelberg, Germany

Printed by Libri Plureos GmbH
in Hamburg, Germany